An Introduction to Oral and Maxillofacial Surgery

An Introduction to Oral and Maxillofacial Surgery

SECOND EDITION

David A. Mitchell, MBBS, BDS, FDSRCPS, FDSRCS (Eng), FRCS (Ed), FRCS (Eng), FRCS (OMFS)
Consultant Oral and Maxillofacial/Head and Neck Surgeon, Bradford Teaching Hospitals NHS
Foundation Trust, Bradford, Yorkshire, United Kingdom
Editor, *British Journal of Oral and Maxillofacial Surgery*
Honorary Tutor, Faculty of Dental Surgery, Royal College of Surgeons of England, London, United Kingdom
and
Anastasios N. Kanatas, PhD, MD, BSc, PGC, MBBS, BDS, MFDSRCS, MRCS, FRCS (OMFS)
Consultant Oral and Maxillofacial/Head and Neck Surgeon, Leeds Teaching Hospitals NHS Trust
Associate Professor, University of Leeds, Leeds, Yorkshire, United Kingdom

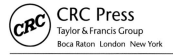

CRC Press
Taylor & Francis Group
Boca Raton London New York

CRC Press is an imprint of the
Taylor & Francis Group, an **informa** business

CRC Press
Taylor & Francis Group
6000 Broken Sound Parkway NW, Suite 300
Boca Raton, FL 33487-2742

© 2015 by David A. Mitchell
CRC Press is an imprint of Taylor & Francis Group, an Informa business

No claim to original U.S. Government works

Printed on acid-free paper
Version Date: 20140818

International Standard Book Number-13: 978-1-4822-4835-7 (Paperback)

Library of Congress Cataloging-in-Publication Data

Mitchell, David A., author.
  An introduction to oral and maxillofacial surgery / David A. Mitchell, Anastasios N. Kanatas. -- Second edition.
    p. ; cm.
  Includes bibliographical references and index.
  ISBN 978-1-4822-4835-7 (alk. paper)
  I. Kanatas, Anastasios N., author. II. Title.
  [DNLM: 1. Oral Surgical Procedures. WU 600]

RK529
617.5'22--dc23   2014028484

Visit the Taylor & Francis Web site at
http://www.taylorandfrancis.com

and the CRC Press Web site at
http://www.crcpress.com

Contents

Basic
Patient
Care

Oral
Surgery

Maxillofacial Surgery

Preface

Oral and maxillofacial surgery is a unique discipline. In the United Kingdom, it was the ninth of the current 10 recognized surgical specialties. In Germany practitioners more often start from a medical base, and in North America they have a dental base. This specialty is internationally recognized as requiring a broad base in both medicine and dentistry and has advanced enormously as a unique surgical discipline since the 1990s.

Partly as a result of the pace of the change, and partly because education tends to lag behind practice in professions, undergraduates and postgraduates – whether medically or dentally based – who wish to grasp the core components of this fascinating discipline are obliged to search far and wide for information and practical guidance. Increasingly, the dental undergraduate curriculum emphasizes restorative dentistry and a (highly likely) career in general dental practice that narrows the focus of many of our graduates to the point of being unable to cope with the basic medical care of hospital patients (a necessity for those wishing any form of oral and maxillofacial surgical experience). The undergraduate medical curriculum barely includes mention of the mouth, and few current basic surgical training rotations include oral and maxillofacial surgery.

In trying to address some aspects of this problem, this book aims to provide the reader with a text that encompasses the full range of oral and maxillofacial surgery while also addressing the core competencies necessary for undergraduates and those in basic specialist training. The initial chapters aim to inform, adding to what is already known, the next section to instruct and the last chapters to provide the detail that those specializing in the discipline require.

It is in all respects a 'generalist' clinical 'specialist' textbook for those anywhere in the world. In this second edition, we have included international perspectives. In those chapters where the UK, US and German perspectives are distinctly different, a section at the end of the chapter has been added. Where there is a general consensus, the views have been integrated into the main body of text.

Whoever chooses to read it, the hope is that they will find it easier to learn something about this exciting and relatively young surgical speciality than has previously been the case. At the end of each chapter, where appropriate, we have included some relevant references and recommendations for further reading. As has been the case with my other books, major input has come from many other colleagues; however, any problems or inconsistencies with the final product remain my responsibility.

David A. Mitchell

Acknowledgements

This book constitutes a complete rewrite of my previous work, *An Introduction to Oral and Maxillofacial Surgery*, with the deliberate intention of making a significant information upgrade and attempting to reflect the diverse approaches to this specialty internationally, at least in the developed world. To this end the input of a younger colleague, recent trainees in the United Kingdom and acknowledged authorities in Europe and the United States have been added. It is hoped that this approach will further disseminate the valuable body of information that has been built up by its predecessor.

That book would, of course, not have been possible without the input of the many collaborators who contributed to that work. These are G. S. Bassi, J. Carey, M. Chan, F. Carmicheal, A. Dalghous, G. Fabbroni, S. Fisher, C. Flynn, P. McCann, K. D. Mizen, T. K. Ong, K. Patel, M. Perry, K. A. Phillips, J. Reid, P. Scott, R. J. Spencer, D. G. Starr, M. R. Telfer and M. Verma.

I would like to thank Laura Mitchell for her usual and unique support and for the support and friendship of Klaus-Dietrich Wolff whose continuing enthusiasm keeps me (and Frank) going more often than he knows. Tas Kanatas, Frank Hölzle and Stephen MacLeod are longtime friends and colleagues whose input has enlivened both me and this book.

List of abbreviations

(We have tried to minimize these, but you will come across some.)

AAOMS – American Association of Oral and Maxillofacial Surgeons

ABC – airway, breathing, circulation

AFB – acid-fast bacillus

AFP – atypical facial pain

AIDS – acquired immunodeficiency syndrome

AJCC – American Joint Committee on Cancer

APTT – activated partial thromboplastin time

ATLS – Advanced Trauma Life Support (course)

BAOMS – British Association of Oral and Maxillofacial Surgeons

BCC – basal cell carcinoma

BIPP – bismuth iodoform paraffin paste

BSE – bovine spongiform encephalitis (prion disease)

BSSO – bilateral sagittal split osteotomy

CCT – Certificate of Completion of Training

CHEOPS – Children's Hospital of Eastern Ontario Pain Scale

CRP – C-reactive protein

CSF – cerebrospinal fluid

CT – computed tomography/tomogram

CVP – central venous pressure

DAHNO – DAta for Head and Neck Oncology (a UK database)

DCIA – deep circumflex iliac artery

DDS/DMD – Doctor of Dental Surgery/Medicine (common basic dental degree outside the United Kingdom and New Zealand [i.e. BDS/BChD]; note in the United Kingdom it can also be a higher degree, similar to a PhD)

DNA – deoxyribonucleic acid (although just as frequently interpreted as do not attempt [cardiopulmonary resuscitation; i.e. DNACPR])

DPT – dental panoramic tomogram

DVT – deep venous thrombosis

EACMFS – European Association for Cranio-Maxillo-Facial Surgery

ECG – electrocardiogram

EMLA – eutectic mixture of local anaesthetics

FAM – facial arthromyalgia

FBC – full blood count

FDS – Fellow in Dental Surgery (of any of four UK Royal Colleges of Surgeons; the highest clinical dental qualification in the United Kingdom)

FNAC – fine needle aspiration cytology

FRCS – Fellow of the Royal College of Surgeons (of any of the four UK Royal Colleges of Surgeons; the highest clinical surgical qualification in the United Kingdom)

GKI – glucose, potassium, insulin

GTN – glyceryl trinitrate

HIV – human immunodeficiency virus

HPV – human papillomavirus

HST – Higher Surgical Training(ee)

IAN (IDN) – inferior alveolar (dental) nerve

ICD – International Classification of Diseases

IMF – intermaxillary fixation

IRM – intermediate restorative material

JVP – jugular venous pressure

KA – keratoacanthoma

LFTs – liver function tests

MCV – mean corpuscular volume

MD – Doctor of Medicine (common basic degree in medicine outside the United Kingdom and New Zealand [i.e. MBBS/MBChB] but also in United Kingdom a higher degree, similar to a PhD)

MFDS – Member of the Faculty of Dental Surgery (intermediate clinical qualification administered by the Faculty of Dental Surgery in the four UK Royal Colleges of Surgeons)

MJDF – Membership of the Joint Dental Faculties (a less demanding version of MFDS, administered by the Faculty of General Dental Practitioners and the Faculty of Dental Surgery of the Royal College of Surgeons of England)

MRCS – Member of the Royal College of Surgeons (intermediate clinical qualification in surgery administered by the four UK Royal Colleges of Surgeons)

MRI – magnetic resonance imaging

MRSA – methicillin-resistant *Staphylococcus aureus*

MTA – mineral trioxide aggregate

NICE – National Institute for Health and Care Excellence (a UK 'arm's length' government body designed to assess new drugs and interventions constantly accused of disguised rationing but probably well meaning)

NSAID – nonsteroidal anti-inflammatory drug

ORIF – open reduction and internal fixation

PATCH – (King's Healthcare) Pain Assessment Tool for Children

PE – pulmonary embolus

PET – positron emission tomography

PHTLS –Prehospital Trauma Life Support

PMHPAT – Princess Margaret Hospital Pain Assessment Tool

PRP – platelet-rich plasma

PSA – pleomorphic salivary adenoma

PT (INR) – prothrombin time (international normalized ratio)

RME – rapid maxillary expansion

SARPE – surgically assisted rapid palatal expansion

SCC – squamous cell carcinoma

SLOB – same lingual opposite buccal

SMAS – superficial musculoaponeurotic (layer)

SSRI – selective serotonin reuptake inhibitor

Super EBA – ethoxybenzoic acid

TB – tuberculosis

TCA – trichloroacetic acid

TENS – transcutaneous electrical nerve stimulation

TGF – transforming growth factor

TMJ – temporomandibular joint

TMJPDS – temporomandibular joint pain dysfunction syndrome
TNF – tumour necrosis factor
TNM – tumour, node, metastasis
TT – thrombin time
U&Es – urea and electrolytes
UICC – Union Internationale Contre Cancer/Union for International Cancer Control
VSS – vertical subsigmoid osteotomy

Tooth notation[*]

FDI

Permanent teeth

R																	L
	18	17	16	15	14	13	12	11	21	22	23	24	25	26	27	28	
	48	47	46	45	44	43	42	41	31	32	33	34	35	36	37	38	

Deciduous teeth

R											L
	55	54	53	52	51	61	62	63	64	65	
	85	84	83	82	81	71	72	73	74	75	

Zsigmondy–Palmer, Chevron, or Set Square system

Permanent teeth

R																	L
	8	7	6	5	4	3	2	1	1	2	3	4	5	6	7	8	
	8	7	6	5	4	3	2	1	1	2	3	4	5	6	7	8	

Deciduous teeth

R											L
	e	d	c	b	a	a	b	c	d	e	
	e	d	c	b	a	a	b	c	d	e	

European

Permanent teeth

R																	L
	8+	7+	6+	5+	4+	3+	2+	1+	+1	+2	+3	+4	+5	+6	+7	+8	
	8–	7–	6–	5–	4–	3–	2–	1–	–1	–2	–3	–4	–5	–6	–7	–8	

Deciduous teeth

R											L
	05+	04+	03+	02+	01+	+01	+02	+03	+04	+05	
	05–	04–	03–	02–	01–	–01	–02	–03	–04	–05	

American

Permanent teeth

R																	L
	1	2	3	4	5	6	7	8	9	10	11	12	13	14	15	16	
	32	31	30	29	28	27	26	25	24	23	22	21	20	19	18	17	

Deciduous teeth

R											L
	A	B	C	D	E	F	G	H	I	J	
	T	S	R	Q	P	O	N	M	L	K	

[*] Because of the difficulties of putting the grid notation in word processed documents it is common practice to indicate the quadrant by abbreviating the arch and side. For example, the upper right second premolar can be labeled UR5 and the lower left second deciduous molar may be labelled LLE.

All tables used by permission. Mitchell D, Mitchell L (2014). Useful information and addresses. *Oxford Handbook of Clinical Dentistry*. Oxford, UK: Oxford University Press.

Contributors

David A. Mitchell, MBBS, BDS, FDSRCPS, FDSRCS (Eng), FRCS (Ed), FRCS (Eng), FRCS (OMFS)
Consultant Oral and Maxillofacial/Head and Neck Surgeon, Bradford Teaching Hospitals NHS
   Foundation Trust, Bradford, Yorkshire, United Kingdom
Editor, *British Journal of Oral and Maxillofacial Surgery*
Honorary Tutor, Faculty of Dental Surgery, Royal College of Surgeons of England, London, United Kingdom

and

Anastasios N. Kanatas, PhD, MD, BSc, PGC, MBBS, BDS, MFDSRCS, MRCS, FRCS (OMFS)
Consultant Oral and Maxillofacial/Head and Neck Surgeon, Leeds Teaching Hospitals NHS Trust
Associate Professor, University of Leeds, Leeds, Yorkshire, United Kingdom

with

Professor Frank Hölzle, MD, DDS, PhD, FEBOMFS (Barcelona)
Head of Department of Oral and Maxillofacial Surgery, University of Aachen, Germany

Professor Stephen P. R. MacLeod, MBChB, BDS, FDSRCS(Ed), FDSRCS (Eng), FRCS(Ed), FRCS (OMFS), FACS
Chief of Oral and Maxillofacial Surgery and Dental Medicine, Loyola University, Maywood, Illinois,
   United States

with contributions from

Ian McHenry, BChD, MFDSRCS
Specialist Registrar in Oral Surgery, Yorkshire, United Kingdom

Louise Middlefell, BChD, MFDSRCS
Specialist Registrar in Oral Surgery, Yorkshire, United Kingdom

Imran Suida, BChD, MFDSRCPS
Specialist Registrar in Oral Surgery, Yorkshire, United Kingdom

Thomas Mueke, PhD, MD, DDS
Oberarzt, Oral and Maxillofacial Surgery, Munich, Germany

1

What is oral and maxillofacial surgery?

The words mean, very simply, surgery of the mouth, jaws and face, and the specialty concerns itself with the diagnosis and treatment of conditions arising in and affecting the mouth, jaws, face, neck and skull and surrounding structures. It is an area of surgical practice that has been largely recognized in European countries as encompassing all the subdisciplines listed in the contents, but internationally the practice of some oral and maxillofacial surgeons may be very much more limited than those of others.

European oral and maxillofacial surgery (OMFS) essentially emerged from surgical dentistry and surgery of the jaws following injuries, particularly in the First and Second World Wars.

From these beginnings a specialty developed that nowadays requires trainees to complete both undergraduate dental and medical degrees. In the United Kingdom this is followed by basic professional training up to the standards of obtaining the membership diplomas in both dental surgery and surgery in general before entering a structured postgraduate training period. It is the youngest of the ten recognized surgical specialties within the United Kingdom and remains unique in requiring this dual base.

As in the United Kingdom, OMFS in Germany is the youngest of the recognized surgical specialties and remains unique in requiring a dual qualification in medicine and dentistry. In Germany, OMFS specialists have two main options after finishing the required 5 years of higher surgical training, namely working autonomously in private practice or pursuing a career in secondary care. The former surgeon's main workload consists of surgical dentistry and implantology. Some minor

skin surgery can be integrated into the daily routine. In practice, this work has much in common with that carried out by oral surgeons – these are dentists completing a 3-year training programme consisting purely of intraoral operations.

With the advent of specialization and specialist lists in the United Kingdom there has been a move toward the creation of specialists in surgical dentistry, which is of course a small but very commonly required area of OMFS. Oral surgery is in effect a form of clinical practice restricting (usually academic) surgeons to a specific range of practice and subdivisions within the overall field of OMFS such as those who specialize in the maxillofacial component of head and neck oncological and reconstructive surgery, cleft lip and palate surgery or craniofacial surgery.

The official OMFS subspecializations that have appeared in the United Kingdom (i.e. head and neck oncology and reconstructive surgery, cleft lip and palate surgery and craniofacial surgery) do not exist in Germany. Every department and in fact every specialist, at least every Head of Department (Chief), is expected to cover the whole range of OMFS. It is still under discussion whether further subspecialization improves the outcome of the surgical treatment or only narrows the experience and surgical skills of the surgeons within the specialty.

In North America the specialty is primarily dentally based (although some training programmes include a formal medical degree) with a career for most oral and maxillofacial surgeons based in an office practice concentrating on dentoalveolar surgery, implantology and sedation and anaesthesia. A hospital-based career is perfectly possible whether with an academic or specialist service and training base; it is simply that, as a proportion of those trained, most of these surgeons are in office rather than full-time hospital practice.

Although these geographic differences illustrate some of the diversity of the specialty internationally, huge areas remain – the Pacific Rim, itself massively variable; the Asian subcontinent; the Sino-Asian regions; South America and Africa, to name a few. My apologies. I hope the differences and similarities within this text at least reflect some of the experiences in these diverse cultural and geographic regions.

Within an international context these artificial subdivisions are recognized as the basic components of the specialty. Fortunately, to date, the specialty encompasses all these potential divisions within the overall remit of OMFS.

From the point of view of the undergraduate student or the early postgraduate studying for a membership diploma, an awareness of the range of the specialty, as well as some factual knowledge and basic skills within the overall field, is what is needed.

The majority of practical skills that will be required of people at this level centre on surgery of the tooth-bearing portions of the jaws and soft tissue surgery in relation to facial trauma. For this reason in this book a large amount of space is devoted to common practical skills and knowledge at the earlier end of training, and surgical detail of the more complex and esoteric areas of the field aims to inform readers of the basics and inspire them to explore further.

At the end of each chapter you will find some guidance for further reading; at the end of some chapters (where there is a clear difference in international perspective) you will find commentaries from North American and German authorities in the field. The final chapter discusses the very substantial differences in training – which often seem greater than the differences in surgical practice.

All any teacher can hope to do is inspire and guide. The rest is up to you.

FURTHER READING

Mitchell DA, editor. *British Journal of Oral and Maxillofacial Surgery.*
Online access is available to the members and fellows of both the British and American Associations of Oral and Maxillofacial Surgery at www.bjoms.com.
www.aaoms.org.
The American Association of Oral and Maxillofacial Surgeons website.
www.bahno.org.uk.
The British Association of Head and Neck Oncologists website.
www.baoms.org.uk.
The British Association of Oral and Maxillofacial Surgeons website, regularly updated and full of useful information.
www.eurofaces.com.
The European Association for Cranio-Maxillo-Facial Surgery website.
www.iaoms.org.
The International Association of Oral and Maxillofacial Surgeons website, for a world view.

2

Basic principles and getting started

Contents

Aim

The aim of this chapter is to introduce you to a series of principles that affect all aspects of surgery.

Learning outcomes

At the end of reading and understanding this chapter, you will have a framework to allow you to plan, think through and carry out an operation in general terms. You should be able to demonstrate this by describing the steps involved in the generic envelope that surrounds each individual operation.

General points

The head and neck in general, and the mouth in particular, are remarkably forgiving areas in which to work. Partly this is because of an excellent blood supply, and partly it is because of the robust and special nature of the tissues in this region. Within the mouth the beneficial effects of saliva and commensal organisms are also seen.

Planning

'Perfect planning prevents poor performance'. This old Armed Forces adage conveys the very essence of sound surgical practice. Every operation should be thought through, even if only briefly, in the mind of the surgeon. If you can think through every step of an operation that you are about to perform you will be in a position to perform that operation safely and competently. If you have no idea how to get from stage to stage in the operation then you will simply be blundering through it. This is no way to conduct surgery. If you have no real idea what you are trying to achieve and the steps involved in doing it, how can you explain the process to the patient for informed consent, explain it to your assistants so that they can do their job or brief the nursing team and anaesthetist? In this way the steps of the operation mirror the generic steps of the patient's journey from initial consultation to discharge. Both sequences are essential to good surgery.

Planning starts with understanding why the operation is being performed and ensuring that the patient has given appropriate consent for the surgery. It is essential that you know the environment in which you are going to carry out the operation and whether this environment is safe and appropriate for that particular operation. This could be something as simple as being aware of good chairside lighting and assistance for the surgical removal of a tooth to having an appropriate level of theatre facility with adequate microscopic capabilities that you understand and can use for a major microvascular procedure. It is paramount that if you feel that your environment is not appropriate for surgery to proceed, then you should not start the operation. Coming to the realization that the operation cannot be conducted successfully because of some problem that was easily foreseeable is unacceptable.

Planning the steps of an operation requires an understanding of the pathology of the disease process, the immediate anatomy through which you will be operating and the procedure by which the patient's pain and anxiety will be controlled, be this local or general anaesthesia.

The background factors such as the patient's medical history and the age or race of the patient may create difficulties in otherwise routine surgery (e.g. very old patients may have osteoporotic or brittle bone and may be using bisphosphonates with the associated risk of osteonecrosis). Heavily built male patients are often described as having particularly robust bone and teeth that are difficult to remove. Irradiated bone is particularly prone to breakdown (osteoradionecrosis) and infection after surgery and should not be operated on (even for extractions) without advice from a specialist.

Environment and equipment

Before commencing any type of surgical procedure, get to know the people you will be working with; your assistants are essential to the progress of the operation and knowing their strengths, weaknesses and limitations is as valuable as understanding the patient's background medical history. You cannot always assume that you are going to have ideal assistance; if this is the case make sure that you can compensate in some other way (Figure 2.1 and Figure 2.2).

Ensure that wherever possible you have gone through the instrumentation and that it is readily available. There are few things more irritating to staff or distressing to the patient than surgeons who are continually flustered because the instrumentation they need is not available and new packs must be repeatedly opened and instruments fetched to the area.

Light is essential, particularly when working in the mouth, which is very much a deep, dark hole. Various specialized lights are designed for both theatre and surgery use. One of the requirements of the light is that it can be adjusted by the operator. Sterile light handles or plastic drapes are used

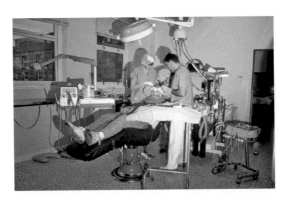

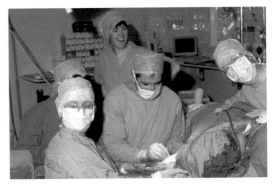

Figure 2.1 All surgery is carried out by a team whether small....

Figure 2.2 ...or large.

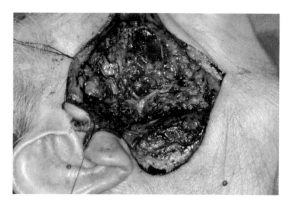

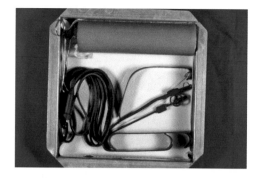

Figure 2.5 Prepacked diathermy kit.

Figure 2.3 In open surgery, such as parotidectomy, suction is less helpful, whereas controlled pressure with a swab is ideal for controlling and localizing bleeding before definitive haemostasis with diathermy or ligation.

to ensure that the light can be easily adjusted. An alternative is a headlight. High-vacuum suction apparatus is routinely available in the dental surgery environment and suction is essential to improve your view, particularly when working in a confined space. When working on open soft tissue it is often more useful to use direct pressure from swabs and diathermy to control bleeding (Figure 2.3).

Pressure followed by accurate diathermy or vessel ligation is the haemostatic technique of choice in open wounds (Figure 2.4 and Figure 2.5).

All instrumentation must be sterilized or disposable, particularly in light of controversy over prion transmission. Instrumentation is covered in Chapter 3. Sutures for intraoral work are usually resorbable. Synthetics such as polyglactin are in common use. The advantage of these sutures is that they do not need to be removed. They do not

resorb in the mouth as quickly as they do when they are buried in soft tissue because of the pH buffering effect of saliva. Patients should be told to expect these resorbable sutures to disappear gradually over a 4-week period. Skin is closed with nonresorbable monofilament synthetic sutures (nylon, polypropylene, polybutester) skin staples or tissue adhesive.

A number of different dressings may be used depending on the type of surgery that is undertaken. Additional dressings such as bismuth iodoform paraffin paste (BIPP) and Whitehead's varnish (a form of iodine in an ether carrier that evaporates) are frequently used to soak gauze to create antiseptic dressings. These dressings can be used to pack cavities of virtually any size. Proprietary dressings such as Alvogyl are designed to be placed in 'dry' sockets. These contain a combination of lidocaine and iodoform that provides analgesia and antisepsis. Sedative dressing materials such as zinc oxide/eugenol and cotton wool glyoxide pastes (e.g. Coe-Pak) are used to relieve pain and cover raw bleeding areas within the mouth such as following excision of hard palate mucoperiosteum. Everyone has his or her own favourite skin dressing, which may range from an antiseptic ointment to sterile occlusive dressings. Few dressings have any strong evidence base.

Special dressings such as vacuum dressings require specialized equipment to be effective. Make sure that this equipment is available before the operation is started.

Thinking through alternatives

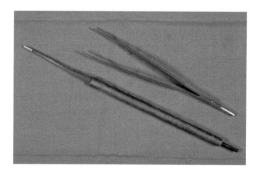

Figure 2.4 Bipolar (top instrument) and cutting (monopolar; bottom instrument) diathermy.

One of the problems with being a surgeon is the natural tendency to think that all problems present before you require surgery. This is manifestly not the case and it is important to remember that many conditions have more than one perfectly acceptable treatment alternative. Just because you own a hammer does not mean every problem becomes a nail.

Always think through the possible treatment alternatives and think what you would prefer to have done to you, particularly if there is a choice between two treatments that have a statistically similar outcome. *Do as you would be done by* is probably the most useful ethical tenet a surgeon can live by, followed immediately afterward by *do no further (net) harm* (thank you, Daniel Sokol, sometime medical ethicist writing in the *BMJ* who coined the 'net' addition).

Medicolegal aspects

Consent is defined as the voluntary and continuing permission of the patient to receive a particular treatment based on an adequate knowledge of the purpose, nature and likely sequelae of treatment including the likelihood of its success, complications and any alternatives to it. Permission given under any unfair or undue pressure is not consent. It seems self-evident that anyone undergoing surgery should understand exactly why he or she is undergoing this procedure and whether it is indeed the right thing to undergo. Being honest with the patient before surgery is a vital component that protects both the patient and the surgeon. The point of obtaining consent is twofold. Clinically it enlists the patient's faith and confidence in the validity of the treatment. Legally it provides those treating the patient with defence to a criminal charge of assault or battery or a civil claim for trespass to the person. Briefly if you advise a patient appropriately, the patient will understand the nature and risks of the procedure, and if you carry it out as a trained person to the best of your ability there should really be no problem. Having a signed consent form that a patient did not understand or carrying out a procedure in a careless or haphazard fashion or performing a procedure you are not trained to do in a negligent fashion is not defensible no matter how complex your consent form may be. No other person can give consent for a competent adult in UK law.

Self-determination

Any adult patient who has a sound mental capacity has an absolute right to choose whether or not to consent to medical treatment. The patient may therefore choose to refuse treatment or to go for one option rather than another even if the doctor believes that choice to be inappropriate. The 'age of consent' is generally held to be 16 years because there is no presumption of competence under this age. The crucial test is the degree of understanding shown by the child. (The age of consent in the United States is 18 years unless the patient is an emancipated minor.)

Consent

Consent can be implied (e.g. when a patient holds out his or her arm to allow blood to be taken), verbal (by spoken agreement) or written. Written consent is usually required for procedures performed with the patient under sedation or anaesthesia. For consent to be valid, three criteria must be met:

1. The consent must be voluntary and obtained without coercion or deceit.
2. The patient must be of sufficient age and mental capacity to be considered competent to give consent. Mentally handicapped and confused patients are thus often incapable of giving consent. In such cases, treatment considered to be in the patient's best interest can be carried out legally without consent, but for routine procedures it is desirable to obtain the assent of the next of kin or carer. Although 16 years is the legal age of consent, a child with sufficient understanding is capable of consenting to or refusing treatment and deserves adequate information, even when a parent signs the consent form.
3. The consent must be informed, meaning that adequate explanation of the procedure must be given, including any alternatives available. The patient should be informed of any serious or life-threatening risks of the operation, even if the probability of such complications is very small (>1%). Warnings given to the patient should be documented in the notes, and it may be advisable to provide additional written information in the form of a

small pamphlet with simple diagrams where appropriate.

In practical terms, to obtain consent involves the following:

- Determine the patient's level of understanding and pitch explanations to the same level.
- Ask the patient to describe what he or she understands about the procedure.
- Describe the procedure in plain language but adequate detail. Explain the benefits and risks, expected postoperative course, wound and scar size and site, drips, drains, monitors and catheters.
- In some institutions it is possible to arrange a visit to the intensive care or high dependency unit or, if the patient is a child, the ward or theatre if appropriate, to familiarize the patient with the surroundings.
- Allow time for the patient to formulate any questions and adequate time to answer them. Most advice suggests that there should be an interval between consent and undergoing a procedure. The period varies with the procedure.
- Obtain verbal and written consent.

In elective surgery in Germany, a minimum of 24 hours should be left between consent and surgery. Although standard consent forms are available for routine procedures, the explanation of the surgical procedure itself always must be conducted individually and can be documented on these forms by drawings or by noting specific questions. In Germany the consent form is a legal document. A copy of the consent form has to be handed to the patient.

Competency

A patient must be competent to give valid consent. A patient is not competent if he or she is premedicated, in labour, under undue stress or being affected by known mental illness or known organic brain disease. A patient who is immature by nature of learning difficulties or who is less than 16 years old is in a similar situation. Consent must be obtained from someone who has been deemed competent; in the case of a child, this is the parent or guardian, although a child with good understanding of the situation can give consent. In strictly legal terms a parent can consent to treatment if a child refuses; however, a parent *cannot* refuse treatment on a child's behalf if the child is 'competent' and consents to treatment. No one can give consent for an incompetent adult. A clinician can proceed 'in the best interests of the patient' but must abide by any preexisting competent declarations made by the patient.

In Germany, a district court has to appoint a legal guardian to look after the medical interests of adults deemed incompetent to consent. This person may be a family member such as a spouse but may even be a friend or a court-appointed custodian.

Who should obtain the consent?

In most areas the practitioner who will or is capable of carrying out the surgery should take the consent.

Warnings

There is a tendency to carry out defensive medicine promulgated by the threat of litigation. In North America this puts a tremendous burden on patients by forcing doctors to explain every last potential risk and complication of any operation, often when the patient has no real valid alternative given the nature of the pathology. This creates significant additional psychological morbidity for patients. The tendency in the United Kingdom is to follow a similar approach. It is generally accepted that if there is a material risk higher than 1:100 then patients should be advised about this. This translates into, for example, when obtaining consent for third molar surgery advising the patients about the risks of lingual and inferior alveolar nerve sensory damage, pain, swelling and trismus.

In Germany, irrespective of whether an operation carries a material risk of greater than 1:100, if said risk can bring significant harm to the patient, the patient has to be informed. For instance, although there is a low risk of mandibular fracture when removing wisdom teeth, the consequence is significant. It is also very rare to suffer blindness following a Le Fort I osteotomy but it is a rare and recognized complication of which it is mandatory to inform patients.

Consent for anaesthesia should be obtained by the anaesthetist, who is the only person in a position to carry out this particular intervention.

Medical notes

It is worthwhile remembering that legible reproducible medical notes are a legal requirement in the management of all patients. Notes should be accurate and complete, dated and timed with an identifiable signature. If your signature is illegible your name should be printed beside it. These notes should be made at the same time or immediately after consulting with the patient and not inserted after the fact. Language should be professional and noncontentious. All efforts should be made to keep the writing legible, and a minimum number of abbreviations and acronyms should be used. Do not write R or L for right and left. Avoid 'personal' acronyms – no one is going to be very impressed if you have to explain in court what KTBO (kick the bugger out) stands for.

If a patient takes a surgeon to court in Germany for malpractice, the prosecuting side must prove that the doctor has made a mistake. If the court finds that the doctor made a severe mistake, the burden of proof is turned upside down. Now the doctor has to prove that he did not make a mistake and worked according to national medical standards. Statistical reports from the association of lawyers in Germany show that in more than 50% of the cases in which doctors are sued, the underlying cause is insufficient documentation.

Once the decision has been made to operate, the environment has been prepared and the patient has been informed and has consented, a surgical plan needs to be formulated. The first step is to indicate on which side or in which quadrant of the mouth you intend to operate. This is done either by marking the patient in indelible ink for surgery to be performed under general anaesthesia or by making absolutely clear which area you are operating on for this particular patient. Imaging in the form of plain radiographs, computed tomography scans, ultrasound scans or magnetic resonance imaging, used to localize pathology or assess their extent, should be available during the operation.

Patient preparation

Most hospitals have a series of guidelines issued by the radiology and anaesthetic departments on the minimum acceptable investigations for surgery. Practically nowhere is it regarded as acceptable to take routine preoperative chest radiographs, and most radiology departments have specific indications for a chest radiograph such as recent acute chest disease, risk of metastases or pathology specific to the chest. Conversely, many hospitals expect any patient who is more than 50 or 55 years old to have an electrocardiogram (ECG) because this is regarded as a useful noninvasive and inexpensive test. The most useful thing you can do is be familiar with your own hospital's protocols and stick to them. If you can work out the justifications for these protocols you will find that you quite quickly understand the reasons for being efficient and thoughtful about preoperative investigations. Preoperative investigation is covered in more detail in Chapter 5.

Preparing a patient for surgery obviously varies widely depending on whether the patient is going to have surgery under local anaesthesia in an outpatient setting, surgery under local anaesthesia with or without sedation in an inpatient setting or surgery under general anaesthesia, which will be in some form of hospital setting either in a day unit or as an inpatient.

A useful way of thinking about how to prepare each individual patient is to walk through in your own head what is likely to happen to the patient. For example, if the patient is a healthy young adult coming in to have a third molar removed under local anaesthesia then the patient will simply be able to walk in, give consent, sit down in the chair, be put into a comfortable position (more of this in a minute), be deemed suitable for anaesthesia, have the surgery, recover from the surgery for a few minutes and leave. In that case all you need to do is have an area where the patient can sign consent, sit down in comfort and undergo surgery. At the other extreme, if the patient has spinal injuries and must be transferred from one ward where the staff members are not used to sending patients to an operating theatre some distance away for salivary gland surgery, then there is a whole series of steps that, if you do not think them through, will create massive problems for all concerned. For example, a patient with spinal injuries presents a handling problem; the nurses on the ward may be aware of this but the staff in theatre may not. The operating theatre staff must be informed and be in a position to make appropriate arrangements to move the patient safely from a trolley onto an operating theatre table into a safe and comfortable position. The type of surgery the patient is going to undergo may require modifications to the anaesthetic regimen. Therefore the anaesthetists need to be aware of the specific operation to be carried out and the type of patient, to allow them to decide what sort of anaesthetic modification they will have to make. A patient such as this may well have other underlying medical problems and is going to need a reasonable range of investigations (e.g. an ECG) and a range of biochemical tests (e.g. urea and electrolytes) at the very least. Because the patient is going to be immobile before, during and after surgery, he or she may well require some form of prophylaxis against deep venous thrombosis.

It is only by thinking about each individual patient separately and working through in your head the kind of steps that will be involved in the surgery that you can adequately prepare the patient. There is little point in using some form of blanket checklist for every patient because it will be overkill for many patients and inadequate for some. The lesson to learn here is to think it through for each individual patient. Even if it does take a little longer it will save you time in the long run.

As part of an effort to avoid surgical errors the World Health Organization has devised a surgical checklist that has been adopted in many guises throughout the world. This checklist basically follows the concepts outlined earlier, with named individuals taking responsibility for each step of the patient's journey from leaving the ward to the anaesthetic room through surgery and back.

FURTHER READING

British Medical Association. *Consent tool kit*, 2001: www.bma.org.uk
This is a source of definitive information.
Deitch EA. *Tools of the trade and rules of the road: a surgical guide*. Philadelphia: Lippincott-Raven, 1997.
This is a fascinating little book full of quirky facts and a sound surgical philosophy.
General Medical Council. *Good medical practice*, 2013: www.gmc-uk.org
This website contains comprehensive guidance and includes an understanding that patients and doctors are making decisions together.
World Health Organization. *World Health Organization surgical checklist*, 2009: www.who.int.
This list aims to improve the safety of surgical care around the world.

3

Asepsis, antisepsis and instruments

Contents

Aims

- To appreciate the nature of asepsis, antisepsis and surgical cleanliness.
- To start to become familiar with surgical instruments and their names.

Learning outcomes

- To be able to describe when sterility is essential and how this can be achieved.
- To be able to describe how surgical asepsis and cleanliness can be achieved and when they are indicated.
- To list the name and use of some common surgical instruments.
- To discuss this as a basis for all further activity in surgery.

Asepsis and antisepsis

Sepsis was an almost universal complication of surgery and carried a high mortality until Joseph Lister, in 1867, in Scotland, proposed his 'germ theory' and put forward the idea of antisepsis to reduce infections in surgical patients as a practical application of the theory. This was one of the major fundamental advances in surgery.

Terminology

- **Sterilization** – a process that results in the complete absence of microorganisms, including bacteria, viruses and bacterial spores.
- **Antisepsis** – a process that results in the absence of most pathogenic microorganisms. However, some bacteria, viruses and spores may still be present.
- **Clean** – a reduction in the total bacterial count.

Cross infection is a potentially serious problem in all patients who are immunosuppressed or who have recently undergone surgery. In hospital this frequently occurs from patient to patient either directly or via the doctor, nurse or some other healthcare professional. Commonly transferred organisms include the following:

- *Staphylococcus aureus.*
- (Multiply) methicillin-resistant *Staphylococcus aureus* (MRSA).
- *Klebsiella.*
- *Streptococcus* species.
- *Pseudomonas* species.

These organisms tend to be transferred by skin contact. Viral infections are more often passed on in the air via microdroplets (*'Coughs and sneezes spread diseases'*).

Sterilization

This is the key process in minimizing cross infection. Unfortunately, sterilization does not guarantee protection against the newly discovered prions, best known for their role in bovine spongiform encephalitis (BSE). Despite this, no recorded case of BSE has been found resulting from the use of sterilized equipment.

There are various ways in which sterilized equipment may be obtained.

- **Disposable items** sterilized by gamma irradiation are available. So long as the pack is not opened the contents remain sterile for a long time.
- **Autoclaving** is the process of sterilization using pressurized steam. The increase in pressure enables much higher temperatures to be obtained. Settings may vary, but the two common ones are 121° Celsius (C) for 20 minutes and 134° C for 3.5 minutes at 32 psi. Items must be mechanically cleaned to remove blood and so forth before they are put in the autoclave. Items are prepacked and wrapped in 'autoclave tape' (Figure 3.1), which indicates when sterilization has been completed.

  Unfortunately, if the drying phase is not complete, metal instruments such as osteotomes and chisels can tarnish, corrode or rust.
- **Dry heat sterilization** – here hot air is applied at 160° C for 60 minutes. This process is useful for multipiece precision equipment such as handpieces, but these instruments need careful lubrication before sterilization.

Boiling in water does not destroy bacterial spores or viruses and is therefore ineffective as a true sterilization technique.

Despite the use of sterilized equipment, cross infection from and to healthcare workers and patients can still occur. To reduce the likelihood of this further, other precautions are necessary. Gloves, gowns, masks and goggles should always be worn when bleeding is likely to occur or when high-speed hand pieces are used because they create an aerosol that can infect the surgeon or the surgical assistant. Chemical disinfection of chairs, lights and so forth and scrupulous hand washing are also essential components of preparation for surgery. Unfortunately, no antiseptic solution exists that can disinfect equipment yet not be harmful to tissues if it accidentally comes in contact with the patient or surgeon.

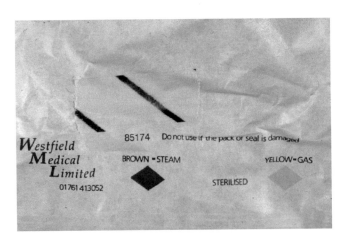

Figure 3.1 Autoclave tape – the tape goes brown, indicating sterilization.

Even if cross infection is eliminated, surgical patients remain at risk of having their wounds colonized by commensal organisms. Skin preparation using antiseptic preparations (aqueous iodine, chlorhexidine, cetrimide) is performed to reduce these organisms. Similar attempts to disinfect the mouth can be made, but this tends to achieve a reduction in overall bacterial count rather than an elimination of bacteria.

Antiseptics and disinfection

An antiseptic can be defined as a nontoxic disinfectant that can be applied to the skin or living tissues and has the ability to destroy vegetative compounds such as bacteria by preventing their growth. Examples of antiseptics include:

- Povidone-iodine.
- Proflavin.
- Chlorhexidine.

Povidone-iodine comes in a wide range of products including antiseptics, skin preparations and mouthwashes. The solution used for wound care is the aqueous solution that contains 1% iodine. It is available in ointment and spray form and is impregnated into a dressing (e.g. Inadine).

Povidone-iodine has been shown to be effective against MRSA, and to date there does not appear to be resistance to it. It is also effective against other bacteria and their spores, viruses and fungi. Because of this, iodine has replaced most topical antibiotics. The main disadvantage is that patients may be or may become sensitive to iodine, and it should be used only in the short term. It should also not be used on large wounds because absorption of iodine may occur, and the iodine is also destructive to human cells (although less than to pathogens). The alcoholic solution is an irritant to wounds and dangerous on the face near the eyes; it is also a fire hazard and is used much less frequently nowadays.

Chlorhexidine is a broadly active antiseptic that is used as an alternative to iodine in allergic individuals and can be used for skin preparation and 'scrubbing up'. It is unusual in that when used in the mouth it binds to both tooth enamel and epithelial cells and leaches out over time, thus providing a longer-acting effect. This may account for the

evidence that suggests chlorhexidine-containing mouthwashes are more effective than others in controlling oral bacterial diseases.

Hand disinfection

'Scrubbing up' should be performed for each case. Fingernails should be kept short and jewellery removed. Gloves are worn after drying. Various disinfectants are available. Commonly used ones are:

- 4% chlorhexidine gluconate (Hibiscrub, Halascrub).
- 7.5% povidone-iodine (Betadine).
- 2.5% chlorhexidine in 70% alcohol (Hibisol) – may be used as an alternative between cases as long as the hands have been thoroughly scrubbed for the first case.
- 0.5% chlorhexidine solution – can be used as a mouth rinse (for the patient) before oral surgery.

Cleaning wounds – 'the solution to pollution is dilution'

Unfortunately, but unsurprisingly, it has been shown that all these antiseptics inhibit fibroblastic activity and therefore interfere with healing. Their use in cleaning infected wounds is not essential because the most important factor is the volume of solution used. Sterile saline in abundance is quite adequate, although a diluted povidone-iodine solution used both to scrub mechanically and irrigate 'dirty' wounds is commonplace.

Antiseptic dressings

Iodine-based medicaments

Whitehead's varnish is a mixture of iodoform, benzoin, storax, balsam of tolu and solvent ether. It is used as an antiseptic dressing in the treatment of dry socket, packing marsupialized cysts and as a postoperative dressing after maxillectomy. Dressings may be left in place for 2 weeks without becoming infected. Alternatively, iodine can be mixed with bismuth to form bismuth iodoform paraffin paste (BIPP). This can be applied to ribbon gauze and used in packing the nose or almost any other cavity. Iodine has a disinfectant action with organic tissue; however, it is also an irritant and may stimulate granulation tissue formation.

Commonly used dressings

Traditional dressings (e.g. gauze and Gamgee) – these are useful as secondary dressings to help to control exudate.

Low adherent dressings (e.g. Mepitel, Melolin, Release, Skintact) – these are useful on wounds that have a low exudate, in securing skin grafts or on burns or abrasions. Some are silicone polymers that may improve scar quality.

Alginate dressings (e.g. Sorbsan, Kaltostat) – these are dry absorbent dressings made from seaweed. The dressing absorbs exudate from the wound and becomes a gel. Alginates are also useful as haemostats. They should not be used on dry wounds.

Charcoal dressings (e.g. Actisorb Plus) – these contain activated charcoal, which is effective in absorbing chemicals released from fungating, smelly and necrotic wounds. Actisorb Plus also contains silver, which helps to reduce bacterial growth.

Foams (e.g. Lyofoam, Cavicare) – these are synthetic dressings of hydrophilic polyurethane that absorb wound exudate and maintain a moist wound healing environment. They can be used on moderately to heavily exudating wounds that are healthy and granulating.

Hydrocolloids (e.g. Granuflex, Tegasorb) – these consist of a hydrocolloid base made from gelatine, cellulose and pectins. They are completely occlusive and provide a moist wound healing environment. Fluid from the wound is absorbed into the dressing and forms a gel. These dressings are useful on necrotic, sloughy and granulating wounds.

Enzyme preparation (e.g. Varidase) – this contains two enzymes (streptokinase and streptodornase) and is used to débride wounds, especially those with a necrotic eschar.

Hydrogels (e.g. Intrasite Gel) – these dressings are made up of a copolymer starch and have high water content. They can be used to débride necrotic tissue or sloughy, granulating and epithelializing wounds.

Impregnated dressings (e.g. Jelonet and Inadine) – Jelonet is woven cotton that is impregnated with paraffin. It is commonly used on minor burns, abrasions, split-thickness skin grafts and donor sites. Inadine is made of rayon mesh impregnated with 10% povidone-iodine. The iodine is released directly onto the wound.

Vapour-permeable films (e.g. Tegaderm, Opsite) – these are semipermeable, adhesive, film dressings that prevent evaporation of water from the wound. They should be used only on superficial low exudating wounds. These dressings can be useful in the prevention of pressure sore formation over bony prominences by reducing friction.

Antibacterials (e.g. Flammazine cream) – Flammazine contains silver sulphadiazine 1% and is a topical broad-spectrum antibacterial that inhibits the growth of nearly all pathogenic bacteria and fungi in vitro. It is particularly effective against *Pseudomonas* and *S. aureus*. It is widely used in the treatment of burns.

Haemostatic agents (e.g. Surgicel, Lyostypt) – these are forms of oxidized cellulose that promote clotting. Flowseal is fibrin foam that is effective on bleeding bone ends.

Glues – a number of fibrin based tissue glues can be used on skin wounds and (as a spray or drops) to stick grafts or flaps to concave wounds.

Vac-Pacs – these are basically adherent dressings that allow the generation of a vacuum (negative) pressure within the sealed area. They promote healing to a sometimes remarkable extent.

Mouthwashes

- Chlorhexidine mouthwash (Corsodyl) is bactericidal. It may be helpful in 'at risk' patients (e.g. osteonecrosis) by reducing the number of bacteria inoculated into the circulatory system if it is used before surgery. The dose is 10 mL rinsed for 1 minute and then expectorated.
- Hot salt water mouthwashes are often advised following surgery. They are helpful in keeping the mouth clean, provide some pain relief and are cheap.
- Benzydamine (Difflam) may be used to relieve the pain associated with oral ulcers or radiation mucositis. The dose is 10 mL twice daily for up to 1 week.

Instruments and sutures

Instruments

The choice of surgical instruments is largely a matter of personal preference and affordability. All instruments must be either disposable or autoclavable. Many different instruments are available on the market. Some of those more commonly used in minor oral surgery are outlined here:

- **Local anaesthetic syringes** – these are usually self-aspirating so that it is possible to tell whether the needle has been inadvertently introduced into a vessel (Figure 3.2).
- **Retractors** (Kilner's cheek, Lack's, Bowdler-Henry in the United Kingdom; Tobold, Wassmund, Langenbeck in German-speaking countries; Army-Navy in the United States) – these are used to retract the cheek, the tongue or soft tissue flaps (Figures 3.3 and 3.4). The main point is to learn what the instrument you need is called wherever you happen to be operating.
- **Scalpel** – dissection can be done with either scissors or a scalpel. Scalpel blades come in a variety of shapes and sizes, depending on their use. Numbers 15, 11 and 10 are commonly used in oral and maxillofacial surgery (Figure 3.5).
- **Periosteal elevators** (Howarth's, Ward's, Mitchell's trimmer) – these are used to lift the periosteum off bone in dentoalveolar surgery or other procedures involving bone

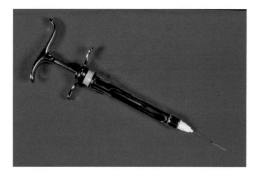

Figure 3.2 Dental cartridge syringe – remember not all local anaesthesia is given using this system. If you are going to use local anaesthesia in an operating theatre, specify what you want.

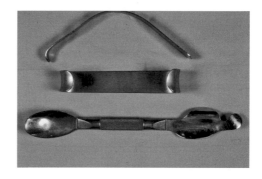

Figure 3.3 From top – Lack's, Kilner's cheek and Rowe's retractors.

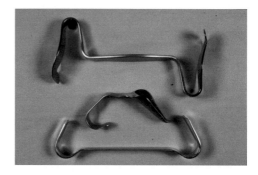

Figure 3.4 From top – Ward's, Laster's and Rowe's retractors.

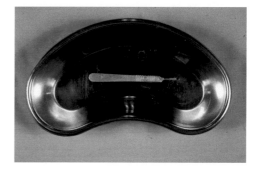

Figure 3.5 A number 5 scalpel handle in a steel kidney bowl for safe transfer.

(Figure 3.6). They need a cutting edge because periosteum is adherent. Careful elevation reduces postoperative swelling.

- **Bone-cutting instruments** – bone can be cut using chisels, osteotomes or burrs on a revolving handpiece. Burrs are probably better in the conscious patient. Rongeurs ('bone nibblers') are useful in removing spicules of bone (Figures 3.7, 3.8 and 3.9). An identical instrument is named after Luer in German-speaking countries.

Forceps and elevators – teeth are removed with forceps and elevators. Elevators are particularly useful when the teeth are buried. Both forceps and elevators come in different shapes to be applied in different circumstances. They include Cryer's, Coupland's and Warwick-James instruments (Figures 3.10, 3.11, 3.12 and 3.13).

Curettes – these are used to scrape soft tissue from bone, for instance in cyst removal.

Artery forceps – these are used for clamping vessels for haemostasis, blunt dissection and holding 'disposable' tissue (Figures 3.14 and 3.15).

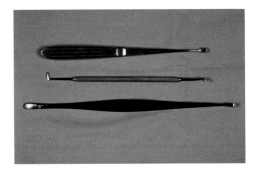

Figure 3.6 From top – Ward's, Mitchell's and Howarth's elevators.

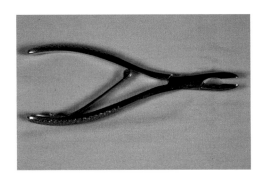

Figure 3.9 Bone rongeurs.

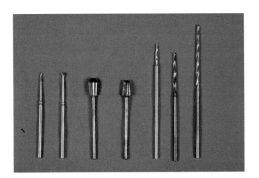

Figure 3.7 Range of surgical burrs.

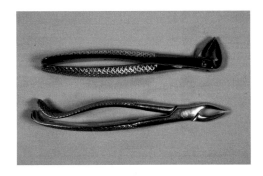

Figure 3.10 From top – lower and upper dental extraction forceps.

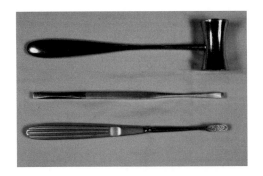

Figure 3.8 From top – mallet, osteotomes, bone file.

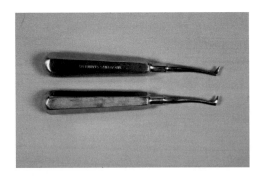

Figure 3.11 Right and left Cryer's elevators.

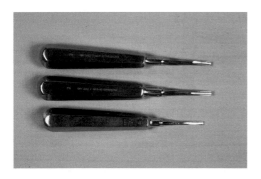

Figure 3.12 Coupland's numbers 1, 2 and 3 elevators.

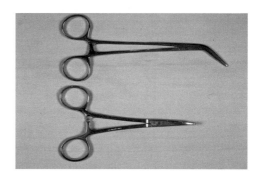

Figure 3.15 Fickling's and Dunhill's forceps.

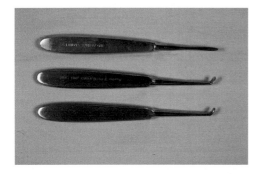

Figure 3.13 Straight, right and left Warwick-James elevators.

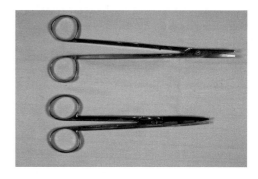

Figure 3.16 Curved and straight scissors.

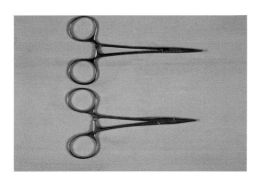

Figure 3.14 Straight and curved mosquito artery forceps.

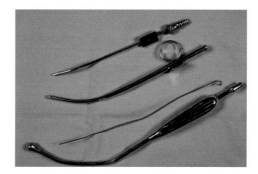

Figure 3.17 Range of suction tips.

Scissors – dissecting scissors come in many forms. All are distinguished by special cutting tips. Suture scissors are not to be used for dissecting and *vice versa* (Figure 3.16).

Suction tips – these vary in size and the presence or absence of a side hole, depending on their purpose (Figure 3.17).

Needle holders and tissue forceps – a wide range exists. Fine needle holders such as the Crile-Wood should be used for delicate sutures; tissue forceps are toothed and nontoothed (Figures 3.18, 3.19 and 3.20).

Mouth props – these are invaluable but are often hard to come by outside the immediate 'dental tray' (Figure 3.21).

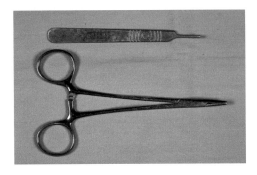

Figure 3.18 Scalpel handle and needle holder.

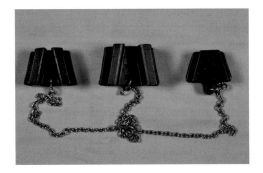

Figure 3.21 Rubber mouth props.

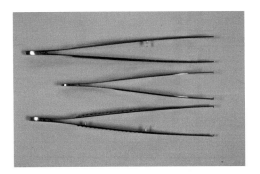

Figure 3.19 A range of dissecting forceps.

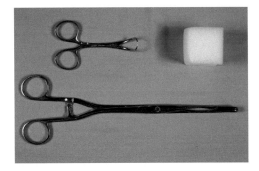

Figure 3.22 Backhaus towel clip (top) and Rampley's sponge-holding forceps.

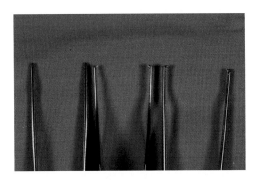

Figure 3.20 Close-up view of the tips of nontoothed and toothed dissecting forceps.

Towel clip and sponge holder – (Backhaus and Rampley's in the United Kingdom) (Figure 3.22).

Sutures

Many different sutures are now available, but they are generally classified as follows:

- Absorbable – polyglactin 910 (Vicryl/Vicryl Rapide), polyglycolic acid (Dexon) and poliglecaprone 25 (Monocryl) and catgut.
  - Vicryl/Vicryl Rapide – these are braided resorbable sutures that are absorbed by hydrolysis.
  - Monocryl – this is a monofilament and is less of an irritant for subcuticular use.
  - Catgut (from sheep) – this has been discontinued for clinical use in the United Kingdom but is available in the United States.
- Nonabsorbable – nylon, polypropylene (Prolene) and polybutester (Novafil).
  - Nylon – this has less memory than Prolene and Novafil but is marginally more of an irritant. These are the usual sutures for closing skin wounds.
  - Silk – this is essentially a temporary suture material nowadays.
- Specially designed skin staples and tissue adhesives are both used in skin closure.

Sutures may also be classified according to structure:

- Monofilament – these minimize infection and produce less tissue reaction. They are the suture of choice for skin.
- Twisted or braided – these have plaited strands, which provide secure knots but may act like a wick causing a focus of infection.

Traditionally, silk has been used in the mouth because it is easy to handle and strong, and the ends are comfortable for the patient. Its major disadvantage is that it must be removed. Vicryl is also popular because it resorbs and does not need to be removed. The use of sutures in different situations is described in later chapters.

North America

The basic instruments used in North America and their purposes are similar to those used in the United Kingdom. However, there are some subtle differences, with a multitude of eponymous instruments just as in the German-speaking countries, particularly periosteal and dental elevators.

Understanding what it is you are trying to accomplish with the instrument will help you in your instrument choice.

Both fast-absorbing and chromic gut sutures are still routinely used in clinical practice in North America.

FURTHER READING

Rather than read about this, ask theatre or outpatient scrub staff to name instruments and describe their use. Many theatres have extensive instrument catalogues, and as there will be incredible variation, it makes more sense to make a note to yourself of the names you are likely to use.

Specific literature includes the following:

Cherian P, Gunson T, Borchard K, Tai Y, Smith H, Vinciullo C. Oral antibiotics versus topical decolonization to prevent surgical site infection after Mohs micrographic surgery: a randomized controlled trial. *Dermatol Surg* 2013;39:1486–93.

Kirby E, Dickinson J, Vassey M, Dennis M, Cornwall M, Mc Leod N, Smith A, Marsh PD, Walker JT, Sutton JM, Raven ND. Bioassay studies support the potential for iatrogenic transmission of variant Creutzfeldt Jakob disease through dental procedures. *PLoS One* 2012;11:e49850.

4

Managing people, pain and anxiety

Contents

Aim

- To gain a basic understanding of psychological (behaviour management) and pharmacological approaches to pain and anxiety control.

Learning outcomes

For undergraduates:

- To be able to describe appropriate techniques for analgesia, sedation and anaesthesia for individuals.
- To be able to describe common complications of analgesia, sedation and anaesthesia.

For postgraduates:

- To be able to discuss the common techniques for analgesia and sedation.

- To be able to prescribe appropriate analgesia for individuals and recognize potential complications.
- To be able to select appropriately patients requiring local analgesia, sedation, a combination of the two or general anaesthesia.

Any patient who attends a healthcare worker is subjected to some form of behaviour management. This is commonly in the form of compassion regarding the patient's problems and a listening ear.

Other techniques include 'tell, show, do' and positive reinforcement. Although mainly used with children, this approach helps to reduce anxiety and builds trust.

Anxiety is an inevitable and probably appropriate response to surgery. Pain is an inevitable response to surgery, and the purpose of pain is to warn the body of damage. Pain has been defined as 'an unpleasant experience associated with actual or potential tissue damage'. It is evident that pain and anxiety are inextricably linked. Anxiety exacerbates the sensation of pain and can promote pain even in the absence of organic stimulus.

There is no single nerve pathway that is devoted exclusively to pain. The peripheral and central pathways of the nervous system associated with pain are complex and heavily influenced by the cerebral cortex.

Most types of dental pain arise as a result of infection or damage to tissue.

The emphasis in this chapter is on how to manage pain. A primary consideration is recognizing that your patient is in pain. Patients who present with extreme anxiety and who describe pains that have no true anatomical or physiological characteristics can be extremely challenging. In such cases it is important to acknowledge that the patient has pain, whether or not an organic cause can be identified. The primary consideration with this kind of patient is to control the pain in the first instance. Patients who are in pain may range from postoperative patients who have been given inadequate analgesia to those who have breakthrough pain despite what would usually be adequate analgesia. In these instances it is often worthwhile resorting to combination analgesics.

Patients with localized or surgical pain can often be helped by deposition of local analgesia or by splinting.

Other patients may attend with very specific pain. Symptoms such as lancinating pain (commonly referred to as an 'electric shock' sensation) originating from a specific sensory nerve are characteristic of trigeminal neuralgia. In this instance both diagnosis and adequate therapy can be achieved by starting carbamazepine. For less typical cases it is worth noting that an alternative, pregabalin, has anxiety-reducing properties.

Patients who attend with bizarre or atypical pain, or long-standing chronic pain, may be helped by a combination of analgesia and antidepressants. If antidepressant use is being considered, it is well worthwhile spending time ascertaining whether the patient has problems with sleeping, in which case a sedative antidepressant taken at night is often helpful. Alternatively if somnolence is a concern, a relatively stimulating antidepressant such as a selective serotonin reuptake inhibitor is of greater advantage.

Local anaesthesia

Local anaesthesia is defined as 'a loss of sensation in a specific area of the body by a depression of excitation in nerve endings'.

Surgery performed using local anaesthesia has a number of advantages:

- Minor treatment or investigation can be offered immediately. Many simple procedures can be carried out using local anaesthesia (e.g. biopsy, exodontia, scar revision).
- It avoids admission or fasting (especially for children and medically compromised patients).
- Local anaesthesia is often safer (in appropriate doses, and sometimes general anaesthesia is actually safer).
- It is more cost effective than admission and general anaesthesia.
- In experienced hands, the block can be easily and quickly performed.
- With the addition of a vasoconstrictor in the local anaesthetic solution, surgical bleeding is reduced.
- Uses can be diagnostic and therapeutic – nerve blocks can be used as a diagnostic test for trigeminal neuralgia or pain thought to be caused by nerve irritation (e.g. neuroma).

The ability to produce effective local anaesthesia in the head and neck, especially the mouth, is an essential skill in oral and maxillofacial surgery. In experienced hands, extensive areas of anaesthesia are possible – almost anywhere in the face, neck, scalp and oral cavity can be effectively anaesthetized. Various techniques can be used, extending from minimally invasive topical anaesthesia to nerve block techniques in which local anaesthetic is placed at sites where large nerve trunks emerge from foramina. When necessary, local anaesthesia may be supplemented with sedation. This is particularly useful in anxious patients or in children. However, it must be remembered that sedation in itself is not a substitute for good local anaesthetic technique – a good working knowledge of anatomy, an adequate dose of local anaesthetic drug, knowledge of drug doses and onset times, and, importantly, patient cooperation are needed. The reward of good technique is good surgical anaesthesia.

Beginning with the technique that requires the least skill, *topical* application allows a local anaesthetic to be absorbed through the skin and mucosa, thus rendering them insensate to further needling.

Infiltration refers to the injection of local anaesthetic close to the area and sometimes through traumatic wound edges, which may be less painful – by diffusion, the sensory nerves are anaesthetized.

Anaesthetizing a peripheral nerve at its most practically reached proximal point results in sensory and sometimes motor block. This is referred to as a *nerve block* (also called a *field block*). Another use of field blocks is the treatment of some types of chronic pain, in which longer-acting local anaesthetic agents are used. (Detailed description of commonly performed dentoalveolar blocks is provided in this chapter.)

With appropriate case selection and good technique the need for admission and general anaesthesia for many minor and intermediate operations can often be avoided. There is a caveat when children, confused patients and psychiatrically unwell patients are being considered for local anaesthetic techniques – good patient understanding and cooperation can mean the difference between a successful and a potentially disastrous outcome.

Local anaesthetic drugs

Classification

1. Chemically – the local anaesthetic agents are either amides or esters.
2. Duration of action – they may be described as short-, intermediate- or long-acting agents, within each of the foregoing chemical groups.

Amide local anaesthetics

- Lidocaine (new internationally recognized name; previously lignocaine)

This is the most commonly used local anaesthetic drug in the United Kingdom.

Presentation – available in dental local anaesthetic cartridges as a plain 2% solution or with 1:80 000 adrenaline. The 2% with 1:80 000 adrenaline is the most commonly used preparation. Proprietary names are Xylocaine, Lignospan and Lignostab. In the United Kingdom, 2.2 mL of solution is present in dental cartridges; each cartridge contains 44 mg of lidocaine.

Uses and routes of administration – infiltration, intraligamentary and regional block anaesthesia for most patients.

Onset of action – anaesthesia is obtained in 2 to 3 minutes.

Duration of action – the plain/hypobaric solution is classified as short acting, its duration of action being 10 minutes. The addition of adrenaline decreases absorption of local anaesthetic from the area, thereby increasing the duration of action 4- to 10-fold, depending on the route of administration.

Although adrenaline is naturally occurring in the body, the concentration present in local anaesthetic/vasoconstrictor combinations is supraphysiological. Adverse effects of high levels of exogenous adrenaline such as tachycardia, hypertension, arrhythmias and cardiac arrest can occur with intravascular injection, necessitating aspiration during injection techniques, particularly around prominent vessels.

Controversy remains about the use of adrenaline-containing local anaesthesia in cardiac patients. Risk/benefit considerations are important – if poor general health precludes general anaesthesia, a procedure using local anaesthesia may be the only alternative, and a lidocaine/adrenaline preparation remains the most effective.

Doses

For *plain* lidocaine – maximum recommended dose is 3 mg/kg (per kg doses refer to the patient's body weight).

For lidocaine and a vasoconstrictor – inclusion of 1:80 000 adrenaline increases the maximum dose to 7 mg/kg.

- Prilocaine
  This is an amide local anaesthetic, as potent as lidocaine, but less toxic. Prilocaine is more rapidly metabolized than lidocaine; this may explain its clinical impression as a less effective local anaesthetic. One of its

metabolites, in excessive amounts, may cause methaemoglobinaemia.

Presentation – available as plain 4% prilocaine or as 3% prilocaine with 0.03 IU/mL felypressin. In the United Kingdom, the solution with felypressin is the usual alternative to lidocaine with adrenaline. Proprietary name – Citanest.
Uses and routes of administration – most effective when infiltrated or as a regional block.
Onset of action – comparable to that of lidocaine.
Duration of action – 1.5 times that of lidocaine.

Doses

The maximum recommended dose is 6 mg/kg (8 mg/kg with felypressin).

- Bupivacaine (proprietary name – Marcain)
  This long-lasting local anaesthetic is not supplied in dental local anaesthetic cartridges in the United Kingdom. (Its stereoisomer, levobupivacaine, is available as Chirocaine. The properties of levobupivacaine are similar to those of Bupivacaine, but with less cardiotoxic potential at higher doses.)

Presentation – available in concentrations of 0.25%, 0.5% and 0.75%. The 0.25% and 0.5% are available with or without 1:200 000 adrenaline. Because of its high degree of protein binding, the duration of bupivacaine is not significantly enhanced with the addition of a vasoconstrictor.
Uses and routes of administration – topically and via infiltration, Bupivacaine is useful for postoperative pain control. It can be delivered using an epidural catheter and filter as a wound irrigant to reduce pain from flap and graft donor sites.
Onset of action – peak effect is achieved in 10 to 15 minutes.
Duration of action – 5 to 10 hours, depending on the route of administration.

Dose

The maximum dose is 2 mg/kg, with or without a vasoconstrictor (Figure 4.1).

Other amides include mepivacaine, etidocaine, and articaine. Articaine is interesting in that it is thought to have the ability to diffuse effectively into bone. It has been suggested that palatal anaesthesia

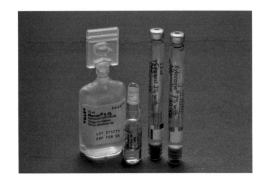

Figure 4.1 From left: a plastic bupivacaine vial, separate glass vial of adrenaline, prilocaine and lidocaine dental cartridges. The latter two can only be used with specific syringes.

may be achieved following maxillary buccal infiltration and that pulpal anaesthesia is possible after infiltrations in the mandible; the evidence for this is inconclusive.

Ester local anaesthetics

- Benzocaine
  Most commonly used in lozenges and topical preparations, it has poor water solubility and is not injectable.
- Procaine
  This is no longer available in the United Kingdom in dental cartridge form. Its only use is when there is a proven allergy to amide local anaesthetics (which is very rare, if indeed it exists). Procaine provides very short-lived pulpal anaesthesia lasting 5 minutes and is therefore not very useful clinically.
- Cocaine
  This produces vasoconstriction and is available as a topical preparation usually used to anaesthetize the nasal mucosa. It is sometimes used topically during nasoendotracheal intubations or before packing a nose to treat epistaxis. The vasoconstrictive effect is the reason habitual recreational use of this drug can lead to septal ischaemic necrosis.

Local anaesthetic techniques

Topical

Anaesthetic agents for topical use are supplied as gels, sprays or ointments.

Intraoral use

- The most common agents used intraorally are lidocaine and benzocaine. Lidocaine is available as a 10% spray (Xylocaine spray) and a 5% ointment (Figure 4.2).
- Benzocaine is normally used as a 20% gel. Different flavours are added to this, to make it popular among children (Figure 4.3).
- These topical anaesthetics penetrate nonkeratinized tissues (reflected mucosa) very well and anaesthetize to a depth of 2 to 3 mm.
- The anaesthetic should be applied for 2 minutes to give maximum effect.

Cutaneous use

- Topical anaesthetics for skin have been developed that penetrate highly keratinized tissues. This is useful before venipuncture or for superficial soft tissue manipulation.
- Preparations include EMLA cream (this is an acronym: Eutectic Mixture of Local Anaesthetics), which is a mixture of lidocaine and prilocaine, and Ametop, which is amethocaine based.

- Both preparations are applied to skin and are covered with a dressing left in place for 1 hour before the procedure (e.g. cannulation) (Figures 4.4 and 4.5).

Injection techniques

A good working knowledge of anatomy is essential. Bone is porous in the maxilla; therefore, infiltration techniques are effective for pulpal anaesthesia. Mandibular bone is denser, infiltration is less effective and regional blocks are needed. The needle, dental local anaesthetic cartridge and syringe are the three components needed to deliver conventional dentoalveolar local anaesthesia.

Needles are supplied presterilized and are single use only. Commonly, two lengths are used (short and long), and they are of a very narrow diameter (Figure 4.6).

Cartridges are prefilled by manufacturers and are sterile. Syringes are usually nondisposable and are sterilized in an autoclave between patients.

Any needle and syringe combination can be used to deliver local anaesthesia, but if using a conventional needle/syringe combination, remember

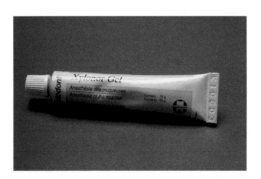

Figure 4.2 Lidocaine (Xylocaine) 5% ointment.

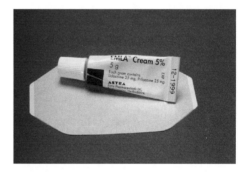

Figure 4.4 EMLA cream.

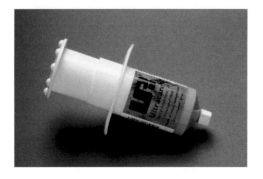

Figure 4.3 Benzocaine 20% gel. Walterberry flavour.

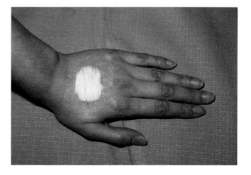

Figure 4.5 EMLA cream applied to skin.

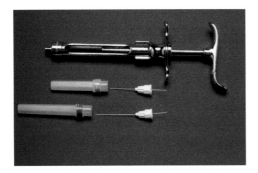

Figure 4.6 Dental local anaesthetic cartridges and needles.

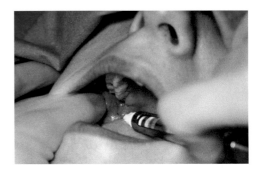

Figure 4.7 Direct method for inferior alveolar block.

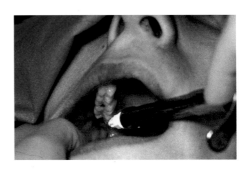

Figure 4.8 Gow-Gates block.

to aspirate and remember to use a Luer-lock system because the pressure exerted can often blow the needle off the syringe.

Common techniques include the following:

Inferior alveolar (inferior dental) nerve block

Local anaesthetic is placed around the interior alveolar nerve as it enters the mandible at the lingula. There are several methods to achieve this:

Direct method
- Administration – the patient's mouth must be wide open. The external and internal oblique ridges are palpated; the line of the pterygomandibular raphe is noted. With the palpating thumb lying in the retromolar fossa, the needle is inserted slightly above the occlusal plane (lateral to the pterygomandibular raphe). The needle is advanced to make contact with the lingula. Once bony contact is made the needle is withdrawn slightly and local anaesthetic is injected after aspiration.
- This provides anaesthesia for most of the mandibular teeth, although the more anterior teeth usually need additional local infiltration because of contralateral supply and sometimes sensory branches from the mylohyoid nerve (Figure 4.7).

Gow-Gates technique
- This method describes the deposition of local anaesthetic close to the head of the condyle. In addition to anaesthetizing the inferior dental nerve (IDN), the lingual and long buccal nerves are anaesthetized.

- Administration – the mouth is wide open. The landmarks are the same as for direct IDN block.
- The needle approaches the puncture point from the opposite corner of the mouth and is slid across the mesiopalatal cusp of the maxillary second molar on the side to be injected.
- The point of bony contact is the neck of the condyle.
- Solution is deposited after aspiration.
- Advantage – it uses one injection to block every branch of the mandibular nerve.
- Disadvantage – it requires wide mouth opening. There is a risk to the maxillary artery winding behind the condylar neck (Figure 4.8).

Akinosi method
- Closed mouth technique – this approach can be advantageous in nervous patients or if the tongue interferes with the direct approach to the IDN. The end point does not rely on bony contact.
- Administration – the tissues of the cheek are retracted with the patient's mouth closed. The needle is advanced at the level of the maxillary

mucogingival junction parallel to maxillary occlusal plane.

- The needle is inserted into the retromolar mucosa and advanced until its hub is at the level of the distal aspect of the upper second molar tooth when the anaesthetic is injected after aspiration.

Indirect method (used in some German universities)

- With the thumb in the retromolar fossa and the index finger holding the angle of the mandible, the needle is inserted slightly above the occlusal plane. Then the needle is advanced almost parallel to the lingula from the midline of the mandible.
- Once bony contact at the lingula is made the needle has to be angled behind the lingula where the inferior alveolar nerve enters the bone. This is done by angling the syringe from midline area to the contralateral premolar region.
- The needle is withdrawn slightly and local anaesthetic is injected after aspiration.

Lingual nerve block

- The lingual nerve is often anaesthetized at the same time as the inferior alveolar nerve, thus producing anaesthesia to the lining of the floor of the mouth and tongue on that side.
- After deposition of solution at the IDN site, the needle is withdrawn to half its length and local anaesthetic is deposited (Figure 4.9).

Long buccal nerve block

This block is achieved by injecting local anaesthetic posterior and buccal to the last molar tooth (Figure 4.10).

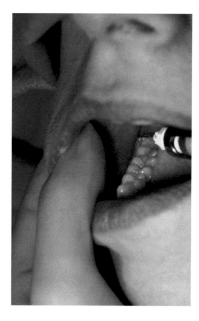

Figure 4.10 Infiltration of local anaesthetic in the region of terminal branches of the long buccal nerve.

Mental nerve block

The mental nerve is the continuation of the inferior alveolar nerve. It leaves the mandible below and between the apices of the first and second premolars at the mental foramen and supplies sensation to the lower lip. Local anaesthetic injected in this region diffuses in through the mental foramen and provides anaesthesia to the ipsilateral lower lip, gingivae and teeth. The lip needs to be placed under tension and the needle is inserted parallel to the long axis of the premolars angling toward bone. Local anaesthetic is then injected.

Bilateral blocks can anaesthetize the entire lower lip and are effective for soft tissue anaesthesia and some restorative procedures (Figure 4.11).

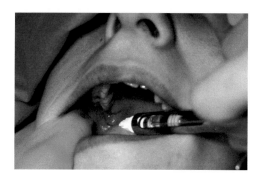

Figure 4.9 Lingual block.

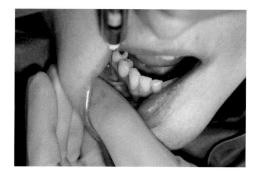

Figure 4.11 Site of injection for mental nerve block.

Infraorbital nerve block

The infraorbital nerve passes along the floor of the orbit and emerges into the cheek about 1 cm below the deepest margin of the orbital rim. This can be infiltrated either directly through the overlying skin or intraorally by lifting the upper lip and injecting in to the depth of the buccal sulcus between the canine and premolar teeth. This block provides anaesthesia to most of the cheek and the side of the nose on the injected side.

Posterior superior alveolar block

This block is rarely needed. The needle is inserted distal to the maxillary second molar and is advanced inward and backward for about 2 cm. Local anaesthetic is deposited above the tuberosity.

Sublingual nerve block

The anterior extension of the lingual nerve can be blocked by placing the needle just submucosally lingual to the premolars.

Intraligamentary analgesia

Individual teeth may be rendered pain free by injecting local anaesthetic directly into the periodontal membrane by using small amounts of local anaesthetic. A specific high-pressure cartridge system is available for this purpose (Figure 4.12).

Infiltration anaesthesia

The aim is to deposit local anaesthetic supraperiosteally, as close to the apex of the tooth to be anaesthetized as possible. The lip or cheek is reflected to place the mucosa under tension, and the needle is inserted along the long axis of the tooth and is aimed toward bone. Local anaesthetic is injected slowly (Figure 4.13).

Palatal infiltrations

These infiltrations are needed when manipulating palatal soft tissue and bone (e.g. during extractions). The palatal mucosa is penetrated directly, and small amounts of local anaesthetic are deposited under force. This is uncomfortable, so the patient should be warned. The discomfort can be minimized by using topical anaesthetic, or infiltrating buccally, then into interdental papillae, then the palatal attached gingivae, thus gradually expanding the area of anaesthesia (Figure 4.14).

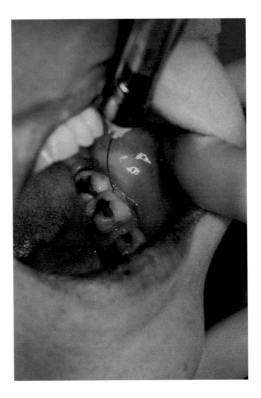

Figure 4.12 Direct intraligamentary injection using a conventional needle and cartridge syringe; specific intraligamentary syringe systems also exist.

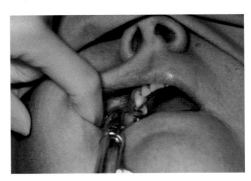

Figure 4.13 Example of local infiltration around the upper molars.

Complications of local anaesthesia

Fortunately, the most common complications are minor. These include the following:

- **Incorrect placement,** resulting in inadequate anaesthesia – this is most likely the result of poor technique, and it tends to occur with

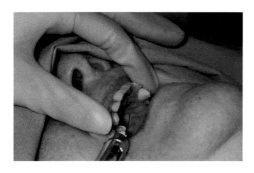

Figure 4.14 Example of palatal injection.

inexperienced operators. It is more likely with regional blocks. To overcome this problem, technique needs to be improved or an alternative method of local anaesthesia sought. IDN blocks can be given either directly or via the Gow-Gates/Akinosi technique.

- Injection of local anaesthetic within the parotid fascia (e.g. caused by incorrect distal placement of the needle tip, thus allowing local anaesthetic to permeate the parotid gland) can result in **temporary facial nerve paralysis.** An eye patch may be required until normal eyelid closure returns.
- **Visual disturbances** – temporary blindness in one eye has been reported following local anaesthesia. This is likely to result from accidental intravascular injection. The local anaesthetic is thought to reach the ophthalmic artery and cause temporary loss of function of the optic nerve.
- **Diplopia** has also been reported, probably from accidental intravascular injection with loss of motor function to the extraocular muscles.
- **Muscle injury** (e.g. medial pterygoid during inferior alveolar nerve injection) can result in muscle spasm (trismus). Usually this is caused by haematoma that resolves spontaneously, but it may require antibiotics and gradual stretching of the muscle. This stretching can be achieved by placing a gradually increasing number of wooden spatulas between the incisors or using a 'trismus screw'.
- **Needle tract infection** – this is surprisingly rare.
- **Postinjection problems** – it is important to tell the patient to avoid smoking, drinking hot liquids or biting the lip or cheek until sensation

is fully returned, to prevent self-traumatizing of the mouth.

- Adjacent vessels may be punctured, resulting in a local **haematoma.** In the majority of cases this is not a serious problem, but beware in patients who are anticoagulated or have bleeding disorders.
- Rapid injection, especially into tight tissues, is **painful.**
- Local anaesthetic should not be injected into inflamed or infected tissues. The altered pH in this environment inactivates the local anaesthetic and results in block failure, and there is a risk of direct spread of infection.

Management of failed local anaesthetic block

Find the cause of the failure, and treat it! Possibilities may include the following:

- **Incorrect placement** – this is described in the previous list.
- **Inadequate volume of local anaesthetic** – however, if the placement is correct, more volume should not improve the block!
- **Impatience** – know the onset time of the local anaesthetic agent, and allow enough time for the drug to take effect.
- **Anatomical variation** – the nerve trunk may be in an unusual position. If this is a suspected reason, infiltrate more widely.
- **Accessory or aberrant nerve supply** – find it and block it.
- **Inability of local anaesthetic during infiltrations to reach the area** – this is usually the result of dense cortical bone. Counteract by using intraligamentary or regional local anaesthesia.
- **Patient understanding** – the importance of choosing patients correctly cannot be overestimated. Some pressure sensation may be felt, and this must be distinguished from pain.
- **Presence of infection** – infection at or around the site is strictly a contraindication to injection of a local block. Do not expect the block to be effective under these tissue conditions.

Major complications include the following:

- Injection of local anaesthetic directly into the venous circulation results in rapid onset of toxic symptoms. These can range from light-headedness and dizziness to confusion. In severe cases, seizures and cardiorespiratory arrest may follow. (In the case of bupivacaine toxicity, cardiac arrest may be refractory to all attempts at cardiopulmonary resuscitation.)

■ Inadvertent intra-arterial injection – local anaesthetic entering the internal carotid artery (via the external carotid artery) is directly delivered to the brain, with dire consequences.

'Self-aspirating' syringes commonly used in dental practice may indicate that the needle is in a blood vessel – Unfortunately, this technique is not foolproof. Nonaspirating syringes (sometimes used in theatre) must be manually aspirated.

Rarely hypersensitivity may occur to preservatives in local anaesthetic preparation – This accounts for virtually all allergic reactions to local anaesthetic agents. Fainting on receiving a local anaesthetic is *not* an allergic response, but it must clearly be distinguished from a seizure.

Sedation

The UK General Dental Council (GDC, 1999) defines conscious sedation as follows:

A technique in which the use of a drug or drugs produces a state of depression of the central nervous system enabling treatment to be carried out, but during which verbal contact with the patient is maintained throughout the period of sedation.

The drugs and techniques used to provide conscious sedation for dental treatment should carry a margin of safety wide enough to render loss of consciousness unlikely.

The level of sedation must be such that the patient remains conscious, retains protective reflexes and is able to understand and respond to verbal commands.

Sedation is a useful technique in anxious patients, children and in those undergoing more lengthy procedures. Patients often experience a sense of disorientation or detachment and may describe the experience as similar to being mildly drunk. In some it can induce sexual fantasies and a chaperone is essential.

Sedation is not a substitute for effective local anaesthesia. If local anaesthesia is inadequate, the patient will still experience pain and may become extremely agitated. Patients do not need to be starved before sedation (although a heavy meal is inadvisable), and any routine medication should be taken as normal. Patients must have an escort to take them home and look after them for 24 hours. Informed consent both for sedation and surgery is required, preferably written.

Sedation can be given in three ways.

Inhalational sedation

This is a relatively safe form of sedation used in dentistry although it has little role to play in more extensive surgery. It is particularly useful in children and can be helpful in quick procedures such as reduction of a dislocated mandible.

A variable percentage mix of nitrous oxide (N_2O) mixed with oxygen (O_2) is used for this technique. N_2O is an extremely potent analgesic, rapidly taken up and excreted by the lungs. The N_2O/O_2 mix has both sedative and analgesic effects. The drug is not metabolized within the body to any significant extent, thus adding to its safety. This technique does not involve the use of injections, and this may be an important factor for some patients.

Note that the terms 'relative analgesia' and 'inhalational sedation' both refer to N_2O/O_2 inhaled techniques. Relative analgesia involves titrating the N_2O, dose whereas inhalational sedation uses a fixed dose of N_2O. Both have a fixed minimum inhaled dose of 30% O_2.

The mix of N_2O/O_2 is used as an adjunct to a local anaesthetic technique and is in no way meant to be used as the sole analgesic. With correct patient selection, adequate local anaesthetic use, combined with reassurance, many dental procedures may be accomplished.

Following administration, patients make a quick recovery with no lasting effects.

Historically, when using N_2O sedation, long-term exposure was thought to lead to vitamin B_{12} depletion and subacute degeneration of the spinal cord. With modern scavenging systems, extensive research has not found this to be a major concern. An additional concern is the potential for abuse of

N_2O by staff for recreational purposes; this should be actively guarded against.

Oral sedation

This is useful in mildly anxious patients and can be administered at home before the appointment. The advantage is acceptability to both patient and surgeon. However, it is essential that monitoring be used during any procedure if the patient has had oral sedation (Figure 4.15).

The disadvantage is that the surgeon has to rely on a compliant patient to self-administer the medication before coming to surgery, within an allotted period of time, for the sedative to be of benefit. This does require a motivated, cooperative patient.

Drugs administered orally take 30 to 60 minutes for any clinical effect to be seen. The dose required to produce sedation is unpredictable, and absorption of drugs from the gastrointestinal tract is also variable. The effects are therefore variable in depth and duration.

There is the potential for complications should multiple doses be administered outside of a monitored environment. It is the responsibility of the prescriber to ensure that all the rules and regulations relating to sedation are applied and strictly followed.

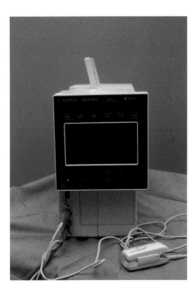

Figure 4.15 A pulse oximeter, which measures the oxygen saturation of haemoglobin by light absorption.

Diazepam is fairly rapidly absorbed from the gut. As a guide, a dose between 0.1 and 0.25 mg/kg of body weight will produce sedation.

Temazepam may be used, 10 to 20 mg 1 hour before treatment.

Intravenous sedation

In the United Kingdom the only recommended intravenous sedation method is the 'single injection of a single drug'. In this country the administration of multiple drugs should be carried out only by fully trained anaesthetists and in a hospital setting, with full monitoring and resuscitation equipment available.

The 'single drug' in question is a benzodiazepine, usually midazolam. The advantages of the benzodiazepines are anterograde amnesia, anxiolysis and a degree of muscle relaxation. Midazolam has a wide margin of safety and is particularly suited to outpatient sedation. It causes minimal respiratory depression, although as patients relax they will often 'forget' to breathe – vigilance is required.

Doses of midazolam for any individual patient are difficult to predict. Most patients reach an adequate degree of sedation with 10 mg or less. Bear in mind that the onset time may be delayed in elderly patients because of a slowed circulation time; patience will avoid inadvertent overdose.

GDC guidelines state that the patient's pulse, respiratory rate and O_2 saturation must be monitored during the procedure. Noninvasive blood pressure recordings must be made at regular intervals, and a defibrillator should be available in the procedure room. All staff involved must be proficient in cardiopulmonary resuscitation in the event of medical emergencies (regulations mandate a 'second appropriate person').

Skills need to be acquired in venipuncture to carry out intravenous sedation (Figures 4.16, 4.17, 4.18, 4.19, 4.20, 4.21 and 4.22).

Flumazenil, a specific benzodiazepine reversal agent, must be available. It rapidly reverses all the effects of the benzodiazepines at a dose of 200 μg intravenously over 15 seconds, followed by 100 μg at 60-second intervals until reversal occurs. Bear in mind that flumazenil has a shorter duration of action, so multiple doses may be required (Figures 4.23, 4.24 and 4.25).

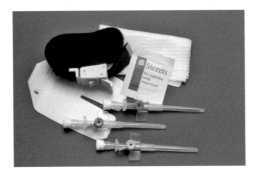

Figure 4.16 Equipment for venipuncture.

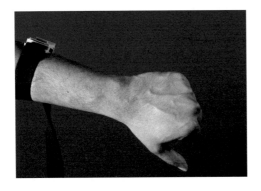

Figure 4.17 Application of a tourniquet and veins on the dorsal hand.

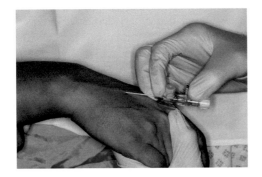

Figure 4.18 Insertion of cannula.

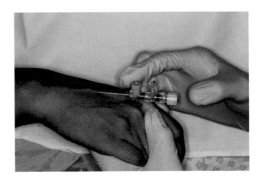

Figure 4.19 Flashback of blood.

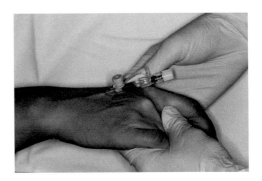

Figure 4.20 Removal of needle.

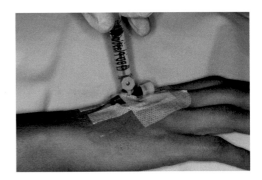

Figure 4.21 Saline flush.

Children may react with the opposite effect; paradoxical stimulation and agitation are well described following intravenous sedation. This method is therefore not recommended in the outpatient paediatric population. Both rectally and orally administered benzodiazepines are popular in paediatric wards for minor procedures such as suture removal.

Analgesia

Dental procedures can be painful, and a sound knowledge of good analgesic prescribing is essential. The principles are simple: give appropriate drugs, in sufficient dose, on a regular basis, at sufficient time intervals. Where possible, use of smaller doses of a combination of drugs will have

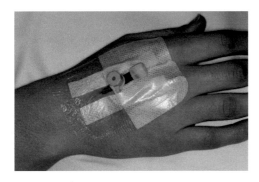

Figure 4.22 Securing Venflon.

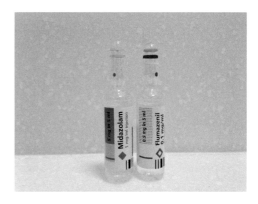

Figure 4.24 Midazolam and flumazenil.

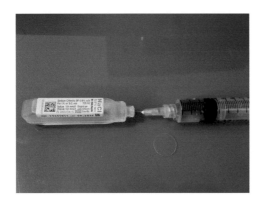

Figure 4.23 Saline drawn up for flush.

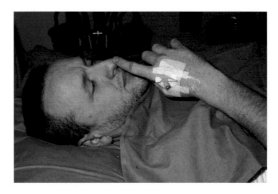

Figure 4.25 Patient attempting to touch nose following administration of intravenous midazolam.

a synergistic effect, while minimizing side effects. When oral analgesics are combined with effective local anaesthetic techniques, the results can be very rewarding.

There are numerous approaches to this end. The simplest is set out in the World Health Organization analgesic ladder on the next page. Devised by the World Health Organization (WHO), it outlines a systematic approach to pain control that will satisfy the needs of the majority of patients.

Simple analgesics

Simple analgesics (e.g. paracetamol) are useful for mild pain. Minimal side effects at therapeutic doses make this an attractive option. Hepatotoxicity is a problem only at toxic doses. Paracetamol has antipyretic and analgesic properties. It is a useful analgesic if nonsteroidal anti-inflammatory drugs (NSAIDs) are contraindicated.

Doses

Adult dose – 1 g every 4 to 6 hours. Maximum daily dose – 4 g.

Paediatrics – dependent on age, consult recent formulary.

Nonsteroidal anti-inflammatory drugs

NSAIDs (e.g. aspirin, diclofenac, ibuprofen, ketorolac) have both anti-inflammatory and analgesic effects; therefore, they are useful particularly when inflammation is the primary cause of the pain. Following oral surgical procedures involving the teeth and bones (e.g. wisdom teeth removal, apicectomies), NSAIDs can be given orally, i.m. or rectally.

World Health Organization analgesic ladder

		Strong opioid ± Nonopioid ± Adjuvant e.g. Morphine ± Paracetamol ± NSAIDs.

Pain persisting or increasing

	Weak opioid + Nonopioid ± Adjuvant e.g. Codeine, tramadol + Paracetamol ± NSAIDs.	

Pain persisting or increasing

± Nonopioid ± Adjuvant e.g. Paracetamol ± NSAIDs.		

±, with or without; NSAID, nonsteroidal anti-inflammatory drug.

These drugs are contraindicated in patients with peptic ulcer disease, renal impairment and coagulation disorders and in patients who have had a previous hypersensitivity reaction to aspirin or NSAIDs.

A note about asthmatic patients and NSAIDs – These drugs are not absolutely contraindicated in asthma. There is, however, a higher chance of allergy and an increased chance of exacerbation of asthma symptoms.

Side effects include gastrointestinal upset, bleeding, hypersensitivity reactions and wheezing. Use with caution in elderly patients – Long-term use can result in severe gastrointestinal haemorrhage.

Doses

Adult dose – Ibuprofen 400 to 600 mg three times daily. Take with food to reduce chances of gastrointestinal upset. Maximum daily dose – 2.4 g.
Diclofenac 50 mg three times daily. Take with food.
Child dose – dependent on weight, consult recent formulary. Avoid aspirin in children with recent flu-like illness – Potentially lethal Reye's syndrome may result.

Minor opioids

These drugs (e.g. codeine, tramadol, dihydrocodeine) are effective for mild to moderate pain.

Given orally or i.m. They can be given in combination with paracetamol.

Side effects include nausea, constipation and confusion, especially in elderly patients.

Doses

Codeine – 30 to 60 mg every 4 to 6 hours to a maximum of 240 mg daily.
Tramadol – 50 to 100 mg every 4 to 6 hours; said to be less likely to interfere with pupillary response in head injury.

Compound analgesic (Co-Codamol [codeine and paracetamol])

This drug is used for mild to moderate pain relief or pyrexia.

Presentations

8/500 – 8 mg codeine phosphate, 500 mg paracetamol. (If Co-Codamol is prescribed with no stated strength, this will be dispensed.) Given orally, constipation and rebound 'analgesic headache' are the main complications.
Adult dose – 1 to 2 tablets every 4 to 6 hours.
Maximum daily – 8 tablets.
Child dose – dependent on age.

30/500 - 30 mg codeine phosphate, 500 mg paracetamol.

> Dose – 1 to 2 tablets every 4 hours. Maximum daily – 8 tablets. Not recommended for children.

60/1000 – 60 mg codeine phosphate, 1 g paracetamol.

> Dose – 1 tablet every 4 hours. Maximum daily – 4 tablets.

Opioids (e.g. morphine, diamorphine)

These are the most potent of the analgesics. The opioids are seldom used after office procedures. The role is analgesia in the postoperative period after major surgery.

Routes of administration – Options include oral (Oramorph), i.m., subcutaneous and intravenous administration and patient-controlled analgesia (PCA). Because of the side effect profile of the opioids, they should be administered only in an inpatient setting, where respiratory monitoring is available.

Side effects – Nausea and vomiting, constipation, sedation, confusion and respiratory depression. Prescription of naloxone, a specific opioid antagonist, and an antiemetic for use alongside the opioid is humane. Consider addition of a laxative, especially in elderly patients or if long-term use is anticipated.

Postoperative pain control

Assessment and measurement of pain

Effective pain management depends on accurate assessment. This can be difficult in children or in patients who cannot speak following surgery. The most reliable indicator of pain is the patient's verbal report or a written equivalent.

By far the simplest tools that rely on the patient's report of pain are Visual Analogue Scale and the Verbal Rating Scale.

For more complex assessment, the McGill Pain Questionnaire explores the sensory, affective and evaluative dimensions of pain. It is a self-administered questionnaire consisting of 21 questions with diagrams for chief pain location and a numerical pain scale.

Assessing pain in children, or in patients with whom we cannot communicate, is particularly difficult. For the paediatric group, several methods are available, depending on each age group. Whereas adolescents can describe their pain in detail, a baby has no such verbal capacity. Vocal expressions, especially crying, and physiological measures, such as tachycardia, are said to be reliable indicators of acute pain. Other methods include the Children's Hospital of Eastern Ontario Pain Scale (CHEOPS), the Princess Margaret Hospital Pain Assessment Tool (PMHPAT) and

---

PAIN SCALES

VISUAL ANALOGUE SCALE (VAS)

No pain – Worst pain imaginable

VERBAL RATING SCALE

0 _ _ _ _ _ _	1 _ _ _ _ _ _	2 _ _ _ _ _ _	3 _ _ _ _ _ _	4 _ _ _ _ _ _
None	Mild	Moderate	Severe	Excruciating

0 = None
1 = Mild
2 = Moderate
3 = Severe
4 = Excruciating

The King's Healthcare Pain Assessment Tool for Children (PATCH).

Other pain control techniques

Cryotherapy

This is the therapeutic use of extreme cold, achieved by using N_2O or liquid nitrogen to freeze tissues. Cell death and subsequent tissue necrosis result in analgesia.

Intractable or recurrent pain from nerve infiltration (e.g. malignancy or physiological conditions such as trigeminal neuralgia) may be treated by cryotherapy.

The diagnosis must be established beforehand, and this is most easily done by a nerve block. In such cases the nerve (e.g. inferior alveolar, infraorbital) can then be exposed and frozen.

Procedure

Informed consent must be gained. In particular, patients must be warned of postoperative oedema and ulceration, which may be quite severe.

A local anaesthetic should be used to anaesthetize the area, followed by selection of appropriate probe tip. A lubricant jelly (such as KY) should be applied to the area to improve contact between probe and tissue. Freeze for 1 minute; thaw for 1 minute is the usual cycle.

During thawing, be careful not to pull the probe from the tissue because this will result in damage to tissue. At least two cycles are used. One may need to overlap ice zones.

Follow up to check symptoms.

The duration of paraesthesia varies, but there is usually an analgesic period after the paraesthesia resolves. If necessary, cryotherapy can be repeated at a later date.

Splinting of fractures

This very simple measure is often forgotten. Displaced, mobile fractures (usually mandibular) should be reduced (after a local anaesthetic has been given) and then immobilized. This can be done simply using a figure-of-eight wire around the adjacent teeth (make sure they are not loose first). This is usually a temporary measure before open reduction and internal fixation of the fractures. This works in the same way that a broken arm is put in a back slab for pain relief. The basic principle is that a broken mobile bone is much more painful than a broken immobile bone.

Adhesive dental materials acid etched onto teeth can aid stabilization of dentoalveolar fractures and reduce pain in the same way.

Transcutaneous nerve stimulation

This technique is thought to work via the 'gate control' theory. Rubbing or massaging a painful area, or the application of a small electrical current to the skin, closes the 'gate' at the spinal cord level and prevents pain fibres from conducting impulses to the brain. Transcutaneous electrical nerve stimulation (TENS) and some types of acupuncture are also thought to promote endogenous opioid release in the brain. In the maxillofacial region this can be effective in postherpetic neuralgia and other forms of deep-seated facial pain.

TENS is contraindicated in patients with pacemakers and should be avoided over the carotid sinus.

Management of cancer pain

Cancer can cause a variety of pain syndromes. However, most of these respond to drug therapy. The WHO analgesic ladder (see the previous box) is a useful guide. This is a step-by-step approach that is effective in the majority of cases. Patients are started on a nonopioid analgesic such as an NSAID or paracetamol. If the pain persists or increases, a weak opioid such as codeine is commenced, with or without the addition of an NSAID. If this proves to be inadequate a strong opioid is substituted for the weak opioid. 'Adjuvant' treatment includes steroids, antidepressants, antiepileptics, some drugs specific for neurogenic pain (e.g. gabapentin, pregabalin) and psychological management. The presence of cannabinoid receptors in epithelial cells has produced a potentially useful role for medicinal cannabis both systemically and topically. The topical preparation (Sativex) is available in the United Kingdom.

Alternative and complementary therapies

Hypnosis

This is thought to produce a state of altered consciousness and relaxation. Hypnosis is generally believed to be an altered state of consciousness. Sleep is the best-known altered state. The aim of hypnosis is to teach people to cope with the situation to the best of their ability.

It has been suggested that in a hypnotic state, patients do not act against their own consciences and always cooperate voluntarily. Always have a chaperone.

Induction of the hypnotic state can be performed verbally by the surgeon, visually or by the patients themselves. Multiple sessions can prepare patients to autohypnotize or respond to posthypnotic suggestion by using key words or procedures.

Acupuncture

Traditionally acupuncture is a holistic approach to the management of disease as well as maintenance of health. It involves insertion of needles into various parts of the body and should be regarded as a supplement to conventional treatment.

It has value in control of postoperative pain and in the management of myofascial pain dysfunction and facial pain. Its value as a sole analgesic for operative treatment is questionable; however, it may play a role in reducing anxiety preoperatively.

The United Kingdom and German-speaking countries are fairly similar in this area. The United States is a little different.

North America

The routine use of office-based, surgeon-administered sedation and anaesthesia is perhaps the most noticeable practice difference in North America compared with the rest of the world.

Oral and maxillofacial surgery trainees in North America spend a significant portion of their training on the anaesthesia service. This is supplemented with considerable clinical training in ambulatory anaesthesia in the clinic. There are rigorous monitoring requirements. The use of capnography to monitor end-tidal carbon dioxide (a marker of adequacy of ventilation) is mandated in addition to the other monitoring mentioned in this chapter.

Benzodiazepines in the form of midazolam are the basis of most intravenous anaesthetic techniques. This provides anxiolysis and amnesia and also helps to attenuate the 'emergence phenomena' associated with dissociative agents such as ketamine. In many cases, particularly those patients with medical comorbidities, this may be the only agent used. Other agents used to deepen the sedation and anaesthesia include fentanyl, a short-acting opioid (its antagonist, naloxone, must be available for use in the event that the patient is rendered apnoeic and requires reversal). Ketamine, a drug that acts on N-methyl-d-aspartate receptors to produce a dissociative anaesthetic state and additional analgesia, and propofol, a short-acting intravenous anaesthetic agent, are regularly used.

All of these agents depend on the presence of good-quality local anaesthesia for painless surgery. They are not a substitute for good local anaesthetic techniques. Most 'rocky' sedations are the consequence of a failure of local anaesthesia. Before using any of these agents, training is required in advanced airway management, including endotracheal intubation, because surgery is being carried out on an unprotected airway and the drugs may produce a deeper level of sedation than planned, resulting in loss of the airway and ventilation.

FURTHER READING

Ghoneum NM, Mewaldt SP. Benzodiazepines and human memory: a review. *Anesthesiology* 1990;72:926–38.
For those who are in need of details about the psychoactive effects of these drugs.
Girdler NM, Hill CM. *Sedation In dentistry.* London: Butterworth-Heinemann, 1998.
A useful overview.
Introduction to acupuncture in dentistry. *Br Dent J* 2000;189:136–40.
Useful basic introduction.

Joint Formulary Committee. *British national formulary.* London: Pharmaceutical Press. Number 48 was the first to contain an amalgamated Dental Practitioners' Formulary. Use the most recent edition.
Definitive text.
Meechan JG, Robb ND, Seymour RA. *Pain and anxiety control for the conscious dental patient.* Oxford: Oxford University Press, 1998.
Hugely detailed; everything you ever wanted to know.
Meechan JG, Robb ND. Sedation in dental practice 3: the role of sedation in management of problems with local anaesthesia. *Dent Update* 1997;24:32–5.
Practical details.
Mitchell DA, Mitchell L. *Oxford handbook of clinical dentistry,* 6th ed. Oxford: Oxford University Press, 2014.
Well obviously!
Specific literature includes the following:
Armfield J, Heaton LJ. Management of fear and anxiety in the dental clinic: a review. *Aust Dent J* 2013; 58:390–407.

El-Kholey KE. Infiltration anesthesia for extraction of the mandibular molars. *J Oral Maxillofac Surg*, 2013;10:1658.e1–5.
Facco E, Casiglia E, Masiero S, Tikhonoff V, Giacomello M, Zanette G. Effects of hypnotic focused analgesia on dental pain threshold. *Int J Clin Exp Hypn* 2011;59:454–8.
Haraji A, Rakhshan V, Khamverdi N, Alisahi HK. Effects of intra-alveolar placement of 0.2% chlorhexidine bioadhesive gel on dry socket incidence and postsurgical pain: a double-blind split-mouth randomised controlled clinical trial. *J Orofac Pain* 2013;27; 256–62.
Oni G, Rasko Y, Kenkel J. Topical lidocaine enhanced by laser pretreatment: a safe and effective method of analgesia for facial rejuvenation. *Aesthet Surg J* 2013; 33:854–61.
Passavanti MB, Grella E, Pace MC, Di Gennaro TL, Aurilio C. Tramadol as a local anesthetic: prospects for use in oncological day surgery. *Plast Reconstr Surg* 2013;131:942e.
Whaley MG, Brooks GB. Enhancement of suggestibility and imaginative ability with nitrous oxide. *Psychopharmacology* 2009;203;745–52.

5

Medical management of the oral and maxillofacial surgical patient

Contents

Aims

For undergraduates:

- To familiarize yourself with the medical aspects of an oral and maxillofacial surgery unit.
- To prepare you to accompany and assist junior trainees in their routine and on-call work.

For postgraduates:

- To provide the background knowledge to enable:
  - Concise clerking and consenting of patients.
  - Organization of investigations.
  - Prescription of fluid regimens and drugs.

- Care for medically compromised patients in the perioperative period.

Learning outcomes

Undergraduates

- To be able to describe the steps in caring for an oral and maxillofacial surgical inpatient.
- To be able to describe the steps taken in treating common complications.
- To be able to describe the steps taken in treating common emergency conditions.

Postgraduates

- To be able to take a relevant history and examination.
- To be able to prescribe relevant and appropriate fluids and drugs.
- To be able to discuss personal roles and limitations with regard to the medical management of inpatients.

Clerking and consent

Clerking is the term used to describe the structured preoperative assessment of patients by means of history taking, examination and relevant special investigations. It applies to all patients admitted for any procedures. This is the time for explanation, answering questions and obtaining informed consent. Additional paperwork (prescription charts, blood request forms, requests for radiographs and electrocardiograms [ECGs]) should be completed, followed by communication with senior colleagues, the anaesthetist and nursing staff should any potential problems need to be addressed.

Preoperative assessment clinics, where patients are clerked several days in advance of their operations, allow adequate time to order investigations and review the results, to anticipate and address medical and social problems. These clinics are in widespread use as part of the process of maximizing 'efficient' use of expensive hospital resources, although how efficient the process actually is warrants careful scrutiny.

As a convention, clerking is a three-step procedure: **history taking** (enquiry), followed by a **physical examination**. Any further **investigations** are dictated by findings in the history and examination.

History taking

- Establish the **reason for admission** as understood by the patient and confirmed from the clinical notes and letters.
- A **medical history** is taken, with particular emphasis on conditions that may pose a surgical or anaesthetic risk. **Drugs** taken (of all types, including creams and those self-prescribed), along with dose and frequency, are recorded in the notes and on the drug card. **Allergies** to medications, plasters and antiseptics are noted. A **family history** of any relevant medical problems (e.g. anaesthetic complications and bleeding disorders) is important.
- The **review of systems** is a systematic enquiry used to assess symptoms and any functional limitation affecting the patient (Table 5.1). It can also reveal any undisclosed conditions that may require further investigation. Assessment of the cardiovascular and respiratory systems is required for everyone. In patients with complicated medical histories, or those requiring major surgery, more intensive history taking is mandatory. The key is to find a systematic approach to questioning that will not miss major symptoms of disease. A guide to the relevant questions is outlined in Figure 5.1. Begin the enquiry by telling the patient that this is a series of routine questions. A positive response to any question should prompt further enquiry and investigation.
- Enquire about any **previous surgery,** its reason, and outcome.
- **Social history** – what does the patient do? Inform the patient of how long to expect to be off work and how to obtain a sick note should this be required (UK patients can sign themselves off for the first week and after this can obtain a sick note from their general practitioner, from the nurses on the ward or at their outpatient review appointment; this will obviously vary worldwide). Family circumstances

Table 5.1 Review of systems

Cardiovascular	Chest pain, previous heart attack, hypertension, palpitations, shortness of breath on exertion, exercise tolerance (how far can the patient walk comfortably? how many stairs can the patient manage?), paroxysmal nocturnal dyspnoea, orthopnoea (how many pillows does the patient sleep on?), ankle swelling.
Respiratory	Cough, sputum, wheeze, haemoptysis.
Gastrointestinal	Weight changes (up or down), appetite, dysphagia, heartburn, nausea, vomiting, abdominal pain, bowel habit, blood or mucus in stool.
Genitourinary	Pain, burning, hesitancy, poor stream, terminal dribbling, incontinence, frequency, nocturia, urgency.
In women	Date of last menstrual period (likelihood of pregnancy?).
Neurological	Fits, faints, blackouts, funny turns, limb weakness, paraesthesia, visual problems, hearing problems.
Musculoskeletal	Joint pain, stiffness, swelling.
Endocrine	Heat, cold intolerance, lethargy, voice change.
Dermatological	Rash, itching, bruising, discoloration.
Psychiatric	Stress, depression, mood swings, sleep disturbance, suicidal thoughts, anxiety.

should be discussed: who will look after the patient? Does the patient have dependent children? Who will care for them while the patient is hospitalized? Present and former **smoking** habit, **alcohol** consumption and recreational drug use are noted.

The physical examination

In clerking before elective surgery, a systematic examination of the patient is performed after taking the history. Start with an overall assessment of the patient, followed by examination of each system and finishing with a detailed local examination of the specific area of pathology.

Each patient admitted to the surgical ward, whether electively or acutely, requires a physical examination. For preoperative patients, the extent of your examination should be tailored to your patient, and this depends on the general health of the patient and the nature of the procedure to be performed.

Knowledge of how to perform a detailed examination of the body is a skill, perfected with practice. Full details of every clinical finding and its significance are beyond the scope of this book – many textbooks on clinical medicine exist should

your interest be piqued on the subject. The aim of your examination is to detect what is normal and what is not. Thereafter, the responsibility is to refer the matter to the appropriate specialist colleague.

Whereas history taking involves assessment of symptoms (that is what the patient complains of), the clinical examination is used to look for signs (what you can objectively detect). Positive findings (e.g. a heart murmur) and important negative findings (e.g. the absence of a wheeze in an asthmatic patient) are equally relevant.

General examination

By convention patients are examined from the right side of the bed. Ensure they have privacy and that you have a chaperone. The patient must be comfortable, lying at about 45° and suitably exposed to allow complete examination of the chest and abdomen (Figure 5.2). Examination begins during history taking, when an overall impression of the patient is formed. Thereafter a systematic examination ensures that each system of the body is examined following a sequence – looking (inspection), touching (palpation), tapping (percussion) and listening (auscultation).

ORAL AND MAXILLOFACIAL (CLERKING PROFORMA FOR ELECTIVE ADMISSIONS)

CONSULTANT:	
PATIENT'S NAME:	UNIT NUMBER:
AGE:	PROPOSED ADMISSION DATE:
DATE:	PROPOSED OPERATION DATE:
DIAGNOSIS:	
OPERATION:	

PAST MEDICAL HISTORY:	CARDIOVASCULAR RESPIRATORY GASTROINTESTINAL GENITOURINARY	NEUROLOGICAL MUSCULOSKELETAL PROGRESSIVE MUSCULAR DYSTROPY
MURMURS MYOCARDIAL INFARCTION ANGINA ANAEMIA HYPERTENSION STROKE DVT/PE	ASTHMA BRONCHITIS TB JAUNDICE DIABETES EPILEPSY/FITS NECK INJURY	OTHER SERIOUS ILLNESS (State below)

DETAILS:

PREVIOUS OPERATIONS (±ANAESTHETIC/SURGICAL COMPLICATIONS):

FAMILY HISTORY:	DRUG HISTORY:
SOCIAL HISTORY:	
SMOKING:	ALLERGIES:
DRINKING:	
HOME CIRCUMSTANCES:	

Figure 5.1 Clerking proforma. BP, blood pressure; CNS, central nervous system; CT, computed tomography; CXR, chest X-ray; CVS, cardiovascular system; DVT, deep venous thrombosis; ECG, electrocardiogram; FBC, full blood count; GP, group; JVP, jugular venous pressure; L, left; LFT, liver function testing; MRI, magnetic resonance imaging; PE, pulmonary embolus; PND, paroxysmal nocturnal dyspnoea; PR, per rectum; R, right; RESP., respiratory; TB, tuberculosis; U + E, urea and electrolytes; URTI, upper respiratory tract infection.

ORAL AND MAXILLOFACIAL (CLERKING PROFORMA FOR ELECTIVE ADMISSIONS)

SYSTEMS REVIEW:		
	COUGH:	DRY
CHEST PAIN		+ SPUTUM
BREATHLESSNESS		HAEMOPTYSIS
RECENT INCREASE IN		CHRONIC
BREATHLESSNESS		
EXERCISE TOLERANCE (1–5)	WHEEZE	
ORTHOPNOEA/PND	CURRENT URTI	
PALPITATIONS		
FAINTING EPISODES		
ANKLE SWELLING		
EXCESSIVE BLEEDING/BRUISING		

DETAILS:

WEIGHT LOSS	DYSURIA	HEADACHE
DYSPHAGIA	NOCTURIA	DIZZINESS/FITS
ABDOMINAL PAIN	FREQUENCY	BLACKOUTS
NAUSEA/VOMITING	HAEMATURIA	HEARING OR VISUAL DISTURBANCE
CONSTIPATION/ DIARRHOEA	URGENCY	WEAKNESS/PARAESTHESIA
BLOOD IN STOOL	INCONTINENCE	ANAESTHESIA
ARTHRITIS	LIMITED MOUTH OPENING	
- NECK	PREGNANCY	
- OTHER JOINTS		

DETAILS:

Figure 5.1 (continued)

ORAL AND MAXILLOFACIAL (CLERKING PROFORMA FOR ELECTIVE ADMISSIONS)

EXAMINATION

GENERAL:

WEIGHT (Kg)			HEIGHT (Metres)		
PALLOR		CYNOSIS		CLUBBING		JAUNDICE	
LYMPHADENOPATHY			DEHYDRATION		

CVS:

TRACHEA: (central to right to left)   RESP. RATE:

EXPANSION: (EQUAL * R > L * L > R)

PERCUSSION:

AUSCULTATION: - Breath sounds
                         - Air Entry
                         - Added sounds

CHEST:	BREAST/SKIN:

PULSE (CHARACTER):   BP: JVP:

HEART RATE: OEDEMA:

APEX BEAT: PERIPHERAL PULSES:

HEART SOUNDS: MURMURS:

ABDOMEN:

SOFT? TENDERNESS?
MASSES:
LIVER:
SPLEEN/KIDNEYS:
BOWEL SOUNDS:
HERNIAE:
GENITALIA:
PR:

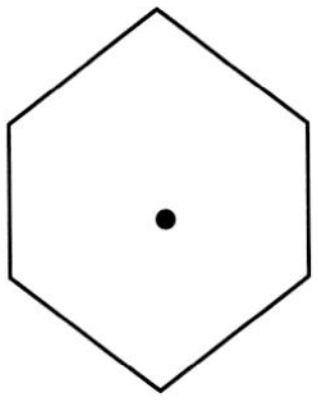

CNS:

CRANIAL NERVES:
PERIPHERAL SENSATION:
PERIPHERAL POWER:
REFLEXES:

CONSENT: SIGNED – YES/NO

INVESTIGATIONS:

	Done		Done		Done	
FBC		U + E		GP+X MATCH		(No. Units)
SICKLE		GLUCOSE		GP+ SAVE		
ECG		LFT		CXR		
CLOTTING				MRI		
RESP. FUNCTION		X-RAYS		CT		
OTHER:				DOPPLER		

Signature .... (Print Name)..

Figure 5.1 (continued)

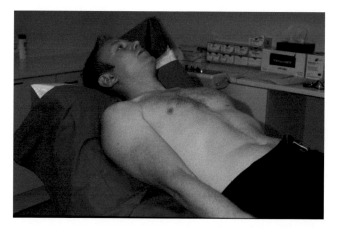

Figure 5.2 A relaxed supine position for clinical examination.

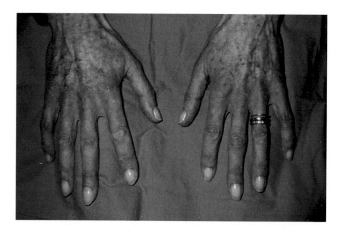

Figure 5.3 Clubbing and koilonychia.

When determining the general status of the patient, the following questions need to be addressed:

- Is the patient well or unwell?
- Is the patient orientated or confused? This is determined from the appropriateness of the patient's responses on general questioning.
- What colour is the patient? Pallor suggests anaemia, jaundice is best determined by looking for yellow sclera, and central cyanosis is identified by looking for bluish discoloration of the lips and undersurface of the tongue.
- What is the hydration status of the patient? Does the patient require fluid resuscitation pre-operatively? (Often the patient will volunteer that he or she is thirsty!) Dehydration is recognized by a dry mouth with cool, poorly perfused peripheries, decreased skin and tissue turgor, sunken eyes and a furrowed tongue.

Look at the hands next for tar stains from heavy smoking, peripheral cyanosis and clubbing (Figure 5.3), as well as for alteration in temperature of the hands and any excess moisture.

Working up from the hands, the radial pulse is taken, assessing the rate, rhythm and character of the pulse. Tachycardia (pulse rate >100 beats per minute) may accompany pyrexia, signify fluid depletion or may simply reflect the patient's anxiety. Bradycardia (pulse rate <60 beats per minute) occurs in patients taking beta blockers or with certain cardiac arrhythmias, but it can also occur in young, fit athletes. If an arrhythmia is

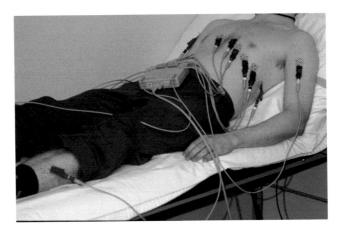

Figure 5.4 Positions for taking a 12-lead electrocardiogram.

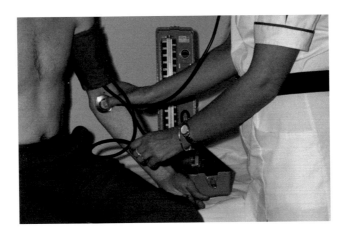

Figure 5.5 Recording blood pressure.

suspected, it can be further investigated with an ECG (Figure 5.4). The rhythm of the pulse is regular, regularly irregular or irregularly irregular (as in atrial fibrillation). The character of the pulse is weak and thready in hypovolaemia, and bounding after exercise or in the presence of a fever.

The blood pressure is taken (Figure 5.5), and the temperature and results of urinalysis are recorded from the nursing observations.

Systematic examination

Cardiovascular system

Inspection

General inspection of the patient may reveal corneal arcus and xanthelasma, indicative of atherosclerotic disease, or clubbing and central cyanosis in patients with congenital cyanotic heart disease. The presence of central cyanosis indicates a reduction in the oxygen saturation of arterial blood and may result from cardiac or respiratory disease (e.g. pulmonary oedema or chronic obstructive pulmonary disease [COPD]). Document scars and know why they are there.

The **jugular venous pressure (JVP)** is estimated as the height in centimetres above the sternal angle of the column of blood in the internal jugular vein. The head is turned to the left to look for filling of the right internal jugular vein, which runs between the heads of sternomastoid muscle inferiorly up to the earlobe superiorly. A raised JVP (>3 cm) most commonly occurs in right-sided heart failure and fluid overload.

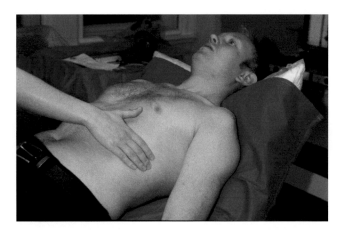

Figure 5.6 Palpating the apex beat.

Palpation

The apex beat is the most inferior and lateral point where the heart can be felt beating. The normal position is the fifth intercostal space in the midclavicular line (Figure 5.6).

The apex may be displaced inferiorly and laterally because of cardiac enlargement. In left ventricular hypertrophy the apex beat is more forceful than normal and is described as heaving. The flat of the right hand is placed on the left anterior chest wall to feel for a parasternal heave, which occurs in right ventricular hypertrophy, and to detect a precordial thrill, which is a palpable heart murmur.

Auscultation

Auscultation of the heart can be notoriously tricky – only with practice will abnormalities in rate, rhythm and the presence of additional sounds in the cardiac cycle be detected. Do not be daunted, however; even the most experienced cardiologists started as novices!

Start at the apex –with the diaphragm and then the bell of the stethoscope, listen for the first and second heart sounds (S_1 and S_2) and then for additional heart sounds and finally for murmurs. The diaphragm of the stethoscope picks up high-pitched sounds; if the bell is lightly applied, it can be used to detect low-pitched sounds. Additional heart sounds are difficult to detect. A third heart sound (S_3) is common and normal in healthy young adults, but in elderly patients its presence indicates impaired ventricular function, especially when accompanied by tachycardia and signs of cardiac failure.

Heart murmurs are divided into systolic, diastolic and continuous murmurs, according to their position in the cardiac cycle, and they can be timed against the carotid pulse. Murmurs arise from turbulent blood flow, which can be caused by regurgitation of blood through an incompetent or leaking valve, by flow through a stiff or stenotic valve or by flow through a septal defect. Additionally, flow murmurs occur when there is increased blood flow through normal valves; such murmurs are common in pregnancy and anaemia. Remember – the aim is to detect an abnormality. It is enough to recognize and refer.

For the interested – commonly heard murmurs:

- **Aortic stenosis** – systolic ejection murmur that increases in intensity after S_1 and decreases before S_2; the murmur is loudest at the right sternal edge, radiating to the carotid arteries and thus can be heard in the neck.
- **Mitral regurgitation** – 'pansystolic' murmur of uniform intensity between S_1 and S_2, loudest at the apex, radiating to the axilla.
- **Aortic regurgitation** – early diastolic murmur heard after S_2, loudest at the lower left sternal edge with the patient seated forward and during expiration.
- **Mitral stenosis** – S_1 is loud, followed by S_2 and then a third heart sound resulting from the opening snap of the stenotic mitral valve, and a low-pitched rumbling mid-diastolic murmur, loudest with the patient rolled into the left lateral position.

Respiratory system

Inspection

General inspection of the patient may reveal signs of respiratory disease including finger clubbing (often from bronchial carcinoma), central cyanosis, laboured breathing or a cough or wheeze; if there is a sputum pot by the bed its contents should be examined. Assess the pattern of breathing, in particular noting any respiratory effort and the respiratory rate (normally 12 to 18 breaths per minute). Look for asymmetry of chest wall movements – a diseased portion of lung leads to reduced movement on the affected side. The remaining examination is completed for the anterior chest and is repeated for the posterior chest, which is examined with the patient seated forward.

Palpation

The trachea is palpated by gently pressing the index fingers into either side of the sternal notch to feel for deviation – this may be uncomfortable so warn the patient. Chest expansion is assessed by placing the hands around the ribs with the tips of the thumbs meeting in the midline at the xiphisternum. The thumbs move apart with inspiration, and the relative contribution of each side of the chest is determined. A similar technique is used when examining the posterior chest. Normal chest expansion is at least 5 cm.

Percussion

The normal percussion note of the chest wall is described as resonant. Percussion of the chest is performed by placing the nondominant hand flat on the chest wall, with the fingers splayed and the middle finger positioned over the area to be percussed. This finger is pressed onto the chest and struck firmly with the tip of the middle finger of the dominant hand, with movement at the wrist. The anterior, lateral and posterior regions of the chest are percussed symmetrically, comparing sides at each level (Figure 5.7). The sounds are described as resonant (normal), dull or hyperresonant (both abnormal).

Auscultation

Breath sounds are assessed by asking the patient to breathe steadily in and out through the mouth. Normal breath sounds (also called vesicular) result from the transmitted sound of turbulent air flow

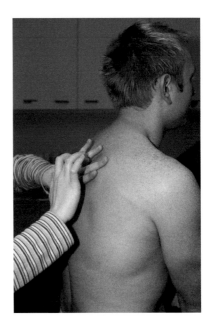

Figure 5.7 Percussing the chest.

in the larynx, through the trachea, bronchi, lung tissue and chest wall. The quality of breath sounds can be reduced in intensity by airflow limitation (e.g. in COPD) or by the presence of a pleural effusion, a collapsed lobe or pneumothorax. Breath sounds become 'bronchial' when lung tissue becomes solidified by consolidation or fibrosis. This sound can be mimicked by blowing over the top of a glass bottle (Figure 5.8).

Any added sounds, namely wheezes and crackles, are noted. Wheezes are musical, like a high-pitched whistle, caused by passage of air through narrow bronchi, and they are characteristic of asthma. Crackles are nonmusical sounds resulting from secretions (in which case they are reduced by coughing) or the opening up of collapsed small airways, usually in the lung bases, on inspiration (e.g. in pulmonary oedema). This sound is compared to the opening of Velcro.

Gastrointestinal system

Physical examination of the gastrointestinal system is confined to the mouth, abdomen and rectum. To examine the abdomen, patients should lie flat with their arms by their sides to ensure that the abdominal muscles are relaxed; nipple to knee exposure is required; otherwise, keep the patient covered (Figure 5.9). Chaperones are advisable.

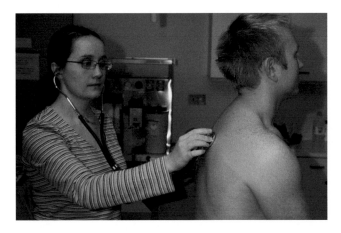

Figure 5.8 Auscultation, listening to the lung fields from behind.

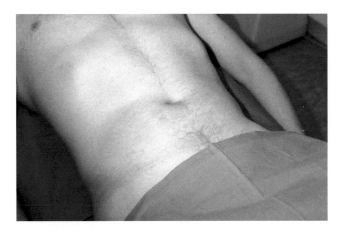

Figure 5.9 The abdomen needs to be relaxed and exposed.

Inspection

General inspection of the gastrointestinal system is used to look for evidence of malignancy, malnutrition and stigmata of chronic liver disease (from heavy alcohol consumption or chronic viral hepatitis) – these signs include jaundice, palmar erythema, leuconychia (white nails from hypoalbuminaemia), bruising and purpura, gynaecomastia in male patients and spider naevi (dilated small arterioles) on the arms, face and upper body.

Inspection is commenced from the foot of the bed while looking at the patient as a whole and at the abdomen for obvious asymmetry, distension, scars or herniae. Cutaneous striae are linear pink or white markings on the abdomen and thighs resulting from pregnancy (stretch marks), obesity and Cushing's syndrome in patients taking steroids on a long-term basis.

Palpation

The abdomen can be divided into nine regions to facilitate description and note keeping (Figure 5.10).

Kneeling at the side of the bed, the right hand is used to palpate each area of the abdomen gently. This must be done while carefully watching the patient's face for any discomfort and asking the patient to report any tenderness. (Ask the patient where maximal pain is felt, and then start your examination on the opposite side of the abdomen. This will engender trust.) Guarding is the term

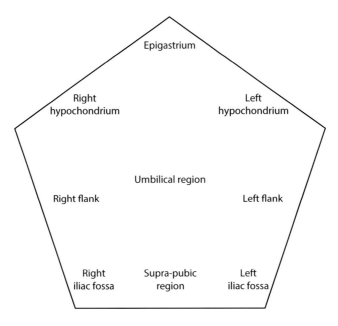

Figure 5.10 The nine regions of the abdomen.

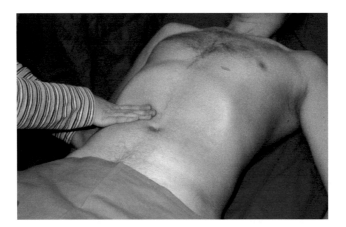

Figure 5.11 Palpation of the liver edge.

used to describe involuntary tensing of the abdominal muscles in anticipation of pain. Rebound tenderness, indicating peritoneal inflammation, is elicited by gently pressing on a region of the abdomen and then releasing the pressure, which causes the pain to increase. This can be simulated by asking the patient to cough, a technique that is particularly helpful in children.

Assess whether the liver, spleen and kidneys are enlarged. Palpation of the liver begins in the right iliac fossa – with the palm flat on the abdomen, the radial border of the index finger is pressed firmly inward as the patient is instructed to take a deep breath (Figure 5.11).

This is repeated while moving the finger up at each breath. Liver enlargement is noted in centimetres below the costal margin. The smoothness of the liver edge, surface characteristics and any tenderness are noted. A common cause of liver enlargement is viral hepatitis, in which the liver is also tender. In cirrhosis, the liver is very hard and may be irregular (although in alcoholic cirrhosis the liver is often shrunken and impalpable). Secondary deposits in disseminated malignancy are associated with a hard, irregular liver surface. The spleen enlarges toward the umbilicus, and palpation is started in the right iliac fossa, moving up toward the left hypochondrium. The tips of the index and middle fingers of the right hand are pushed inward and upward on inspiration. Splenic enlargement occurs in a number of conditions, including glandular fever and leukaemia.

The kidneys are palpated bimanually in the loins, with one hand under the patient and the other on top, by pushing the hands together to trap the kidney between them. Kidney enlargement may be compensatory after nephrectomy or may be caused by obstruction, cystic disease, amyloidosis, myeloma or tumour. Generally an easily palpable kidney is abnormal.

Percussion

Organ enlargement can be confirmed by percussion, proceeding from resonant to dull; the percussion note is dull over an enlarged liver or spleen, but it remains resonant over an enlarged kidney because of the overlying bowel filled with gas. In the presence of ascites (fluid in the peritoneal cavity), fluid accumulates in the flanks, thus leaving the resonant bowel floating centrally. To elicit ascites, percussion is commenced in the centre of the abdomen (Figure 5.12), while working toward the left flank until the percussion note becomes dull. At this point, the finger is kept in the same position and the patient asked to roll to the right. The fluid

redistributes by gravity, and after a few moments the percussion note over the same area becomes resonant. This is known as shifting dullness (also an unkind reference to a group of students).

Auscultation

Bowel sounds are the result of peristalsis, commonly detected by listening over the abdomen with the stethoscope. Absence of bowel sounds occurs in paralysis of the bowel wall (known as ileus) – this is a fairly common postoperative complication or effect of opioid use. Bowel sounds are increased and tinkling in bowel obstruction.

Digital rectal examination

This part of the examination is rarely indicated in the patient with a head and neck condition except in the presence of symptoms of bowel disease or polytrauma, and it is best left to medically qualified staff. On occasion, rectal examination may be required to diagnose constipation, another complication in patients using opioids regularly. Before the examination, the procedure and its importance should be explained. A glove, some gel lubricant such as KY jelly and a piece of gauze are required. The patient should be as relaxed as possible, to minimize discomfort, and reassured that the examination, although unpleasant, should not be painful. The patient is positioned lying in the left lateral position, with the buttocks at the edge of the bed and the knees curled up to the chest. The perianal skin is examined for lesions such as fissures, tags and warts. The

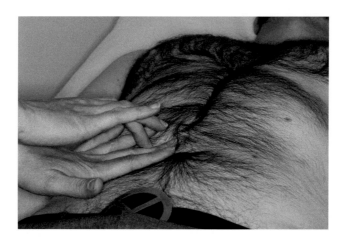

Figure 5.12 Percussion of the abdomen.

gloved index finger of the right hand is lubricated and inserted along the posterior wall, with gentle pressure, into the rectum. The finger is then slowly rotated to enable examination of the anterior rectal wall. Any mucosal abnormality is noted. In male patients the size and characteristics of the prostate are assessed. Prostatic enlargement is extremely common in older men and frequently contributes to postoperative urinary retention – it is important to anticipate this because catheterization may prove difficult in such circumstances. On withdrawal, examine your finger for the presence of blood.

Nervous system

Examination of the nervous system begins during history taking, when orientation, intellectual function and speech are assessed, and any obvious neurological deficit (e.g. facial palsy or hemiparesis) will be apparent. The examination requires cooperation and must be adjusted to the individual patient's problem, understanding, behaviour and intellect. If there is a suspicion of a dementing illness or confusional state, a 10-point abbreviated mental test is a useful tool to test memory and intellect. A point is scored for each fully correct response, with an acceptable score being 7 or more.

ABBREVIATED MENTAL TEST (AMT)

1. What is your full name?
2. Where are you? (hospital/ward name).
3. Two person recognition. For example, point to a uniformed nurse and doctor and ask the patient what their jobs are.
4. What is your date of birth?
5. Give the patient an address, for example '42 West Register Street' and ask the patient to repeat it immediately and then at the end of the test.
6. What time of day is it?
7. What year is it?
8. Ask the patient to count backward from 20 to 1.
9. What are the dates of the First/Second World War?
10. Who is the current monarch?

Cranial nerves

Ask a senior colleague to demonstrate cranial nerve examination, which should then be straightforward; the following list is merely a reminder of the action of each nerve:

I. Smell.
II. Visual acuity and fields – funduscopy requires individual skill teaching.
III. Eye movements – ask about diplopia.
IV. Eye movements – ask about diplopia.
V. Motor – muscles of mastication; and sensory – corneal reflex and facial sensation.
VI. Eye movements – ask about diplopia.
VII. Muscles of facial expression.
VIII. Hearing and balance.
IX. Gag reflex.
X. Speech, soft palate movement.
XI. Sternomastoid, trapezius movements ('shoulder shrug' action).
XII. Motor – tongue movements.

Peripheral nerves

Checking the tone, power, reflexes, sensation and coordination of each limb assesses peripheral nerves. Again a senior colleague is best to demonstrate this examination.

Assessing head injury

This is an essential component of the medical management of the maxillofacial trauma patient (see Chapter 16).

A change in the level of consciousness is the earliest and most reliable sign of brain injury in patients not affected by drugs. A combination of pupillary response to light, limb movement and the **Glasgow Coma Scale (GCS)** (see box) is normally used.

A GCS score of less than 6 in the absence of drugs indicates a very poor prognosis. A change of GCS by more than two points (usually a drop) signifies brain injury, and action is required; contact a senior colleague or obtain neurosurgical advice.

Other things to look for Pupils – the size ranges from 1 to 8 mm. Pupils should constrict when exposed to light. A fixed, dilated pupil in association with a fall in GCS equals brain injury and mandates that you get help. Decreasing pulse and rising blood pressure (Cushing's response) and decreasing respiratory rate are late signs of raised intracranial pressure.

GLASGOW COMA SCALE

Eyes open

- Spontaneously – score 4.
- To speech– score 3.
- To pain – score 2.
- Do not open –score 1.

Best verbal response

- Orientated – score 5.
- Confused – score 4.
- Inappropriate – score 3.
- Incomprehensible – score 2.
- None – score 1.

Best motor response

- Obeys commands – score 6.
- Localizes pain – score 5.
- Normal flexion – score 4.
- Abnormal flexion – score 3.
- Extension – score 2.
- None – score 1.

Scoring

Minor head (brain) injury – 13–15.
Moderate head (brain) injury – 9–12.
Severe head (brain) injury – <8.

Also be aware that unequal limb movements, open skull fractures, depressed skull fractures, worsening headache and unequal pupils are all signs and symptoms associated with intracranial injury.

What can you do? Get help.
Provide high-flow oxygen and mechanically ventilate if the patient is not breathing. Leave hyperventilation to experts. Control any accessible bleeding and give intravenous (i.v.) fluid (2 L Hartmann's (aka Ringer's lactate or alternatively 0.9% saline solution) immediately, and then be guided by the patient's response); give blood if needed. Once the patient is stabilized (if that is possible) and help has arrived, then obtain a computed tomography scan in conjunction with neurosurgical advice. Remember that if the patient is in shock he or she is much more likely to be bleeding from the chest, abdomen or pelvis than the face or head. Ensure that such bleeding has been addressed (this may mean going to theatre for the patient's spleen to be removed before neurosurgery) before you take responsibility for the patient. In haemodynamically normal patients with face, head or brain injuries, you may be responsible for primary stabilization and contact with neurosurgery and anaesthetics (the latter are essential for transfer, intubation and ventilation).

Facial palsy

Causes of unilateral facial weakness include the following:

- Head injury.
- Herpes zoster infection (shingles).
- Bell's palsy.
- Multiple sclerosis.
- Parotid or intracranial tumours.

It is important to determine the cause accurately because treatment for each cause is completely different. Upper motor neuron facial palsy tends to spare the temporal branch to a limited extent (Figure 5.13).

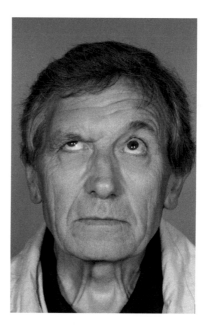

Figure 5.13 Right-sided facial palsy, an example of lower motor neurone palsy (complete). Upper motor neurone palsy spares the temporal branch.

Head injury Facial weakness following a head injury usually indicates a fracture involving the temporal bone. Diagnosis is usually clinical with a history of significant trauma. In addition there may be:

- Bleeding from the ear.
- Haemotympanum (blood visible behind the ear drum).
- Deafness.
- Vertigo.
- Nystagmus.
- Herpes zoster infection (Ramsay Hunt syndrome). This is a viral infection affecting the geniculate ganglion. In addition to facial weakness, vesicles are visible on the ear canal, pharynx and face. Management is with aciclovir.

Bell's palsy Idiopathic facial palsy (Bell's palsy) should be a diagnosis of exclusion. All other causes must be eliminated clinically or following investigations. A thorough examination of the head and neck, especially the cranial nerves, is essential, and, if necessary, magnetic resonance imaging is performed before the diagnosis can be made. Treatment involves high-dose steroids. Evidence does not support the use of aciclovir. The prognosis for Bell's palsy is generally good.

Investigations – where, what, why and how?

Investigations are used as an aid to diagnosis, preoperative assessment and postoperative management – they should be ordered only after adequate clinical history taking and examination. The results should be interpreted in the context of clinical findings. Do not order a test without interpreting the results and *acting* on abnormalities, even if this simply means informing someone else. Each hospital has guidelines for preoperative investigations.

It is the responsibility of the clinician clerking the patient to inform the surgeon, anaesthetist and theatre staff if problems are anticipated or if special arrangements need to be made. For example, frozen sections may be needed, or the photographer may be required in theatre. If any doubt arises during the clerking or preoperative management of patients, a few minutes spent discussing the matters with an appropriate colleague are always preferable to ignoring problems or leaving them for others to discover.

Bedside investigations

There are several important tests that are performed at the patient's bedside and charted by the nursing staff on a regular basis. It is important to look at the results and trend in these observations because consistent abnormalities usually signify a problem (Figure 5.14).

Temperature – axillary temperature is about 1°C less than oral temperature; an oral temperature above 37.5°C is pathological. Pyrexia is usually caused by infections, although noninfected collections of secretions in the alveoli after an anaesthetic (a condition called atelectasis) can do this. Pus collections cause swinging pyrexia with daily spikes. Postoperative pyrexia may be the first sign of deep venous thrombosis (DVT), chest wound, urinary tract infection or transfusion reaction. Detecting pyrexia means that you should identify the cause and treat it.

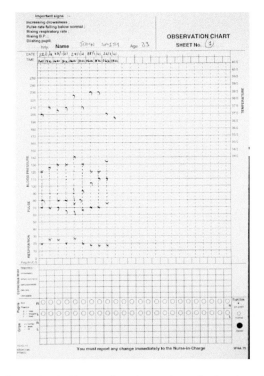

Figure 5.14 Observation chart; always look at it and question what you do not understand.

Blood tests

Commonly requested blood tests are full blood count (FBC), urea and electrolytes (U&E), coagulation profile, blood group and cross-match, and liver function tests (LFTs). Other biochemical tests are used when clinically indicated and include thyroid function tests, cardiac enzymes and a bone profile.

The following box gives a reference range for the most commonly requested tests. Remember the range varies slightly with each laboratory, and local values should be used. Similarly, request forms vary, but all must be filled in accurately with adequate clinical data, signed and dated.

ADULT REFERENCE RANGES

Sodium	135–145 mmol/l
Potassium	3.5–5.0 mmol/l
Creatinine	60–120 µmol/l
Urea	3.5–7.0 mmol/l
Glucose	3.0–6.0 mmol/l (fasting)
Haemoglobin	11.5–16.0 g/dl (women)
	13.5–18.0 g/dl (men)
MCV	76–96 fl
White blood cells	4.0–11.0 × 10^9/l
Platelets	150–400 × 10^9/l
TT	10–15 seconds
PT	0.9–1.3 seconds
APTT	34–45 seconds

APTT, activated partial thromboplastin time; MCV, mean corpuscular volume; PT, prothrombin time; TT, thrombin time.

Full blood count and film

The FBC looks at haemoglobin concentration, white blood cell count, platelets and the red blood cell (RBC) parameters and gives a differential white blood cell count. An FBC is required as a baseline for any patient who is having surgery that will involve significant blood loss, for patients who are clinically anaemic or polycythaemic and for patients with suspected infections, malignancy or lymphoreticular disorders.

Haemoglobin concentration is reduced in anaemia, and the mean corpuscular volume (MCV) can give an indication of the type of anaemia – in iron deficiency anaemia, the MCV is low; in vitamin B_{12} and folate deficiency, the MCV is raised. The haemoglobin concentration is increased in polycythaemia. Patients with anaemia and polycythaemia may need treatment or require further investigation before anaesthesia.

The white blood cell count is increased in infections and leukaemias and in conditions involving an inflammatory reaction, such as after surgery or trauma; in septic patients and patients taking immunosuppressive drugs and steroids, this white cell response may be suppressed.

Platelets – very low platelet counts predispose to intraoperative and postoperative bleeding problems. Unexplained abnormal platelet counts should be referred to haematologists.

Urea and electrolytes

U&Es enable measurement of the plasma sodium, potassium, urea and serum creatinine concentrations. Uncorrected electrolyte abnormalities, especially potassium, pose a risk of cardiac dysrhythmias and cardiac arrest. Abnormalities in urea and creatinine concentrations may reveal renal insufficiency – under the additional stress of surgery or major blood loss this may precipitate acute renal failure.

Not every patient requires preoperative U&E measurement. Indications include the following: baseline for patients who are to undergo major surgery; patients with cardiovascular disease, diabetes and renal disease; or patients taking medications that may alter their renal function. Regular U&E monitoring is required for patients receiving i.v. fluid infusions to aid clinical assessment of fluid and electrolyte requirements.

An abnormality in **sodium** concentration usually reflects hydration status, by increasing in dehydration and decreasing when patients are fluid overloaded or in congestive cardiac failure. Diuretic therapy is a common cause of sodium derangement – all patients taking diuretics require U&E measurement. Many dispersible drugs contain excess sodium.

Potassium – low potassium is commonly caused by diuretic therapy, diarrhoea and vomiting, and it also occurs in patients who abuse laxatives. A high potassium value may be erroneous as a result of a haemolyzed blood sample, and in an asymptomatic patient, the test should be repeated. More ominously, it occurs in renal failure, in patients taking potassium-sparing diuretics and in patients given excessive amounts of potassium in i.v. fluid regimens. Plasma potassium is tightly maintained within a relatively narrow range – outside this range serious cardiac instability can occur. Correction of plasma potassium levels is not for the occasional practitioner – consult and refer.

Plasma **urea** is produced in the liver, as a product of protein breakdown, filtered by the glomerulus and eliminated in the urine. Urea levels increase in patients with renal insufficiency. However, urea concentration is influenced by a number of factors such as protein intake, the absorption of additional amino acids following gastrointestinal bleeding, dehydration and hypermetabolic states. Conversely, **creatinine** levels give a more accurate indication of renal function because they are mainly dictated by the patient's muscle mass. The urea concentration is raised in dehydration before renal insufficiency supervenes.

Blood glucose

For patients with known diabetes or patients whose urine is positive for sugar, random blood glucose testing should be requested. If the value is high, a sample should be taken after an overnight fast, and if it is still elevated, referral to diabetologist is required.

Liver function tests

LFTs include tests of some of the *functions* of the liver, such as bilirubin and albumin production, and tests for *liver cell integrity,* measuring liver enzymes released into the circulation by damaged hepatocytes, such as alkaline phosphatase, plasma aspartate and alanine transaminases (aspartate aminotransferase [AST] and alanine aminotransferase [ALT], respectively). These enzymes are not specific to the liver and are not reliably diagnostic of liver disease, although abnormalities should prompt further investigation.

In surgical patients, LFTs are often requested for patients with malignant disease, although metastases can be present without significantly affecting the results. Plasma alkaline phosphatase may be raised in the presence of liver metastases, and hypoalbuminaemia is a common finding related to malnutrition, cachexia and liver metastases. Plasma gamma-glutamyl transpeptidase is a good indicator of heavy alcohol consumption, even in the absence of liver damage.

Coagulation tests

These tests measure thrombin time (TT), prothrombin time (PT or international normalized ratio [INR]), and activated partial thromboplastin time (APTT). Indications for testing – patients taking medication that alters normal coagulation; patients undergoing major surgery; and patients with known or suspected coagulation disorders or liver disease (including suspected metastases). For patients taking warfarin – before surgical procedures the INR should be checked. The normal reference range is between 2 and 4. Exodontia is generally safe in patients with an INR of less than 4, provided local haemostatic measures are taken. For more major surgery or in patients with an INR greater than 4, warfarin should be stopped and an alternative, usually heparin, started. Heparin infusions and subcutaneous injections are used as a substitute because the action of heparin is easily reversed should life-threatening haemorrhage occur. In bleeding patients or in those with seriously elevated INR, reversal with fresh frozen plasma or vitamin K may be needed. Take advice from haematologists.

'Group and save' and cross-match

A group and save procedure is required for patients undergoing surgery in which there is a moderate risk of significant blood loss (e.g. single jaw osteotomies or superficial parotidectomy). If transfusion is required within 48 hours of the sample, a request can be made to the laboratory without further blood sampling, and blood can be available within a short time. Cross-matching is costly and should be requested only if there is a high risk of significant operative blood loss. The number of units requested varies according to the procedure.

Cardiac enzymes

These values are used to aid in the diagnosis of myocardial infarction. The enzymes measured are creatine kinase, aspartate transaminase, lactate dehydrogenase, the cardiac isomer of creatine kinase (CK-MB) and the troponins. The troponins are now considered the most relevant. The enzymes should be measured in patients presenting with acute chest pain at the time of suspected infarct and after the suspected event. Serial ECGs are performed at the same time to look for the typical changes of a myocardial infarction. Some of the enzymes are not tissue specific to cardiac muscle. Troponin levels are used as a more specific enzymatic indicator of myocardial infarction.

Blood gas analysis

Arterial blood is sampled from the radial, brachial or femoral arteries to assess oxygen and carbon dioxide concentrations. This is a painful procedure for patients, so perform it only if absolutely necessary. Indications – patients who are clearly not able to maintain their oxygen saturation greater than 95% on room air or patients with marked respiratory disease who may require postoperative ventilation. Consult a senior colleague or the anaesthetist if in doubt whether to perform this test (Figure 5.15).

Blood cultures

Patients with septicaemia or patients who develop sudden pyrexia require at least two samples to be

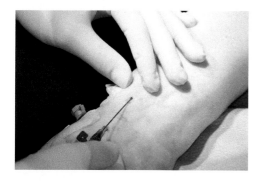

Figure 5.15 Arterial line; arterial blood gases can be sampled from this or a separate arterial puncture.

taken from separate sites and placed in bottles for aerobic and anaerobic culture. Ideally, samples should be taken before 'blind' antibiotic therapy is instituted, and therapy should be altered if the results, available at 24 to 48 hours, indicate antibiotic resistance.

Venous access and blood taking

These techniques are essential skills that are best acquired during daylight hours; acute situations are not the ideal setting for first attempts. Anaesthetists can be helpful at demonstrating peripheral venous cannulation, and the anaesthetized patient is the ideal subject on whom to learn. Similarly, an hour or so spent with a phlebotomist provides an ideal opportunity to acquire blood taking skills.

Venous cannulae come in various sizes and are colour coded. Commonly used codes are as follows: green (18 gauge), ideal for i.v. fluids and antibiotics; yellow (24 gauge), blue (22 gauge) and pink (20 gauge), which are smaller and are useful when venous access is difficult or in children; and grey (16 gauge) and orange/brown (14 gauge), which are larger and are required when large volumes and/or blood products are to be transfused.

How to insert a cannula

1. Collect and have at the bedside all the equipment required. In children local anaesthetic cream (e.g. EMLA) can be applied an hour before elective cannulation. If inserting a large-bore cannula, 0.5 mL intradermal lidocaine should first be inserted at the site of skin puncture, using a fine-bore (orange) needle. If using lidocaine, allow enough time for it to work.
2. Place a tourniquet around the arm. This inhibits venous return, thus dilating the superficial forearm veins.
3. Select a suitable vein by inspecting and palpating the lower forearm and dorsum of the hand. Veins have a tendency to move when the cannula approaches, and the least mobile site is at the confluence of two veins. Swab the area clean with an alcohol wipe.
4. Stabilize the patient's hand and arm and make the skin taut in the region of the vein by using your nondominant thumb. Puncture the skin, then the vein. At the time of venous entry, a

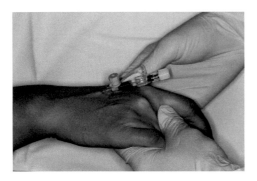

Figure 5.16 Siting of an intravenous cannula in a straight segment of vein.

flashback of blood is seen in the hub of the needle. Slowly and carefully advance the cannula a farther 3 mm along the vein, withdraw the needle slightly and then advance the cannula along the vein, aiming the cannula in the direction in which the vein appears to be running.

5. Release the tourniquet and elevate the arm slightly, and with a finger placed over the vein to occlude flow, remove the needle and discard it safely. Place the plastic bung into the end of the cannula. Flush the cannula through with normal saline to ensure it is patent and free of stagnant blood.

6. Adequately secure the cannula with an adhesive dressing to prevent it dislodging (Figure 5.16).

How to take blood

1. Collect together all equipment and take it to the patient (Figure 5.17).
2. Place a tourniquet above the elbow and ask the patient to straighten the arm.
3. Palpate the antecubital fossa because veins in this region are often easier to feel than to see.

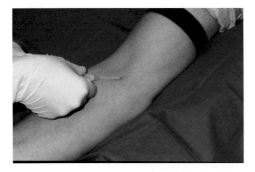

Figure 5.17 Taking blood from the cubital fossa.

4. Swab the area clean and insert the needle, at an angle of 45°. If vacuumed syringes are used, the sample for biochemistry should be taken first, and that for coagulation last; the needle is held still in the vein while further tubes are applied in turn.
5. Release the tourniquet and place a piece of cotton wool over the puncture site as the needle is withdrawn; apply pressure for a few minutes to obtain haemostasis. Dispose of sharps in the appropriate sharps bin.

Radiographs

Chest radiographs

These studies should not be used as preoperative screening tests. In cases where a chest radiograph is desirable, it is useful to ask patients whether they have had a recent chest X-ray (within the last 6 months), and if so to obtain this to avoid unnecessary duplication. A posteroanterior chest radiograph is indicated in the following situations (Figure 5.18):

- Preoperative patients with a history of cardiovascular disease (e.g. hypertension, ischaemic heart disease and heart failure).
- Patients with malignancy. This is to look for metastases or a synchronous primary tumour.
- Patients with diagnosed chronic obstructive and restrictive pulmonary disease or patients whose history or examination may be suggestive of respiratory disease (e.g. long-standing smokers with productive cough or wheeze) (Figure 5.19).

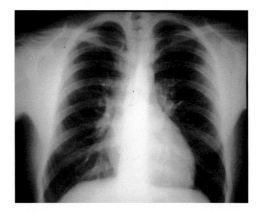

Figure 5.18 Normal posteroanterior chest X-ray.

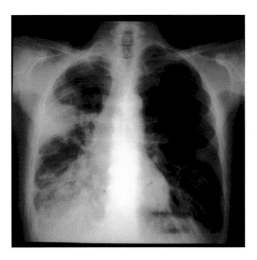

Figure 5.19 Abnormal chest X-ray showing collapse and consolidation of the right lung.

- Patients who are recent immigrants from countries in which tuberculosis is endemic and who have not had a radiograph in the preceding 12 months.
- A mobile chest radiograph can be requested urgently in patients who become acutely breathless, develop severe chest pain or are being managed in the intensive therapy unit.

Cervical-spine radiographs

Any patient with a suspected upper airway injury should have a cervical spine X-ray (Figure 5.20). Patients with rheumatoid arthritis are at risk of atlantoaxial joint subluxation. Clinical assessment of neck movements and cervical spine radiographs in flexion and extension should be obtained to aid the anaesthetist in deciding the appropriate means of airway control. (For trauma and the cervical spine, see Chapter 16.)

Cardiovascular and respiratory system investigations

- **ECG** – a standard 12-lead ECG should be obtained preoperatively in patients with known or suspected cardiovascular disease or diabetes. In patients with ischaemic heart disease, the preoperative ECG may prove invaluable for comparison should the

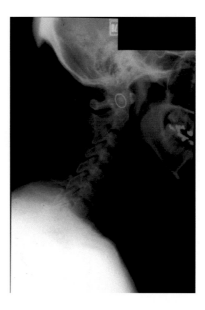

Figure 5.20 Normal lateral cervical spine X-ray (spine views are essential in polytrauma).

patient develop postoperative chest pain. If abnormalities are present, the ECG should be discussed with a senior colleague and the anaesthetist.
- **Echocardiography** – this investigation is a noninvasive ultrasound study of the blood flow through the heart. The indication for this test should be discussed with a cardiologist before the test is requested.
- **Pulmonary function tests** – these tests are used preoperatively to assess lung volumes and flow rates in patients with chronic obstructive and restrictive respiratory diseases. The degree of reversibility of the disease to medications such as inhaled salbutamol and steroids can be assessed, and appropriate therapy can be maximized before elective operations. (Should there be more than a 15% improvement in forced vital capacity after inhaled bronchodilators, it is inferred that the current therapy is suboptimal.)

Drugs

Filling in the prescription card

Each hospital pharmacy produces a slightly different drug card, but all follow a similar pattern, with spaces for regular medication, medications to be given when required (prn) and once only medications such as premedications. Each entry should be legible, with the generic name of the drug written in full, dated and signed. For prn medications, the maximum dose or the dose interval should be written, along with the indication for administration (e.g. for nausea, pain or constipation).

Medications to stop and the risk of deep venous thrombosis

- Oestrogen-containing oral contraceptive pills (OCPs) increase the risk of DVT in patients undergoing major surgery, and for 2 weeks postoperatively, or until patients are fully mobile. Advice on the use of alternative contraception should be given.
- Warfarin is discussed in an earlier section. The dose of heparin is adjusted based on the 6-hourly APTT. Desired level – 2 to 2.5 times the control level.
- Other oral anticoagulation – aspirin needs 12 days if platelet function is to return to normal, clopidogrel and similar drugs need a similar length of time. Do not stop treatment without thinking whether this puts the patient at a greater or lesser risk.
- DVT is common in patients in the following groups:
  - Obese patients.
  - Patients more than 40 years old.
  - Patients with malignant disease.
  - Patients with a history of DVT or pulmonary embolus (PE).
  - Patients undergoing prolonged or major surgery, with prolonged periods of postoperative bedrest.

Prevention of DVT involves generalized measures to reduce venous stasis, including physiotherapy, early mobilization, graduated compression stockings (thromboembolism deterrent [TED] stockings) and pneumatic calf compression.

At-risk patients should be prescribed TED stockings and low-dose subcutaneous heparin. Standard fractionated heparin requires a twice daily regimen (5000 units 2 hours preoperatively and a further 5000 units twice daily until the patient is mobile). Newer low-molecular-weight heparins (e.g. tinzaparin) can be given as once daily injections. Familiarize yourself with your hospital's policy.

Antiemetics

Prochlorperazine, cyclizine, metoclopramide and ondansetron are the most commonly used antiemetics. In children and in elderly patients, prochlorperazine and metoclopramide can cause acute dystonias and oculogyric crises, which can be aborted with procyclidine. Cyclizine is commonly used in conjunction with systemic opioids (e.g. morphine) and ondansetron for children and for recalcitrant nausea.

Cytoprotection

Patients undergoing major surgery are at risk of stress ulceration, which can result in major gastrointestinal bleeding. Such patients may benefit from the prescription of a mucosal protecting agent such as sucralfate (2 g orally twice daily) to cover the immediate postoperative period. The disadvantage of this drug is that it occludes nasogastric tubes. An alternative is an i.v. H_2 antagonist such as ranitidine or a proton pump inhibitor such as omeprazole. The disadvantages of this treatment are the loss of the gastric pH barrier and the risk of ascending infections caused by gram-negative aerobic bacilli.

Antibiotics for infection prophylaxis

Local protocols dictate which antibiotics are to be given in the preoperative period to prevent postoperative wound infection. These are usually prescribed for administration at or before the induction of anaesthesia, to obtain maximum blood levels at the time of surgery and for up to 24 hours postoperatively. In patients with conditions of the head and neck, commonly used drugs are amoxicillin, metronidazole and co-fluampicil (a 50/50 mixture of ampicillin and flucloxacillin). Always check local protocols.

Analgesics

See Chapter 4.

Patients on steroids

Patients taking corticosteroid preparations on a long-term basis for conditions such as severe asthma, chronic inflammatory conditions or adrenal cortical insufficiency or following organ transplants have a risk of atrophy of the adrenal cortex that can persist for years after steroid withdrawal. In the presence of increased physiological stress (e.g. trauma, surgery or infection), these patients are unable to produce sufficient endogenous corticosteroids – profound hypotension, collapse and death may mark the onset of acute adrenal insufficiency.

Patients who regularly take oral steroids require steroid coverage in the perioperative period. For major surgery a typical regimen is i.v. hydrocortisone, 100 mg at induction and then repeated every 8 hours. The dose is then halved every 24 hours until the normal maintenance dose is reached on about the fifth postoperative day. At this point, the patient reverts to his or her normal regimen. For ambulatory surgery a single prophylactic IM dose of 100 mg hydrocortisone 30 minutes preoperatively, an i.v. dose immediately preoperatively or doubling the normal oral dose suffices.

Fluids

Fluid therapy covers three main areas:

- Replacing daily maintenance fluids in the perioperative nil by mouth patient.
- Rehydration of the dehydrated patient.
- Resuscitation of the critically ill patient.

Not every patient requires i.v. fluids – in the lucid, cooperative patient, all fluid requirements are taken orally, within the dictates of the patient's thirst. However, in ill, preoperative, or unconscious patients, i.v. replacement with salt or glucose solutions becomes necessary. The idea is to replace what the normal intake would be (maintenance) or what has been lost (rehydration and resuscitation).

The most commonly used monitor of adequate hydration is urine output – called 'the poor man's CVP', it infers that if the kidneys are being perfused, there is adequate intravascular volume and pressure. The magical amount of 0.5 to 1 mL/kg patient body weight is the desired urine output in adults.

When prescribing fluids the following information should be remembered:

- The average daily requirement for fluid is 2500 to 3000 mL for a 70-kg adult. This is the *total* amount of fluid in solid and liquid intake.
- The daily sodium requirement is 70 mmol; the daily potassium requirement is 50 to 60 mmol.
- 0.9% saline contains 150 mmol/l sodium and chloride, no potassium; 5% glucose contains 50 g/l glucose, no salts. Once the glucose is used, essentially i.v. water is being administered.
- Dextrose/saline solution contains 30 mmol/l sodium and 4% glucose.
- An i.v. fluid regimen of 1 litre normal saline and 2 litres 5% dextrose in 24 hours, with the addition of 20 mmol/l potassium after the first 36 hours, provides 3 litres water, 150 mmol sodium and 60 mmol potassium. An alternative regimen is to give 3 litres of dextrose/saline.

This is a simplistic view of fluid management. There are many patients who require that this regimen be altered to avoid fluid overload or who have specific nutritional needs that are not met using the foregoing 'recipe'. Consult if in doubt.

Monitoring fluid balance

For older or medically compromised patients, detailed fluid balance monitoring is essential, using a fluid balance chart to monitor losses – urine, surgical drainage and gastrointestinal losses – which should then be replaced. A urinary catheter may be required. In addition, the pulse, temperature and plasma U&E should be monitored. Pyrexial patients need increased fluids to allow for loss of salt and water in sweat. In the postoperative period, the physiological response of the body is to conserve fluid and salt; thus the urine output is initially decreased. The most common cause of inadequate urine output in surgical patients is inadequate fluid replacement. Hypovolaemia is often accompanied by tachycardia and reduced peripheral perfusion.

The blood pressure is an insensitive indicator of fluid status because a normal reading may represent relative hypotension in an elderly or chronically hypertensive patient, and young healthy patients can tolerate an acute blood loss of up to 20% of their blood volume with neither tachycardia nor hypotension as accompanying signs.

In rare circumstances, maxillofacial surgical patients may suffer acute blood loss of sufficient quantity to cause shock. This is a surgical emergency, and its initial management is to address airway, breathing and circulation (see Chapter 16), as well as to get help as soon as possible. Remember, however, that it is extremely rare for a facial injury to cause haemorrhagic hypovolaemic shock; this is much more likely to be caused by bleeding from the chest, abdomen or pelvis.

Catheterization and monitoring

How to insert a urinary catheter

Nurses usually catheterize female patients, but it is not uncommon to be asked to insert a male urethral catheter for fluid balance monitoring or for the relief of acute urinary retention. An aseptic technique is essential (Figures 5.21, 5.22 and 5.23).

1. Set up a sterile trolley with a catheter pack, sterile gloves, a 16- or 18-gauge Foley catheter and catheter bag, antiseptic solution, sterile

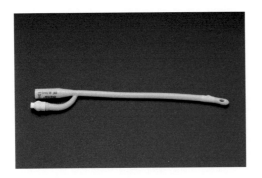

Figure 5.21 Urinary catheter.

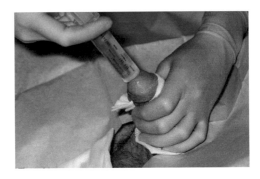

Figure 5.22 Instil adequate local anaesthetic or lubricant gel.

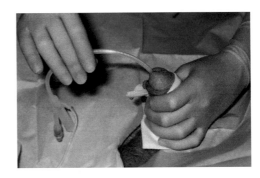

Figure 5.23 Pass the catheter using aseptic technique, and insert full length before inflating the balloon.

lignocaine gel, a syringe and 20 mL sterile water. Explain the procedure to the patient, and expose the patient's genitalia.

2. Wearing sterile gloves, hold the shaft of the patient's penis wrapped in a gauze swab, away from the scrotum, retract the foreskin and thoroughly clean the glans with gauze and aqueous antiseptic solution.

3. Apply sterile drapes; then hold the penis elevated and straight to insert the anaesthetic gel through the meatus. Massage along the length of the urethra and wait.

4. Place the kidney dish from the catheter pack between the patient's legs. With the right hand, pick up and insert the catheter tip, passing it gently along the urethra until it enters the bladder. Insert the full length of the catheter to ensure it is in the bladder before inflating the balloon. The catheter may stick at the prostatic urethra; in this case raise the penis

to right angles to the body and rotate the catheter while advancing. The catheter usually then passes. Collect the urine in the kidney dish, inflate the balloon with the sterile water and connect the catheter to the catheter tubing and bag. If the bladder is empty or gel is blocking it, irrigate with sterile water using a bladder syringe.

5. Ensure the foreskin is replaced, to avoid congestion of the glans (known as paraphimosis).

Blood products and transfusion

The transfusion of blood and blood products is not without complication and should be done only when it is believed that the benefits outweigh the risks. Most serious transfusion reactions are caused by avoidable human errors in labelling, sampling and administration.

Blood is usually given as **packed cells;** 1 unit of packed cells contains 450 mL of blood and 63 mL of preservative. This increases the haemoglobin concentration by 1 g/dl in the adult patient. **Whole blood** (when available) is used in emergency situations where there is uncontrollable haemorrhage. If there is not enough time for a full cross-match (~45 minutes), type-specific (~10 minutes) or un–cross-matched O negative blood (immediate) is initially used.

For elective surgery, in which a transfusion is unlikely but possible, a preoperative group and save procedure is performed; where transfusion is anticipated a cross-match for a specific number of units is requested. For elderly patients and those with heart failure or impaired renal function, transfusions should be performed slowly (>4 hours), and these patients may require a diuretic (frusemide 40 mg orally or 20 mg intravenously) to prevent fluid overload.

Postoperatively, the decision when to transfuse depends on the operative blood loss and the patient's preoperative condition. The young and healthy are able to cope with haemoglobin as low as 6 g/dl. In patients with ischaemic heart disease, this does not apply, and the threshold to transfuse is usually around 10 g/dl.

- **Platelet transfusions** are rarely indicated, but they may be necessary in patients undergoing surgery with a platelet count of less than 20 × 10^9/l. Consult with haematologists – unnecessary request for this blood component is very costly.
- **Fresh frozen plasma** is used when urgent correction of clotting defects is required (e.g. to control acute haemorrhage in patients taking warfarin).
- **Autologous transfusion** – patients scheduled for major elective surgery may donate blood over a period of weeks preoperatively and can thereby be transfused with their own blood intraoperatively. This service is not available universally, it is not cheap and many patients may still require additional donor blood.

Complications of blood transfusions

1. ABO incompatibility – this causes rapid-onset pyrexia, breathlessness, headache and loin pain and rapidly leads to shock and renal failure. The condition requires emergency resuscitations with oxygen and fluids, with adrenaline and hydrocortisone used in a similar sequence to anaphylaxis treatment (discussed later).

2. Mild febrile reactions – these are usually the result of non-RBC immune incompatibility. They are indicated by pyrexia and tachycardia and treated by slowing down the transfusion; if this fails, chlorpheniramine 10 mg may help. If the temperature continues to climb, or the patient develops systemic symptoms such as rigors, stop the transfusion, return the blood to blood bank, and repeat the cross-match. Consider using leucocyte-depleted blood for future transfusions. Use of a white cell filter can decrease the risk of this complication.

3. Transmission of infection from the donor – UK blood is screened for human immunodeficiency virus (HIV), hepatitis B and C and syphilis; however, other viral, bacterial and protozoal infections may be contained in blood products. Modern viricidal treatment of blood products should virtually eradicate the infection risk.

4. Rate-related complications – if cold blood is transfused rapidly, hypothermia is a serious risk. In addition, RBCs continue to undergo

normal cellular activity in the bag, and this makes transfused blood high in potassium, citrate (a preservative) and lactate.

Diabetes mellitus

Diabetes mellitus (DM) is an extremely common condition with a prevalence of 3% to 7%, which increases with age. Complications of DM result from large and small vessel disease affecting the cardiovascular, renal and neurological systems, including the eyes. The danger in the perioperative period is that diabetic patients are at increased risk of wound infection and poor wound healing. In addition, surgical stress and the ensuing increased cortisol levels make control of DM more difficult.

Diabetic patients fall into two categories – insulin-dependent (type 1) DM and non–insulin dependent (type 2) DM, the latter being controlled by diet alone or by diet and oral hypoglycaemic tablets. The complications of DM are unfortunately not always prevented by tight glucose control – there is no such thing as mild DM. The adequacy of long-term glucose control can be measured by the HbA1C test, in which RBC glucose levels are used as a marker.

If a diabetic patient requires surgery, the anaesthetist should be informed; it may be prudent to inform the diabetic team if major surgery is planned. The patient should be admitted 24 hours before the operation, to allow assessment and optimization of diabetic control.

Preoperative considerations

Preoperatively, investigations should include FBC, U&Es, random blood glucose, ECG, chest X-ray and regular bedside finger-prick glucose monitoring (BMs). Schedule the patient first on the theatre list.

Insulin-requiring patients should be started on some form of glucose, potassium and insulin (GKI) infusion from the time the patient is starved. Finger-prick glucose measurement should be done 4 hourly.

There are two recognized ways of delivering GKI. It is important to understand that they are quite different and that each hospital has its own preferred method.

Glucose, potassium and insulin

A GKI infusion is set up as follows:

- 500 mL 5% dextrose.
- Plus x units of insulin run at 100 mL/hour.
- Plus x mmol of potassium chloride (KCl).

For patients with adequate diabetic control (i.e. blood glucose 6 to 11 mmol/l), 15 units of short-acting soluble insulin (e.g. Actrapid) with 10 mmol KCl is used. If values are outside these parameters, the DM team should be involved. The infusion, which is in effect a best guess of the diabetic patient's requirements, is run through a single i.v. cannula via a controlled-rate infusion device.

Sliding scale

A sliding scale is an infusion of glucose and potassium in the same mixture as the GKI, **but** the insulin is delivered in an adjustable format as 50 IU Actrapid insulin dissolved in 49 mL of normal saline via a syringe driver (Figure 5.24). It is essential that although the insulin and glucose and potassium come from two separate sources, they go into the patient through a single cannula. The risk to this approach is that if the tubing of one of the solutions becomes blocked, the patient may receive unopposed insulin or glucose.

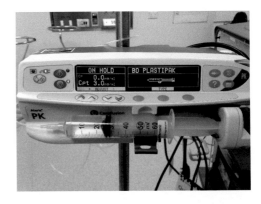

Figure 5.24 A syringe driver; such controlled infusion devices are essential when delivering powerful drugs such as insulin or morphine in small quantities.

An example of a sliding scale (relating how much insulin is given in relation to the blood glucose) is shown here:

- Glucose (mmol/l)
- More than 20   Ask for advice from diabetic team.
- 15–20   3 IU/hour.
- 10–15   2 IU/hour.
- 5–10   1 IU/hour.
- 2–5   **Stop**.
- Less than 2   Give glucose.

Postoperative care

Postoperatively, a bedside blood glucose test is performed and repeated at 1- to 2-hourly intervals. A sliding scale is prescribed to determine insulin requirements.

When the patient is eating and drinking, the patient's normal evening insulin can be given before the evening meal.

Patients with non–insulin-dependent DM whose treatment consists of diet alone should have a random blood glucose test to assess DM control and regular bedside glucose monitoring. For those taking long-acting hypoglycaemic drugs (e.g. metformin, chlorpropamide), this medication should be changed several days preoperatively to a short-acting agent (e.g. tolbutamide). No diabetic patient should be presented for surgery if the glucose concentrations are outside the normal range. On the day of surgery, the oral hypoglycaemic drug is withheld because the patient omits breakfast, and it is recommended when the patient is eating again. Regular bedside blood glucose monitoring is performed, and if the blood glucose rises to more than 13 mmol/l, 6 units of short-acting subcutaneous insulin are given.

The bleeder

Bleeders can be grouped into two kinds: iatrogenic and congenital. All patients who fall into this category require an FBC and clotting screen/INR/APTT/PT, depending on local protocol. The risk is obviously in the perioperative period, when intraoperative or postoperative haemorrhage complicates management.

Anticoagulated patients

By far the most common group of patients presenting for surgery with bleeding disorders consists of patients taking oral anticoagulants.

Warfarin

Warfarin is a vitamin K antagonist and affects production of clotting factors II, VII, IX and X. The drug is used to prevent thromboembolic events in high-risk patients such as those with prosthetic metal heart valves, patients in atrial fibrillation and patients with recurrent PEs. It is important to remember that certain drugs interfere with or increase the risk of bleeding with warfarin. Aspirin, other nonsteroidal anti-inflammatory agents and steroids should be avoided, as should co-codamol and certain antibiotics including metronidazole.

If urgent reversal of warfarin is needed, fresh frozen plasma may be used to replace clotting factors. Intravenous vitamin K should not be used unless the patient is *in extremis* because reestablishing anticoagulation control can prove very difficult for several weeks after its administration. Some haematologists now recommend low doses of oral or subcutaneous vitamin K – consult earlier rather than later.

Other oral agents

There are a bewildering number of antiplatelet agents on the market, predominantly prescribed by cardiologists for prevention of coronary thrombosis. These include, among others, low-dose aspirin, adenosine diphosphate antagonists and glycoprotein IIb/IIIa antagonists. The importance is that their use is documented, particularly if two or more of these agents are being taken simultaneously. Consult with haematologists if in doubt whether or not to stop these agents preoperatively – the risk of coronary clot formation must be weighed against the potential for perioperative haemorrhage.

Congenital coagulation defects

All these defects require consultation with haematologists. Despite this, most of these patients are managed using self-delivery of cryoprecipitate and can often be managed essentially the same way as patients without bleeding disorders.

- **Haemophilia A** (factor VIII deficiency) is the most common congenital clotting defect. It is an X-linked recessive condition, predominantly affecting males, with female carriers. In one-third of cases there is no family history. The disease varies in severity, depending on the level of factor VIII. Characteristically, the patient will initially appear to stop bleeding after a surgical insult but will then start to ooze uncontrollably several hours later.
- **Christmas disease** is identical in its clinical presentation to haemophilia A, but is caused by factor IX deficiency. Most patients with haemophilia can be treated using factor VIII cryoprecipitate with factor IX. Discuss any proposed surgery with the haematologist, and ensure that adequate prophylactic measures, including the use of clotting factor concentrates and DDAVP, are instituted. Unfortunately, many patients with haemophilia were infected with HIV and hepatitis C before the routine screening of blood and blood products in 1985. Acquired immunodeficiency syndrome (AIDS) is now the most common cause of death in patients with severe haemophilia.
- **Von Willebrand's disease** is a condition caused by von Willebrand factor deficiency, leading to defective platelet function. The clinical presentation ranges from mild to moderate bleeding following surgery or trauma, although it is rarely as severe as in patients with haemophilia. Management is similar to that of mild haemophilia.

Platelet disorders

These disorders result from abnormal platelet *function* (e.g. from aspirin therapy, chronic renal insufficiency and myeloproliferative diseases) or from abnormal platelet *number* (thrombocytopaenia), which may be caused by immune system destruction, bone marrow failure or drugs or may be part of a coagulation syndrome such as disseminated intravascular coagulation and idiopathic thrombocytopaenic purpura. The results are excessive bruising and purpura, mucosal haemorrhage including epistaxes and postextraction bleeding.

Management must include consultation with haematologists. Assuming normal platelet function, levels greater than $50 \times 10^9/l$ are preferable for surgery. Should platelet transfusion be required, this should be performed by the anaesthetist in the immediate preoperative period. The management of postoperative bleeding includes local measures and the use of tranexamic acid, which is effective as a mouth rinse for intraoral haemorrhage.

The 'deranged' patient

Acute confusion is a common problem, especially in elderly patients. The patient may display confusion with decreased responsiveness, agitation, aggression, delusions or hallucinations. The causes are varied – it is important to exclude the most likely by looking for pointers in the history, examination and review of the recent blood results. Some possibilities include the following:

- Hypoxia (check the oxygen saturation with a pulse oximeter).
- Alcohol/drug withdrawal.
- Metabolic upset, particularly hypoglycaemia.
- Hypothermia.
- Infection (urinary tract, chest and wound are likely suspects).
- Drug reaction (even mild opioids such as co-codamol can cause problems in elderly patients).
- Disorientation to unfamiliar surroundings.
- Constipation.
- Acute retention of urine.

As for management, treat the underlying cause! The patient should preferably be nursed in a well-lit side room. Administer facemask oxygen if saturations are reduced. Resist the urge to sedate confused patients without carefully exploring treatable, reversible causes. Attempt to settle the patient with sympathetic nursing care; if that fails, consult with physicians specializing in care of elderly patients.

Postoperative problems

Abnormal symptoms or signs in the postoperative period may indicate complications. This finding warrants a detailed history, thorough examination and appropriate investigations, not wishful thinking. The most common problems are outlined here.

- **Pain** – adequate pain control is of paramount importance in the postoperative period (see earlier).
- **Nausea and vomiting** – anaesthetic agents, opioid analgesia, swallowed blood and pain all contribute. Ensure that all patients are prescribed an antiemetic (e.g. cyclizine or ondansetron).
- **Fever** – common causes are basal atelectasis with or without chest infection, wound infection and urinary tract infection. Sputum and blood cultures and midstream urine specimens are usual investigations. Usually empirical antibiotic treatment is started if there is a likely culprit – prescribe according to the local guidelines until sensitivities are available. Other important causes are DVT and PE, reaction to blood transfusion and drug reactions.
- **Tachycardia** – this is a physiological response to pain and sepsis. In older patients consider heart failure or a dysrhythmia, which may result from myocardial infarction or fluid overload. In the absence of an easily identifiable cause, an ECG and chest radiograph can aid diagnosis.
- **Hypotension** – in elective maxillofacial surgical patients, this is very rarely caused by excessive blood loss or hypovolaemia. Treatment consists of elevating the foot of the bed and administering i.v. fluids. Always exclude the possibility of myocardial infarction as a cause!
- **Urinary retention** – this exists almost exclusively in male patients. The risk increases with age as the prostate hypertrophies, causing a tendency toward urinary outflow obstruction. Prevention is by early mobilization and adequate analgesia. Treatment is urinary catheterization.

Critical care

Patients who undergo major surgery involving the head and neck, especially those with preoperative cardiorespiratory disease and those in whom surgery compromises the airway, often require a period of intensive monitoring and treatment in the immediate postoperative period. This can be in a high-dependency unit, or, if ventilation is required, in the intensive care unit (these are sometimes referred to as levels 1, 2 and 3, in order of intensity of care, with 3 being highest). Whatever the setting, no amount of monitoring equipment is a substitute for thorough and regular clinical examination by clinicians who know what they are doing.

Monitoring and care of such patients involves the following:

1. Maintenance of the airway – this involves regular humidification and suction if an artificial airway is in place.
2. Oxygenation – all patients require oxygen; the aim is to maintain oxygen saturations at an acceptable level without causing carbon dioxide retention, especially in patients with COPD. Regular clinical examination of the chest, measurements of arterial blood gases and pulse oximetry are the means of monitoring. Chest physiotherapy is used to help prevent atelectasis (collapse of small airways), which reduces oxygenation and predisposes patients to chest infections.
3. Circulatory support – this maintains a blood pressure adequate to perfuse tissues. A cardiac monitor is used to assess heart rate and rhythm, and invasive (arterial line) or non-invasive (blood pressure cuff) blood pressure monitoring is used. In maxillofacial microvascular surgery, circulatory support is mainly achieved with i.v. fluids because there has been controversy over the risks of the vasoconstrictive effects of inotropes on flaps. This risk has probably been overstated.
4. Fluid balance – this involves monitoring and charting input and output (urinary, faecal and insensible losses plus extra losses, e.g. from haemorrhage, drains, vomiting or sweating), aiming to match input to output. This usually requires urinary catheterization, especially if the patient is sedated. Regular clinical examination to determine fluid status is vital; where fluid management is difficult, central venous pressure monitoring helps.

5. Temperature control – this prevents hypothermia and maintains tissue perfusion.
6. Nutritional support – this should be instituted after several days if prolonged periods of critical care are anticipated. Nasogastric feeding can often be started 24 hours after major head and neck surgery.

Emergencies

An emergency requires urgent management to limit serious morbidity and prevent mortality. By following certain basic principles, it should be possible to manage any emergency regardless of the cause until expert help becomes available.

Syncope

If a collapsed patient is breathing spontaneously and has a pulse, the most common cause is a simple faint. Often the patient will anticipate the event by feeling nauseated and lightheaded before the collapse. The treatment is to lay the patient flat and loosen constrictive clothing; if the patient fails to recover very rapidly, rethink the diagnosis.

Collapse

When called to see a collapsed patient, the basic principles of resuscitation are required.

HHH (Hazards Hello Help) – check for any potential hazard to you or other rescuers. This may include exposed electrical wires! Call the patient's name. Call for help.

ABC – if there is no response, lay the patient flat, and work through the **ABCs** of resuscitation. The airway is patent and secure if feasible, checking for evidence of spontaneous breathing and ventilating with oxygen if not; establish that a pulse is present, and compressing the heart 100 times per minute if not, thereby maintaining adequate circulation to perfuse the vital organs. See the detailed description of cardiopulmonary resuscitation (CPR) in the next section. Only then is it necessary to establish and treat the underlying cause. The unconscious (but breathing with a pulse) patient should be nursed in the recovery position, with the airway protected.

Cardiorespiratory arrest

Suspect cardiorespiratory arrest in a collapsed patient with no spontaneous breathing and absence of a pulse (Figures 5.25 and 5.26). The initial management is as noted earlier: Alert the crash team. Management of the airway involves extending the neck and opening the mouth. If the airway is blocked, use suction to clear debris, blood and secretions. Next look for chest movement and listen for breath sounds; if absent give two rescue breaths (ones that elevate the chest wall). Feel for a carotid pulse for 10 seconds; if absent begin CPR.

CPR involves delivering 100 chest compressions per minute in tandem with 15 breaths per minute in a ratio of 15:2. This is a practical skill that needs to be practised regularly on a manikin. It is vital to realize that CPR only buys time; if a patient is in ventricular fibrillation, defibrillation is the immediate treatment and optimally needs to be delivered within 90 seconds. Asystole will require further drug treatment (adrenaline 1 mg i.v., atropine 3 mg i.v. and some others); pulseless electrical activity requires treatment of the underlying cause for any hope of recovery. All these activities, in reality, can be accomplished only by trained teams, so **get help.**

Hypoglycaemia

In diabetic patients, consider hypoglycaemia as a cause of collapse. Often the patient anticipates the onset of hypoglycaemia – feeling anxious, sweaty and irritable – and at this stage an oral glucose drink should abort the attack. Occasionally the patient's ability to detect hypoglycaemia is lost. Thus, following basic resuscitation, IM glucagon 1 mg or 50 mL of i.v. 50% dextrose should be urgently administered to any collapsed diabetic patient.

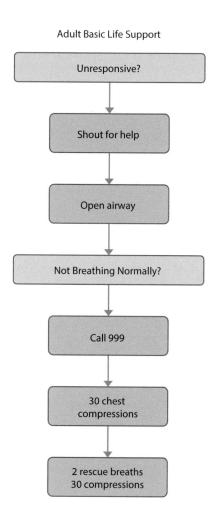

2010 Resuscitation Guidelines

Resuscitation Council (UK)

Adult Basic Life Support

Unresponsive?

Shout for help

Open airway

Not Breathing Normally?

Call 999

30 chest compressions

2 rescue breaths 30 compressions

Figure 5.25 Adult basic life support algorithm. Reproduced with the kind permission of the UK Resuscitation Council.

Addisonian crisis

As discussed, patients who take corticosteroids on a long-term basis have a suppressed adrenal response to stress and are at risk of hypotension and collapse when exposed to stress (e.g. surgery or trauma). If collapse occurs in such a patient, management is to lay the patient flat, maintain the airway and administer 100 mg of i.v. hydrocortisone, which can be repeated up to a dose of 500 mg.

Seizures

In an epileptic patient who is having a seizure, the priority is to ensure safety by maintaining the airway and preventing any unintentional self-harm. Place the patient in the recovery position (if possible) and wait for spontaneous recovery. If the fit is prolonged, rectal diazepam 5 mg or i.v. diazepam 5 to 20 mg should stop the seizure. If the fit persists, call for expert help.

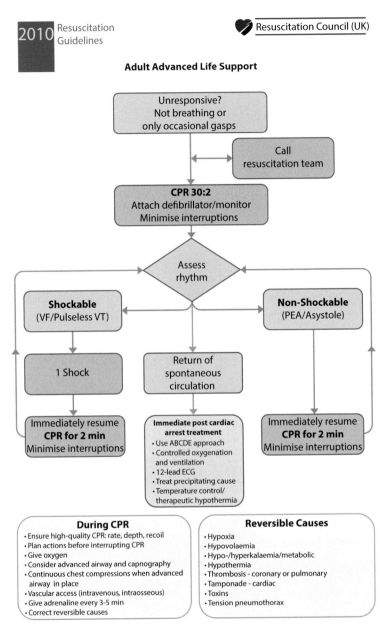

Figure 5.26 Adult advanced life support algorithm. Reproduced with the kind permission of the UK Resuscitation Council.

Chest pain

Sudden, severe central chest pain may be caused by angina or a myocardial infarction. The pain is often described as gripping, heavy or like a tight constricting band around the chest, and it may be associated with panic, sweating and breathlessness. If the patient is known to have angina, nurse upright, give oxygen and administer a sublingual glyceryl trinitrate (GTN) tablet, which should relieve pain resulting from angina. Try and obtain an ECG during the episode – it may confirm the diagnosis. If the pain is unrelieved by GTN, establish i.v. access, give 5 to 10 mg morphine with an antiemetic and telephone for help from the on-call medical senior house officer or resident medical officer.

Difficulty breathing

Acute breathlessness may occur in patients with a background of airway disease such as asthma or chronic bronchitis or unexpectedly.

If an **asthmatic patient** becomes breathless and wheezy, sit the patient upright and give nebulized salbutamol 5 mg with oxygen and 30 mg oral prednisolone. If the attack is not quickly aborted, or there are features of life-threatening asthma (the absence of breath sounds, cyanosis, bradycardia or exhaustion), **call for help,** repeat the nebulizer, check the arterial blood gases and arrange for a portable chest radiograph.

In cases of unexpected breathlessness, there are several causes:

- PE.
- Acute pulmonary oedema.
- Hyperventilation from anxiety.
- Anaphylaxis.

Regardless of the underlying cause, the management principles are the same because the basic principles of resuscitation apply. Check that the airway is patent, measure the oxygen saturation and give oxygen. Inspect and auscultate the chest for symmetrical movements and bilateral breath sounds. Listen for added sounds such as a wheeze or crackles. If the oxygen saturations are low (<94%), check arterial blood gases and ask someone to arrange an urgent portable chest radiograph.

Hyperventilation is recognized by tachypnoea and anxiety, with an otherwise normal respiratory examination. The patient may describe paraesthesia and extreme fear. Pulse oximetry shows normal oxygen saturations, but a low carbon dioxide is present on arterial blood gas sample. Carpopedal spasm can develop. Management consists of reassuring the patient in a calm environment, accompanied by having the patient rebreathe into a bag if needed.

Anaphylaxis is a hypersensitivity reaction following exposure, usually injection or ingestion, of an allergen. It is recognized by facial oedema and flushing, itching, cyanosis and wheezing, which can result in collapse resulting from hypotension. **Call for help.** Lay the patient flat, maintain the airway, give high flow oxygen and administer 0.5 mL of 1:1000 IM adrenaline, which may be repeated every 10 minutes until the patient recovers, 100 mg of i.v.

hydrocortisone, i.v. chlorpheniramine 20 mg and an infusion of i.v. crystalloid to maintain the blood pressure. Following recovery the patient must be informed of the possible allergy, and arrangement is made for confirmatory testing (Figure 5.27).

Acute pulmonary oedema is usually caused by fluid overload in elderly patients, those with preexisting cardiovascular disease or those with left ventricular impairment. It may accompany an acute myocardial infarction, which should always be considered as an underlying diagnosis. It is recognized by breathlessness, tachypnoea, cyanosis, tachycardia and fine inspiratory crackles on chest auscultation. The treatment is to sit the patient upright and give oxygen, 2 to 5 mg of morphine and 40 mg of i.v. frusemide. Check the U&Es and arterial blood gases and arrange a portable chest radiograph. Following the administration of frusemide, the urine output should be monitored to ensure an adequate diuresis – this may require catheterization.

A nonfatal PE may manifest as acute breathlessness and collapse, classically following major surgery, but often following a period of reduced mobility (e.g. long flights or bus trips). The patient may complain of chest pain that is worse on inspiration; there may or may not be evidence of DVT. Signs include tachypnoea, cyanosis, hypotension, haemoptysis, raised JVP and tachycardia. The diagnosis is initially clinical, and management consists of basic resuscitation, high flow oxygen, and i.v. heparin or an equivalent treatment dose of subcutaneous enoxaparin. A chest radiograph and ventilation-perfusion scan can then be arranged to assist in the diagnosis.

Foreign bodies in the upper aerodigestive tract – objects in the mouth and nose may be swallowed or inhaled, usually in young children. Usually the cough reflex prevents objects from lodging in the upper airway. However, this reflex may be lost, particularly if the patient is obtunded in some way.

Foreign bodies may lodge in the following sites:

- **Pharynx and oesophagus** – the pharynx is the site where teeth, dentures, blood and so forth tend to collect following trauma. Fishbones commonly wedge in the tonsils or the back of the tongue. Sharp, localized pain on swallowing is highly suggestive of this condition, and these bones can often be removed using topical anaesthesia. If not, an examination with

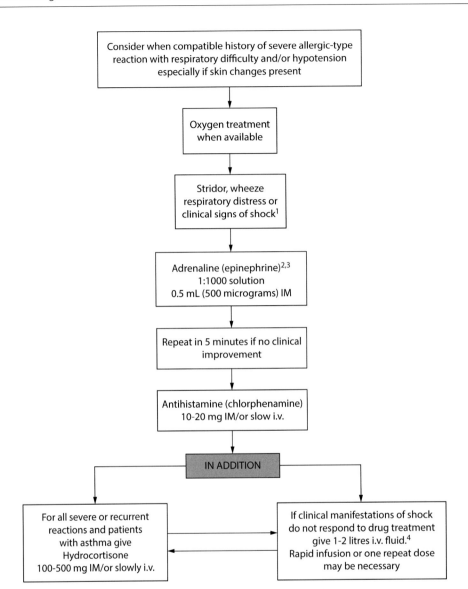

Consider when compatible history of severe allergic-type reaction with respiratory difficulty and/or hypotension especially if skin changes present

Oxygen treatment when available

Stridor, wheeze respiratory distress or clinical signs of shock[1]

Adrenaline (epinephrine)[2,3] 1:1000 solution 0.5 mL (500 micrograms) IM

Repeat in 5 minutes if no clinical improvement

Antihistamine (chlorphenamine) 10-20 mg IM/or slow i.v.

IN ADDITION

For all severe or recurrent reactions and patients with asthma give Hydrocortisone 100-500 mg IM/or slowly i.v.

If clinical manifestations of shock do not respond to drug treatment give 1-2 litres i.v. fluid.[4] Rapid infusion or one repeat dose may be necessary

1. An inhaled heta₂-agonist such as salbutamol may be used as an adjunctive measure if bronchospasm is severe and does not respond rapidly to other treatment.
2. If profound shock judged **immediately** life threatening give CPR/ALS if necessary. Consider **slow** i.v. adrenaline (epinephrine) 1:10 000 solution. This is **hazardous** and is recommended only for an experienced practitioner who can also obtain i.v. access without delay. Note the different strength of adrenaline (epinephrine) that may be required for i.v. use.
3. If adults are treated with an Epipen, the 300 micrograms will usually be sufficient. A second dose may be required. Half doses of adrenaline (epinephrine) may be safer for patients on amitriptyline, imipramine, or beta blocker.
4. A crystalloid may be safer than a cotloid.

Figure 5.27 Anaphylaxis algorithm.

the patient under anaesthesia may be necessary. In elderly patients, dry food may become stuck in the oesophagus and cause severe retrosternal discomfort (which may mimic cardiac pain) and dysphagia. This should always raise the suspicion of a stricture (possibly malignant) and further investigations should be carried out.

- **Larynx** – this can result in severe respiratory distress, and patients usually have stridor. It requires immediate attention (either the Heimlich manoeuvre in a mobile patient or a surgical airway if the patient is obtunded).
- **Tracheobronchial tree** – here foreign bodies tend to lodge in the right main bronchus. If not removed, they will lead to collapse of the associated lung. Removal using a rigid bronchoscope with the patient under general anaesthesia is necessary.

The airway is simply assessed by asking the patient 'What happened?', and any foreign bodies are looked for and are removed with a finger or with suction. In all cases, where teeth, dentures, crowns and so forth are missing, they *must* be accounted for. If they are still not found, radiographs of the chest and soft tissues of the neck must be taken. A foreign body found at either site must be removed. Remember, when looking for fishbones, radiographs are not 100% reliable because many 'bones' are in fact cartilage and will not show up.

Vomiting in the drowsy patient is a particular problem, especially after heavy drinking. Aspiration can occur if the patient is left lying on their back, which can lead to obstruction and pneumonitis. If vomiting does occur, patients need to be turned on their side. If a spinal injury is suspected (all significant injuries above the clavicle), the patient must be immobilized and turned en bloc – the 'log roll' manoeuvre (Figure 5.28).

Another aspect to consider includes pulmonary aspiration following surgery. This is an infrequent but potentially serious anaesthesia-related complication that carries a considerable mortality,

Prepare to Log Roll

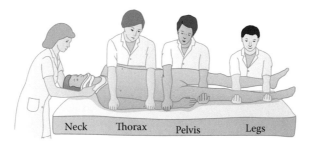

Log Roll

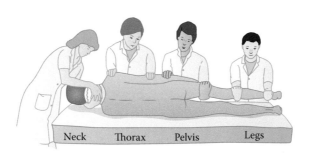

Figure 5.28 A safe log roll needs four people to move the patient and one to examine them.

especially in elderly patients. The management of aspiration includes the following:

- Position the patient head down to limit pulmonary contamination and suctioning to clear the oropharynx.
- Administer 100% oxygen.
- Apply cricoid pressure and ventilate.
- Use rapid sequence anaesthesia.
- Intubate the trachea and perform trachea suction and bronchoscopy.
- Administer bronchodilators if necessary.
- Chest radiograph is useful (but in approximately 25% no changes are noted).
- Observe after extubation for 2 hours.
- If well, discharge from recovery.

No evidence supports the use of antibiotics or steroids in these patients.

Paperwork and relationships

Paperwork

Accurate note keeping is essential both for continuity of patient care and because medical records are legal documents. It is essential to document the salient features of each ward round, review of the patient and any discussions with patients or relatives. Each entry should be legible and include the date and a note of the senior staff present. To ensure the salient points are documented, the mnemonic **SOAP** is useful:

S – Subjective (i.e. what the patient complains about).
O – Objective (i.e. the important clinical findings on examination, including any abnormalities in the observations).
A – Assessment of the problem.
P – Plan.
Finally, sign the entry and print your surname.

Relationships

Hospital practice can be daunting, and on-call work can make it especially tough. Teamwork and communication are the keys to success, and good relationships among colleagues can make life considerably easier and happier. Teamwork should bring with it a sense of camaraderie and a system of communication among colleagues to ensure potential problems can be swiftly sorted out.

Never be afraid to ask for help or feel too proud to admit to finding it difficult to cope. There should be at least one sympathetic listener in the team. The pressures imposed by unfamiliar duties, stressful clinical situations and long hours can be too much for some people. If someone in the team is showing signs of excess stress, try talking to the person about possible solutions, such as arranging teaching from the more senior colleagues, altering the timetable to give a fair division of labour, or making provision for a change of shifts. If this fails, talk in confidence about the problem to a trusted senior colleague. The formal mechanism for this should be your appraisal, although these are often too distant to be of direct help.

If it is collectively believed that aspects of the job are unacceptable or excessively demanding, form a delegation and approach senior colleagues with a plan for how things could be improved. If this fails, approach the hospital junior doctors' representative for help.

Bad news

Breaking bad news is a skill requiring sensitivity and empathy, but also practice and confidence, and it is usually the responsibility of a senior clinician. It is useful to 'sit in' with a consultant to get a feel for how, or how not, to talk to patients about difficult issues. It is likely that at some point, patients will ask junior staff questions about their diagnosis or prognosis, and with certain basic principles, it should be possible to deal with these appropriately.

- Always set aside adequate time for interviews with patients and relatives.
- Treat the patient as you would expect your closest relative or friend to be treated.
- Speak to the patient in a quiet room, away from the busy ward, and where you are unlikely to be interrupted (Figure 5.29). Leave your bleep with someone else.

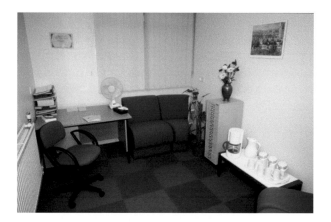

Figure 5.29 A relaxed, nonthreatening environment for breaking bad news.

- Assess how much the patient understands about the tests that have been performed and the possible diagnosis. Avoid being too brusque; instead introduce the subject gently, leading the patient to the diagnosis or result. An example is given here:

Clinician: 'I understand you had a biopsy recently, do you know what it was we were looking for?'

Patient: 'I'm not sure; they think I may have a growth.'

Clinician: 'I have the results here. You were right, there is a type of growth, but some of the cells in the sample looked abnormal.'

Patient: 'What do you mean "abnormal"?'

Clinician: 'Some of the cells were cancerous.'

Patient: 'Do you mean I have cancer?'

Clinician: 'Yes, you have a type of cancer; I'll explain what we can do to help in a minute. How do you feel about that news?'

Note: Although it seems silly to ask patients how they feel about such news, this gives them the opportunity to absorb the information and express themselves. You will always be surprised at some of the responses.

- Allow time for the information to sink in and answer questions honestly and openly; if you do not know the answer, say so, but explain that you will find someone who does, and do so.
- Patients rarely remember many of the facts of the conversation, so write down the salient points.

- Allow the patient time to digest the information. Suggest that the patient have some time alone and with the family, and that he or she write down any questions that arise. Explain that you or a senior colleague will return to discuss the treatment options and answer any questions at a definite time in the near future.

FURTHER READING

American College of Surgeons. *Advanced trauma life support course: student manual,* 6th ed. Chicago: American College of Surgeons, 2009.

This manual is available as part of the ATLS course and is updated regularly, details are available from the ATLS office RCS in England and the American College of Surgeons in the United States. Whatever your opportunities, you must go on one of these courses if you have any serious interest in working at even a fairly basic level in postgraduate oral and maxillofacial surgery.

Deitch EA. *Tools of the trade and rules of the road: a surgical guide.* Philadelphia: Lippincott Williams & Wilkins, 1997.

A slightly quirky view of an American house surgeon's life but full of gems.

Donald A, Stein M, Muthu V. *The hands-on guide for house officers,* 2nd ed. Oxford: Wiley-Blackwell, 2002.

A nice and very practical alternative to the Oxford Handbook of Clinical Medicine emphasizes practical survival at the junior medic level.

Longmore M, Wilkinson I, Baldwin A, Wallin E. *Oxford handbook of clinical medicine,* 9th ed. Oxford: Oxford University Press, 2014.

(Get the most recent, it's updated regularly.) This is the one all preregistration house officers (and medical students) use, so why don't you?

Waybright RA, Coolidge W, Johnson TJ. Treatment of clinical aspiration: a reappraisal. *Am J Health Syst Pharm* 2013;15:1291–300.

6

Exodontia and its sequelae

Contents

Aims and learning outcomes

For undergraduates:

Understanding of this chapter should enable you to:

1. Describe when it is appropriate and when it is inappropriate to remove teeth.
2. Select the appropriate instruments for removing teeth.
3. Describe and demonstrate the importance of patient positioning and self-positioning during tooth extraction.
4. Be able to describe the body movements required to remove the majority of teeth under usual circumstances.
5. List and understand the reasons for postoperative instructions after tooth extraction.

6. Identify preoperatively and deal with postoperatively common complications of tooth extraction.
7. Describe the steps involved in the transalveolar removal of retained roots.

For postgraduates:

This chapter should enable you to refresh your memory and reemphasizes the importance of this often denigrated but essential oral surgical procedure. In addition some of the hints and tips regarding transalveolar tooth removal should augment your current knowledge.

'Exodontia' refers to the extraction of teeth (sometimes referred to as the simple extraction of teeth; however, the ability to remove a tooth with forceps and elevators is an acquired skill that you will have to work at to achieve).

Patient assessment

Assessment of patients is essentially covered in Chapter 5, and controlling pain and anxiety is covered in Chapter 4. These are clearly essential prerequisites to actually removing teeth; however, this chapter concentrates on the removal and problem solving required in the process of exodontia.

The anticoagulated patient

Patients 'anticoagulated' with aspirin or most other antiplatelet drugs rarely present a problem that cannot be dealt with by simple pressure, oxidized cellulose packs or suturing (see later).

Patients taking warfarin have been a source of concern for a long time (see Chapter 5). There is, however, evidence to show that for a small number of extractions all that has to be done is:

1. Plan the extraction.
2. Check the international normalized ratio (INR), either by testing it yourself or via the patient's anticoagulation clinic.
3. If the INR is less than 4, carry on as normal but pack and stitch the socket.
4. If the INR is greater than 4, complex extractions are anticipated or the patient is a medical 'high risk', refer.

Assessment of the need for tooth removal

It is worthwhile considering the justification and need for tooth removal. This procedure may be indicated or contraindicated along two broad lines – the patient and the tooth itself.

Patients may require removal of restorable teeth because of underlying medical problems (e.g. infective endocarditis) or before radiotherapy of the jaws or face. Other patients may require a modification or support to the medical condition (e.g. supplementary oxygen). Yet other patients may be medically healthy but require anxiolysis because of an inability to cope with what you would perceive as a relatively straightforward procedure.

These situations need to be addressed individually with the background knowledge that you have already obtained in patient management, and they are best worked through by case example and repeated exposure to patients.

Clinical and radiographic assessment of individual teeth

Clinical assessment is often all that is required for the extraction of a non–broken down, but carious or periodontally involved tooth. A patient who has adequate mouth opening with a visible crown and has no coexisting medical problems presents little problem. Patients without these factors become increasingly more difficult to manage. Teeth that are significantly displaced from the arch, or are lingually inclined, may be impossible to remove with conventional forceps, and the application of brute force and ignorance will not help in this situation (Figures 6.1 and 6.2).

Bone density

Bone density increases and elasticity decreases with increasing age, and teeth become increasingly brittle with increasing age. This can result in the sensation of removing a milk bottle embedded in concrete in some older patients (Figure 6.3).

Extensive restorations or abrasion cavities, particularly associated with root fillings or extensive caries, make teeth more likely to shatter on application of forceps (Figure 6.4).

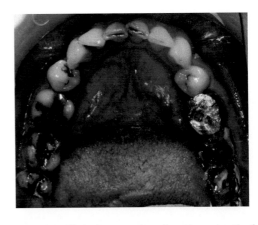

Figure 6.1 Clinical example of carious tooth for extraction.

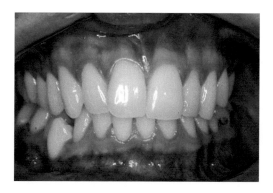

Figure 6.2 Clinical example of a displaced lower premolar.

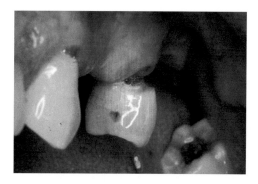

Figure 6.4 An example of abrasion cavities.

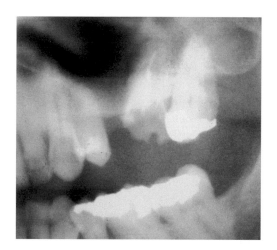

Figure 6.3 Radiograph of a root filled upper molar with sclerotic bone, likely to be a difficult extraction.

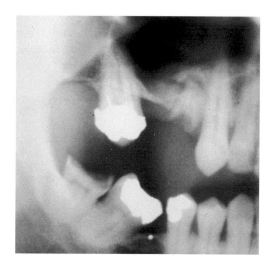

Figure 6.5 Radiograph showing several teeth and roots – which are the difficult ones?

In instances where you have doubts about your treatment plan or some of the foregoing features apply (e.g. extensive periapical infection, heavily restored or root-filled teeth, single standing upper molar teeth), or if the patient volunteers previous difficulties with extractions, it is worthwhile taking a radiograph. For single teeth, often all that is required is a periapical radiograph; for multiple teeth, a dental panoramic tomogram is better (Figures 6.5 and 6.6).

Once you have satisfied yourself that the tooth can be removed under whichever form of anaesthesia is deemed appropriate and you have the relevant investigations to hand, it is time to remove the tooth.

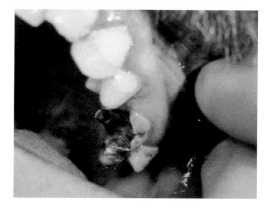

Figure 6.6 Beware the grossly broken down upper molar.

Elevators

These instruments are discussed in Chapter 3. Elevators are instruments that are designed to wedge a lever between tooth and tooth or between tooth and bone to mobilize the tooth. They may be used for removing roots or third molars in isolation, or they may be used in standing teeth by introducing the elevator between the bone of the socket and the root of the tooth or into a point of application created in the root of the tooth.

Three groups of elevators are commonly used in the United Kingdom: Warwick-James right, left and straight; Coupland's 1, 2 and 3; and Cryer's right and left (Figure 6.7). In Germany a universal elevator called Bein, a lower third molar elevator (Barry) and an upper third molar elevator (Flohr) are used. Periotomes are increasing in popularity.

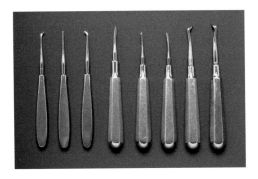

Figure 6.7 Range of elevators – from left, Warwick-James (three), Coupland's (three), Cryer's (two).

Elevators are used as rotational levers around their long axis. They should not be used as first class levers along their length. If you are using another tooth as a fulcrum, it has to be accepted that the other tooth will move, and therefore this technique is appropriate only if the tooth against which it is being used as a fulcrum is also being removed. In all other cases, the bone of the socket should be used as the fulcrum. Elevators need to be handled, and it would be useful to obtain some elevators and hold them in your hand to identify the manner in which you can produce a finger rest to stop the elevator from slipping when in use and to learn to hold it appropriately (Figure 6.8).

Use of elevators

From the point of view of straightforward tooth removal, elevators are principally used when removing multiple teeth, and the adjacent teeth can be used as the elevator's fulcrum to loosen and mobilize the teeth before extracting them with forceps. Heavily broken down teeth, particularly those that are periodontally involved, may be removed using elevators only. A bifurcation can be engaged by the point of an angled elevator such as Cryer's or Warwick-James. On occasion very broken down multirooted teeth can be split by placing a straight elevator such as Coupland's between the bifurcation, separating the roots this way and

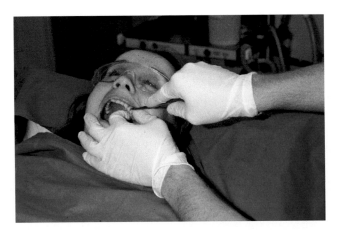

Figure 6.8 The way to use an elevator appropriately.

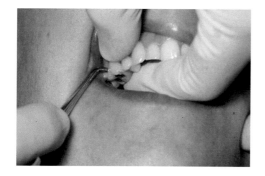

Figure 6.9 Warwick-James elevator in use.

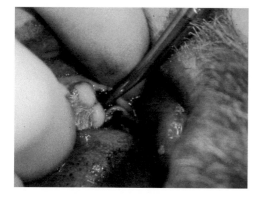

Figure 6.10 Coupland's elevator in use.

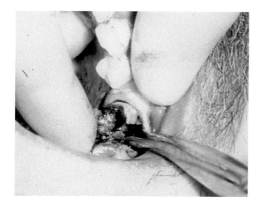

Figure 6.11 Cryer's elevator in use.

then elevating the roots using the opposite root as a fulcrum. An angled elevator such as Cryer's can then be placed into the now empty socket of the first root and used to elevate the second root (Figures 6.9, 6.10 and 6.11).

The other main indication for the use of elevators is in elevating unerupted teeth or third molar teeth that are either partially erupted or unerupted. These are principal areas in which forceps are either less useful or potentially dangerous.

Dental extraction forceps

Upper extraction forceps are designed as straight-handled, straight-beaked forceps with a variety of designs on the beak. These may be slightly off-set as in bayonet forceps or designed to engage bifurcations of multirooted teeth (Figure 6.12).

Lower extraction forceps are designed with the beaks at right angles to the handle. The controlled force used to extract teeth is directed down along the root of the tooth (Figure 6.13).

The angulation and design of dental extraction forceps carry with it an implication that you and your patient must be appropriately sited to make

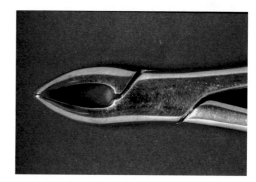

Figure 6.12 Upper extraction forceps.

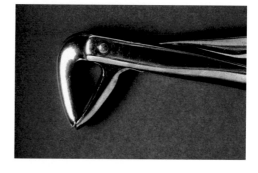

Figure 6.13 Lower extractions forceps.

use of this instrument. There is a large amount of body positioning technique involved in dental extractions, and it most certainly is not simple application of brute force. In some respects it is akin to the martial art of Aikido, in that positioning and precise application of force are crucial.

General principles of forceps

Essentially all extraction forceps consist of two blades and a set of handles attached to a hinge. The blades fit in a concave fashion around the tooth root. The tips of the blades are sharp, to divide periodontal ligaments and wedge into the socket in an attempt to dilate the socket as they engage the root of the tooth so that both the dilating action and the force needed to mobilize the root before lifting it out can be generated (Figure 6.14).

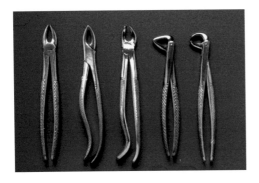

Figure 6.14 Range of extraction forceps.

Removal of upper teeth

After appropriate assessment and provision of local analgesia, the patient is positioned semisupine with the chair elevated so that the patient's face is at the approximate level of the surgeon's elbow (Figure 6.15).

Upper extraction forceps come in universal, premolar and molar patterns.

The forceps are positioned as shown (Figure 6.16).

Force is then generated using a straight arm. The blade of the forceps is driven through the periodontal membrane into the socket to dilate the socket and firmly engage the root. Upper anterior teeth can then be removed by a rotating motion that disrupts the periodontal membrane, enlarges the socket and then allows the tooth to be lifted from the socket while the rotating motion is continued.

Upper premolar teeth have a more oblong pattern to the root and can seldom be rotated, particularly the often two-rooted first premolar. In this instance the driving force is the same, but the motion to remove the tooth is more of a buccal 'bend', which can be repeated to 'wiggle' the tooth before either 'bending' it buccally out or 'pulling' it straight down.

Upper molar teeth are usually removed using molar forceps. These are designed as left and right because the buccal beak of the forceps is pointed to fit into the bifurcation or trifurcation of the molar teeth. Maxillary molar teeth are removed by applying a vertical force up along the roots into the socket, in this instance manipulating the

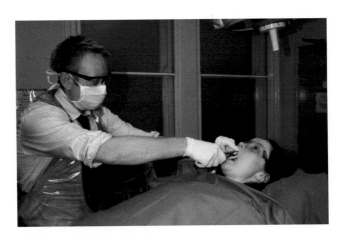

Figure 6.15 Positioning of patient for extraction of upper teeth.

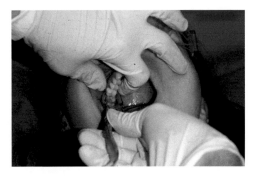

Figure 6.16 Positioning of upper extraction forceps on upper tooth.

tooth buccally. Actual buccal palatal movement with the final buccal movement accompanied by downward force will usually deliver maxillary molars, but it is not uncommon for the buccal roots to fracture or indeed for the bone on the buccal plate, which is very thin, to fracture with the removal of the tooth.

Removal of mandibular teeth

Mandibular teeth are removed using lower extraction forceps. Again these may be straight bladed for incisors, canines and premolars and modified to engage the bifurcation with molars. Removing mandibular teeth on the patient's right, the patient is in a sitting position with the surgeon standing behind the patient using lower extraction forceps widely used in the United Kingdom and continental Europe (Figure 6.17).

For lower left teeth the patient is again in a sitting position, and the surgeon in this case is standing in front of the patient (Figure 6.18).

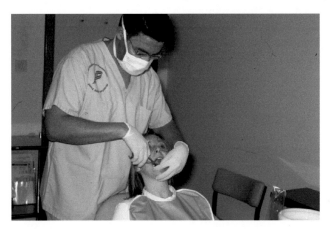

Figure 6.17 Positioning of patient for extraction of lower teeth on right.

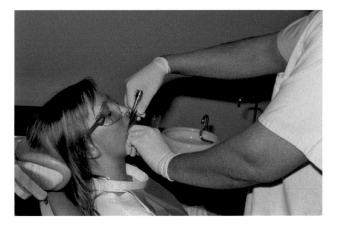

Figure 6.18 Positioning of patient for extraction of lower teeth on left.

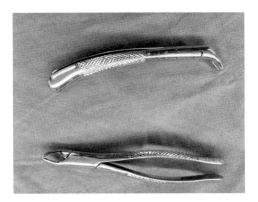

Figure 6.19 US adult extraction forceps.

Angled forceps designed to have blades that are angled to come straight out of the mouth (Figure 6.19), sometimes used in North America, require a different extraction technique. The operator is positioned in front of the patient on the operator's dominant side to perform the extractions. The movements used to deliver the tooth are as described in the following subsections.

Mandibular incisors

The mandibular incisors have roots that are not sufficiently conical to allow rotatory movement. These teeth are delivered by buccolingual force, again by 'wiggling' the tooth buccolingually until it is mobilized and then delivering the tooth with either a small rotatory and significant amount of buccal force or a purely buccal force.

Mandibular canines

Mandibular canines are delivered using a similar technique, but both maxillary and mandibular canines are often long rooted and frequently ankylosed teeth that require considerably more force to deliver than incisors.

Mandibular premolars

These teeth have conical roots and can be delivered by rotation.

Mandibular molars

Again as with maxillary molars these multirooted teeth have to be displaced by force acting buccally, and the teeth are mobilized buccolingually. However, generating a figure-of-eight motion can mobilize the roots of these teeth and allow considerable mobility before the teeth are eventually delivered with a buccal movement.

Attempting forceps extractions of lower third molars that have partially erupted or are awkwardly angled is potentially dangerous because of the risk of generating fracture-inducing forces through the angle of the mandible.

Removal of deciduous teeth

All the information with regard to body and patient positioning described for adult teeth applies to deciduous extraction. There are, however, some small but specific differences.

Deciduous extraction forceps

These forceps are essentially miniature versions of adult extraction forceps. The molar forceps, particularly lower molar forceps, have a slightly more rounded appearance that allows them to circumvent the more bulbous aspect of the crowns of deciduous teeth and engage the root. It is possible to remove deciduous teeth with adult extraction forceps, but the main risk in doing so is that the side of the forceps will be difficult to use in the smaller child's mouth, and you have a higher risk of engaging an underlying permanent tooth and damaging it while removing the deciduous tooth. Therefore, deciduous extraction forceps should be used (Figure 6.20).

Anatomy and physiology of deciduous teeth

The important point here is that most deciduous teeth have an underlying successor that must not be damaged in the process of removing the deciduous tooth. This is particularly a risk in removing deciduous molars when the underlying premolar may lie between the very thin, fragile roots of the deciduous molar. The way to avoid this is to try

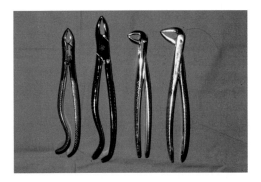

Figure 6.20 Comparison of adult (left) and deciduous (right) extraction forceps.

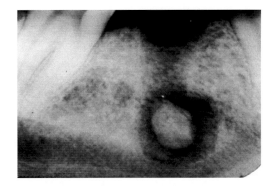

Figure 6.21 Root displaced into an infected cystic apical cavity.

to engage the roots of the deciduous tooth as you remove it. In addition these very thin roots are quite liable to break, and it is not at all uncommon to fracture the roots of deciduous teeth. These roots can be removed by the use of a small curved elevator in much the same way as the roots of adult teeth can be removed. Once again you have to remember you are working in a socket that probably contains a permanent successor that must not be damaged.

Submerged deciduous teeth

See Chapter 9. These teeth usually require the transalveolar approach if they are being removed.

Complications of extractions

Failure to obtain adequate anaesthesia is described in Chapter 4. The fracture of a tooth is the most common complication. If a segment of root larger than approximately 3 mm is left in place, particularly if the reason for removing the tooth was the presence of infection, then this should be removed by a transalveolar procedure (Figure 6.21). Small fragments (<3 mm) of a tooth removed for reasons other than established infection can often reasonably be left *in situ*.

Transalveolar removal of teeth and retained roots

Once you have removed a few teeth, there will be no mistaking the sickening crack that is heard when you break a tooth root. This is no real cause

for shame and happens to everyone. The cause for shame would be either ignoring the fact or doing nothing about it. If there is a significant root fragment that exceeds more than the apical third or is being removed for reasons of infection, either locally or because the patient is at serious risk from a distant infection or the retained apex has been significantly mobilized within the socket, then it has to be removed. Tiny, otherwise healthy fragments can quite reasonably be left *in situ*. If the tooth is going to be removed, the sensible thing to do is to advise the patient what has happened, give a little more local anaesthetic and prepare your equipment for a transalveolar surgical approach while the additional anaesthesia is working and the patient is settling down.

Transalveolar technique

Having carried out the previous procedure, it is often worthwhile making a single attempt to elevate a fractured or retained root by using an elevator as discussed before. If Coupland's elevator can be driven along the socket between the roots and the bone, it is sometimes possible to displace the root coronally, or it may be possible to place an angled elevator (e.g. Cryer's or Warwick-James) into an empty root socket and engage a retained root to lift it up and out.

It is however, psychologically important both for you and the patient to define a limited amount of time during which you are going to attempt to do this. If the root does not come up immediately, accept that you are going to have to adopt a transalveolar procedure. This is not a disaster. It is simply a progression in the overall procedure of removing the tooth. By this time the additional local analgesia will have worked and you can get on with the job in hand.

Transalveolar approach – raising the flap

For transalveolar surgery the flap to be elevated is a full-thickness mucoperiosteal flap. This means that the bone is directly visualized and the plane of dissection of the flap is between the bone and the periosteum. This is a very safe area to be working in, gives excellent visualization and access to retained roots with relatively minimal bleeding. Only a small number of vital structures will lie in this plane; tiny vessels and the mental nerve emerge just below the apices of the first and second mandibular premolars. This is why relieving incisions are not made in this region. In the palate the main problem is the course of the greater palatine artery; for this reason, vertical relieving incisions are not made in the palate. When a flap is raised without vertical relieving incisions, it is known as an envelope flap.

For exposure to palatal roots, an envelope flap is always raised, and this runs from the distal aspect of the upper molar tooth behind the retained root to the canine on the contralateral side if length is required to gain access.

In the region of the mandibular first molar and second premolar where a relieving incision cannot be made, the envelope flap extends at least two teeth on either side of the retained root. In all other instances a vertical relieving incision can be made. If a relieving incision is to be made, it is only necessary to extend the incision one tooth width behind and one tooth width in front of the retained root in question because mobilization of the flap is obtained by the vertical relieving incision, which is designed immediately before or after the interdental papilla so that this is not split in two.

The incision is carried out in the gingival crevice and down to bone. If you are making a vertical relieving incision, it continues down on bone into the reflection of the alveolar mucosa. This always blunts the scalpel blade, and the blade should be discarded after a full-thickness flap has been raised. The second relieving incision may be

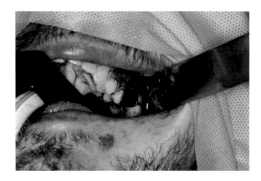

Figure 6.22 The transalveolar approach, raising a mucoperiosteal flap.

made behind the area of the retained root. This is seldom required because access is usually adequate with a single anterior relieving incision or the long envelope flap. The flap is elevated in a subperiosteal plane (Figure 6.22). This is most easily identified in the area of the loose alveolar mucosa by placing an elevator (e.g. as Howarth's) into the incision and down onto bone; a small scraping movement will expose bone, and it is directly onto the bone that you want to work with your instruments. The alveolar mucosa area is more easily peeled off, and it is worthwhile doing this and then working up to the more densely bound down attached gingiva to avoid tearing the flap. This can be achieved in a few seconds. A retractor can then be placed to hold the flap back, and this should give you a good view of the alveolar bone, the area that contains the retained root and the tooth in front and behind the area of interest. It is essential when learning how to make these incisions that you first watch someone doing this and then are taken through it step by step because simply reading this information will not teach you a safe transalveolar approach.

The next thing stopping you from removing a retained root is the enveloping bone. In most cases this is buccal bone, which is removed with a surgical burr (Figure 6.23). A number 8 tungsten carbide burr is usually used for this purpose. The burr should be cooled with saline irrigant, which not only cools the burr but also prevents bone overheating and washes away bone debris.

The bone to be removed is that lying buccal to the retained root to provide a point of application for an elevator. You start coronally and remove 2 or 3 millimetres of buccal bone to expose the root (Figure 6.24). Once the root is

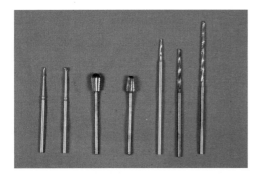

Figure 6.23 A range of burrs for bone removal.

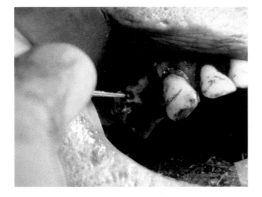

Figure 6.24 Bone removal for retained roots.

visualized it may be possible to drill into the root to create a point of application or identify a point of application, in which case an elevator is placed and the root is elevated from the socket. If it is a two-rooted tooth that is retained, again remove some coronal bone and then change to the fissure burr and divide the roots so that an elevator can be placed between the two roots and controlled force used, by having one retained root as a fulcrum to elevate the other and then using an angled elevator in the then empty socket to create a point of application with the burr if need be in the other root to elevate it.

What is very important is not to cut into the tooth root as you drill away the coronal bone. This leads to a loss of root anatomy and makes it quite difficult to distinguish the root from the bone (although usually root is more yellow than the bone and bone will bleed, even if only slightly). If it becomes impossible to remove the root despite removing several millimetres of coronal bone, it is sometimes worthwhile placing a fissure burr

vertically inside the socket to cut the bone away around the root to mobilize it. There is an advantage in preserving alveolar bone height because simply completely destroying the buccal cortex will result in significant bone resorption in this area with inevitable problems for prosthesis (see Chapter 15). Following the removal of the roots, any sharp spicules of bone should be smoothed, although excessive reduction of alveolar bone should be avoided because again this will reduce bone height unnecessarily early in the patient's life. Remember to wash away any bone dust; collection of bone dust underneath the mucoperiosteal flap is probably one of the most important causes of persistent, inexplicable discomfort following transalveolar surgery. The flap is then repositioned and sutured with interrupted sutures across the socket, with a single suture holding the relieving incision. Resorbable synthetic sutures such as polyglactide are the most appropriate for this purpose. Suture materials such as catgut have been withdrawn from use in most countries (although not the United States), and nonresorbable sutures (e.g. black silk), although very easy to use, necessitate further appointments for removal of sutures and frequently become extremely dirty in the mouth.

Suturing is a skill best learnt by practice. You should use a needle holder with a suture with a reverse cutting or cutting needle if at all possible, carrying a 3-0 or 4-0 resorbable synthetic suture.

The suture should be passed through the free edge of the flap and then through the fixed site to which it is being sutured (Figure 6.25). The flap is then mobilized to its resting position, and the position is controlled by tightening of the first knot of the suture. This is achieved by passing the thread

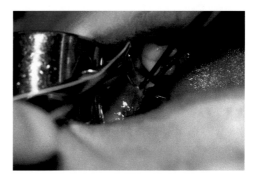

Figure 6.25 Suture the edge of the free tissue to fixed.

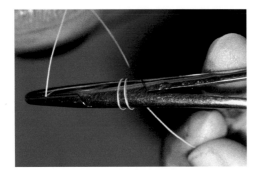

Figure 6.26 Loop the suture material twice around the needle holders to create the first part of the knot.

twice around the needle holder, grasping the free end and pulling it through (Figure 6.26). This creates a first knot that has some resistance to loosening and allows you to position the flap. This is then tightened, and the procedure is reversed with a single throw in the opposite direction to lock it; then this is repeated to ensure that the lock is secure.

Patients who have had transalveolar surgery are at a higher risk of wound infection and most certainly have postoperative discomfort. All such patients should be provided with adequate analgesia such as ibuprofen 400 to 600 mg three times a day with or without paracetamol 100 mg four times daily with or without codeine (8 to 30 mg depending on anticipated degree of pain) four times daily, and an antibiotic such as amoxycillin 250 mg three times daily or metronidazole 400 mg three times daily.

Patients taking antiresorptive medication (bisphosphonates, denusomab) should have an attempted watertight mucosal closure with as little periosteal disturbance as possible.

Postoperative instructions

The following advice should be given to patients who have had operations on their mouths.

Following your operation you can expect to have the following difficulties:

1. Some swelling of the face.
2. Stiffness of the jaws, particularly when lower wisdom teeth have been removed.
3. Slight oozing of blood. This may last for 12 hours or longer.
4. Pain.

If you have had a general anaesthetic (that is to say you have been put to sleep) you should:

1. On arriving home, go to bed for the remainder of the day.
2. You must NOT drive a car or operate machinery for at least 24 hours.
3. You must NOT consume alcohol in any form for at least 24 hours.
4. You must be supervised by a responsible adult for 24 hours.

The day after your general anaesthetic you may experience some stiffness of the limbs and feel 'under the weather'. This is common following general anaesthesia and usually goes away in 1 or 2 days. You may have a dry or sore throat, which will be eased by frequent drinks.

After care – local anaesthetic and general anaesthetic

It is important to keep your mouth clean. We recommend gentle mouth washing with salt and warm water. After meals, any remaining teeth should be carefully brushed. There is no limitation on eating or drinking.

You may have stitches in your mouth and will be instructed when you leave hospital about whether these stitches will dissolve or need removal later.

Complications and how to deal with them

- **Bleeding** – if the bleeding is from one small area or tooth socket, take a clean handkerchief, knot one corner and firmly apply it to the bleeding area. Do NOT keep rinsing out your mouth because this will make the bleeding worse. Any blood accumulating in the mouth should be gently spat out.
- **Pain** – it is normal to have pain after oral surgery that will be controlled by simple pain-killing tablets taken on demand. If pain becomes more severe 3 or 4 days after operation, you may be developing an infection and you should seek advice.

- **Swelling** – this will normally settle after 3 days, but if it is getting worse after 3 days you should seek advice.
- **Bruising** – this can vary with the individual and gradually goes away.

What to do when postoperative instructions "have not helped"

Patients do develop complications following both straightforward extractions and transalveolar surgery. The important thing for you is to recognize when these are genuine complications or simply the expected sequelae of the procedure. First it helps if you ask yourself *'Is the problem real?'* You can improve things by asking patients to describe the pain that they may have. The classical pain of a dry socket is that they had toothache before the tooth was removed, and the toothache has not gone away at any point and in fact is now worse. This is a typical *complaint* from somebody with a dry socket, and this can be an extremely painful condition in which the blood clot has broken down and they have superficial inflammation of the bone of the socket.

Patients may describe localized pain made worse when they bite their teeth together or an abnormality in their bite. This is a classical description of a fracture, which is a very rare occurrence but can happen following tooth removal.

They may describe a tense swelling that has become increasingly painful, the kind of pain experienced with an infected haematoma; or it may be the most terrible pain they have ever experienced and that goes all over their head and down their arms and over their body and is stopping them sleeping at night, and the family pet has left as a result. This is a fairly typical blunderbuss approach to the description of pain seen in patients who are grossly exaggerating their symptoms for a variety of different reasons. This kind of symptomatology is not an emergency.

In addition you should ask patients to describe any bleeding they may be experiencing. If they describe chunks of blood clot rather like liver coming out of their mouth, this is almost certainly genuine and is describing persisting bleeding from the socket that needs immediate attention.

Alternatively, patients may describe fresh red blood coming from their mouth. This is unlikely, and rare, but it can occur if a small vessel has been cut in a transalveolar procedure. Again this needs to be seen immediately.

Patients could also describe blood on their pillow, or blood that they keep on spitting out. Often this is simply blood-stained saliva, and the patient has not paid attention to the postoperative advice that had already warned them about this.

It is also helpful to ask patients to describe swelling. If they have had rapid onset of swelling that is hard, then this is usually a haematoma, and you will need to see these patients immediately. If it was of delayed onset, but is hard and painful, then this is often a collection of pus, which can be very painful and certainly will need to be seen immediately. Rapid onset of soft swelling is usually oedema and does not mandate immediate attention.

After you have had a description of their problems, and decided whether or not there is a real problem, check that the patients have followed the postoperative instructions. If they have not followed the postoperative instructions, they should do so and then recontact you after half an hour to see whether this has solved the problem.

If patients have followed postoperative instructions and the problem from the description of symptoms appears to be real, then see them immediately. The main genuine problems centre around haemorrhage, infection, and pain, and these may be interrelated. The common conditions are as follows:

Dry socket

This condition has a number of different names, and it occurs in approximately 3% of routine extractions and in up to 20% of surgical extractions (Figure 6.27 and 6.28). The pain is localized to the site of extraction and is often throbbing and very severe. It will often keep the patient awake at night, and the classical description is of a toothache that never went away when the tooth was removed. Some dry sockets may start after the tooth is removed, and the pain does not commence until the clot has completely broken down and established bony inflammation has started. Although some patients benefit from the use of nonsteroidal anti-inflammatory drugs (NSAIDs) such as ibuprofen, the pain can often be so severe that these analgesics do not really help.

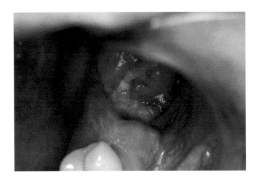

Figure 6.27 'Dry socket' – a painful osteitis of the tooth socket.

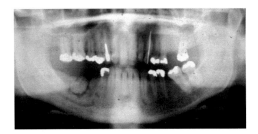

Figure 6.28 At the extreme end of the 'dry socket' spectrum sequestration can occur.

Examination of the socket shows either a yellow sloughy clot or a completely denuded socket of exposed bone. The surrounding gingivae are often erythematous, and the entire area is very tender. There is often associated halitosis, and the role of anaerobic bacteria in the infective component of dry socket has been well described.

Established localized alveolar osteitis such as this is best treated by local means. If the patient can tolerate the application of a local anaesthetic, then cleaning out the socket and dressing it with either commercially available resorbable antiseptic or an analgesic pack (Alvogyl) will often be all that is needed. If this approach has already been tried and is ineffective, and particularly if a number of other treatments have been tried, including analgesics, then applying a local anaesthetic, cleaning out the socket and placing a pack made up of cotton wool, a small amount of zinc oxide powder and eugenol will provide complete pain relief. This pack will have to be removed and sometimes has to be replaced, but it is almost unique in providing complete pain relief in patients with really intractable dry socket pain.

If the patient is not prepared to tolerate a local anaesthetic, then provision of antibiotics (particularly an anaerobicidal drug such as metronidazole) and of systemic analgesics (NSAID with or without codeine/paracetamol) with an antiseptic mouthwash is just about all that can be achieved.

The aetiology of dry socket has been subject to a number of studies. It is generally considered to be more common in the following patients: women taking oral contraceptives; smokers; patients who are more than 40 years old and are having molar teeth, particularly lower molar teeth, removed using local anaesthesia. Curiously dry socket has a diurnal variation, with a higher spring and autumn prevalence.

It is most likely a condition that is instigated by a susceptible patient whose blood clot undergoes a local fibrinolysis possibly because of an opportunistic infection with anaerobic bacteria, although the causative rather than associative role of bacteria has not been conclusively established.

It is well worth noting that patients who advise you that they have postoperative problems with dry socket are almost certainly correct, and some people do seem to be much more prone to this condition than others.

Postextraction haemorrhage

Once the tooth is removed, bleeding should stop after approximately 10 minutes. Bleeding that occurs after this time or continues beyond it is usually the result of small vessels bleeding from mucosal tear or, very occasionally, significant bleeding from the bone of the socket.

Reactive haemorrhage

Reactive haemorrhage following resolution of the vasoconstrictor in local anaesthesia is sometimes seen. This is often caused by small tears in the mucosa that allow little capillaries previously in spasm to open up.

Secondary haemorrhage caused by secondary infection of the clot is comparatively rare and occurs after a number of days.

Bleeding from the socket

Bleeding from the socket can be dealt with first by pressure, and patients are always advised to do this in their postoperative advice sheet. If this does not work, you need to see the patient, remove any established clot and identify the source of bleeding. If the bleeding is coming from the socket, the socket itself will need to be packed in some way to apply direct pressure to the bleeding site. This can be done with ribbon gauze dipped in antiseptic such as bismuth iodoform paraffin paste or Whitehead's varnish, which will provide a tamponade effect within the socket and stop the bleeding, but it does need to be removed and will mean that the socket will heal very slowly. Oxidized cellulose agents can be placed in the socket; this approach is designed to provide scaffolding for normal clotting, rather than creating an actual tamponade effect within the socket, and many low-grade bleeding sockets will respond to this.

If the bleeding is from the gingival margins or mucosal tears, then suturing the socket will be effective. Almost any form of suture – simple interrupted, figure of eight or mattress sutures – will be effective in swaging the mucosa to the bone and effectively strangling minor capillary bleeding and preventing further haemorrhage.

Patients who have been bleeding for hours, particularly if they attend with a large number of relatives, should be moved to an area where you can work with them in peace. Always wear protective clothing because these patients will often have swallowed a fair amount of blood and are likely to vomit on you as blood is an extreme irritant to the stomach. You need to have some decent light and suction. Remove the clot, clean out the socket and use a combination of oxidized cellulose within the socket and suturing and pressure. If patients continue to ooze beyond, get them to the hospital and keep a pressure pack, in addition to the other measures, on overnight. Patients can then be provided with antiemetics and, if need be, intravenous fluid, which will make them feel considerably better.

This combination will always prove to be effective unless the patient has a significant bleeding diathesis. This may be either iatrogenic, caused by anticoagulants such as warfarin, or undiagnosed, such as haemophilia. Patients who have had

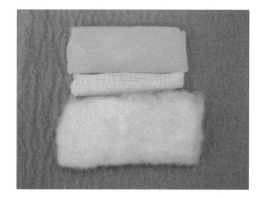

Figure 6.29 Woven and fibrillar oxidized cellulose and bone wax, examples of the aids to haemostasis.

palatal flaps may bleed from perforating vessels from bone. This is particularly likely around the incisive foramen and papillae. This bleeding can be effectively controlled by a material known as bone wax, which is massaged into the bleeding site. This is a very effective way of stopping bleeding from bone. Unfortunately it tends to form a small granuloma in the long term at this site because it is not resorbable. It should therefore be used in the smallest possible quantity (Figure 6.29).

Very rarely, significant vessels such as the palatine artery may be cut. This should be controlled by conventional methods such as diathermy or ligation. For other information regarding the management of patients who have either iatrogenic or congenital bleeding diatheses, see Chapter 5.

Fractures

The most likely fracture to occur is fracture of the maxillary tuberosity or buccal plate of the jaws (Figure 6.30). Most often this is seen at the time of extraction, and nothing more than dissecting the piece of bone free and closing the mucosa are needed. If a tooth has been removed and fracture of the buccal plate or the alveolus has not been noted, then this may sequester and become loose, painful or infected. The sequestrum will need to be removed.

Fracture of the mandible or maxilla following tooth removal is comparatively rare but can occur in the third molar region if excessive force

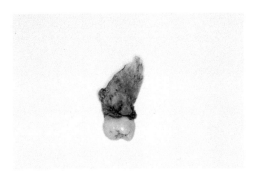

Figure 6.30 A fractured tuberosity with upper molar.

is used, particularly in patients who have had forceps extraction of lower third molars. It is difficult to justify carrying out such a procedure because of the known risks of fracture. In this instance patients may present with malocclusion, pain on biting or persisting infection and pain in the region of the extraction. Fractures of the mandible are managed as described in Chapter 16.

FURTHER READING

Moore U. *Principles of oral and maxillofacial surgery,* 3rd ed. Oxford: Blackwell Science, 2010.
An update of an old established basic text mainly concerned with traditional oral surgery.

Pedlar J, Frame JW. *Oral and maxillofacial surgery: an objective based textbook,* 2nd ed. Edinburgh: Churchill Livingstone, 2009.
This is a nicely written and well thought out introductory text with a good section on exodontia and transalveolar surgery.
Specific literature includes the following:
Bajkin BV, Bajkin IA, Petrovic BB. The effects of combined oral anticoagulant-aspirin therapy in patients undergoing tooth extractions: a prospective study. *J Am Dent Assoc* 2012;143:771–6.
Lillis T, Ziakas A, Koskinas K, Tsirlis A, Giannoglou G. Safety of dental extractions during uninterrupted single or dual antiplatelet treatment. *Am J Cardiol* 2011;108:964–7.
Morimoto Y, Niwa H, Minematsu K. Risk factors affecting postoperative hemorrhage after tooth extraction in patients receiving oral antithrombotic therapy. *J Oral Maxillofac Surg* 2011;69:1550–6.
Morimoto Y, Niwa H, Minematsu K. Hemostatic management of tooth extractions in patients on oral antithrombotic therapy. *J Oral Maxillofac Surg* 2008;66:51–7.
Powless RA, Omar HR, Mangar D, Camporesi EM. Management of antithrombotic therapy before full-mouth extraction. *J Calif Dent Assoc* 2013;41:417–20.

7

Surgical endodontics

Contents

Aims

For undergraduates and postgraduates:

- To understand the rationale of surgical endodontics.
- To understand the various procedures of surgical endodontic treatment.
- To appreciate the importance of conventional root canal therapy (RCT).

Learning outcomes

- To describe the indications and contraindications for surgical endodontics.
- To be able to outline surgical endodontic procedures.
- To be able to describe the stages of endodontic surgery and give guidelines on best current practice.

Surgical endodontics

Surgical endodontics may be divided into the following categories:

- Incision and drainage.
- Periradicular surgery.
- Corrective surgery.
- Extraction and reimplantation.

Indications and contraindications

The consensus report of the European Society of Endodontology suggests that endodontic surgery is indicated when:

- A canal is obstructed (e.g. with a separated instrument), and there are associated symptoms.
- Extruded material is present with clinical symptoms (e.g. pain) that continue over a significant time period (at least 1 week).

- Conventional RCT has failed and retreatment is inappropriate.
- Perforation of the root or the floor of the pulp chamber has occurred, with radiological findings or clinical symptoms, and where repair from within the pulp cavity is not possible.

In almost all situations, conventional RCT should be attempted first, and after a sufficient time period the tooth should be reassessed for further treatment (Figures 7.1 and 7.2). If the nonsurgical RCT has been performed to the highest practicable standard but symptoms persist, then surgical endodontic therapy may be appropriate. If, however, there have been procedural errors or there are technical deficiencies in the RCT, then conventional retreatment, if practical, is indicated before considering surgery. In some situations it is impossible to revise the existing root filling, particularly when some of the older pastes have been used, even though ideally one would wish to do so. In these circumstances endodontic surgery is the only viable option to extraction if the patient is symptomatic, but the patient should be fully informed of the lower success rate.

Where a tooth has been restored with a post crown, the principles outlined earlier still apply,

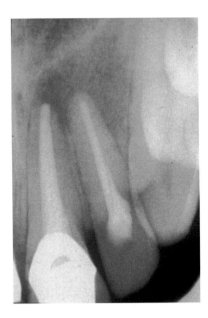

Figure 7.2 Lesion almost completely healed 6 months later with conventional endodontics. Periradicular surgery was not indicated.

and attempts should usually be made at dismantling the post crown and performing conventional retreatment. Occasionally, however, removal of a post may carry a significant risk of root fracture, and in such cases it may be preferable to leave the post *in situ* and carry out surgical endodontic therapy (Figures 7.3 and 7.4).

Contraindications to surgical endodontic treatment include:

- Anatomical factors such as an inaccessible root end.
- A tooth with a hopeless prognosis (e.g. advanced loss of periodontal support) that cannot be made functional or does not contribute to aesthetics.
- A patient who does not provide informed consent to undergo the procedure.
- A patient with a compromised medical history, such as uncontrolled systemic disease (e.g. diabetes, haematological disorders) (see Chapter 5).

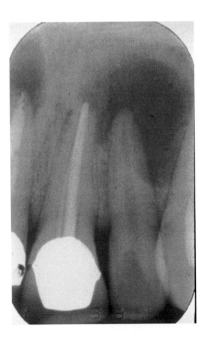

Figure 7.1 Large periapical radiolucency associated with UL2.

Success rates

For nonsurgical endodontic treatment, success rates of 86% to 96% have been reported,

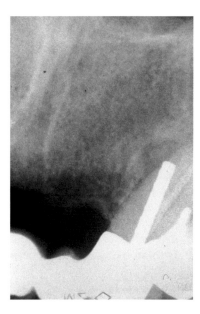

Figure 7.3 Lateral perforation of UL3 by a post. The canine is a bridge abutment, and dismantling it is not in the patient's best interest.

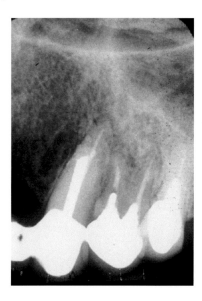

Figure 7.4 Appearance 3 months after perforation repair with mineral trioxide aggregate. It was decided to leave the post *in situ* and surgically repair the perforation because of the significant potential for root damage during post removal attempts.

and for retreatment, reported success rates are 60% to 98%. Clinical success following surgical endodontic therapy has been reported to vary between 58% and 96%. The wide range of reported success rates may reflect differences in evaluation criteria, diagnoses, operator skill and length of follow-up.

Bacteria are the main causes of periradicular disease. *Enterococcus faecalis* has been found to be the predominant microbial in treatment failures, and *Actinomyces* species is able to survive in periapical tissues. An effective coronal seal is thought to improve success rates by reducing the viability of bacteria in the root canal system and the apical area.

Factors thought to improve success include:

- Position of the tooth in the arch that favours anterior teeth.
- A well-condensed orthograde root canal filling.
- A small apical lesion (<6 mm).
- Use of a microtip.
- First attempt at apical surgery for the tooth.
- Use of an endoscope.

Assessment for endodontic surgery

A history and clinical and radiological examinations should be performed when surgical endodontic treatment is being considered. The patient and the tooth are assessed for suitability for surgery and conventional endodontic treatment should always be considered first. If this has already been done, then the RCT is assessed and a decision made on its effectiveness. Local anatomical factors (e.g. the proximity of the surgical area to the maxillary sinus or neurovascular bundles) need to be taken into account, as does the feasibility of surgery. Be honest with yourself and your resources.

Once endodontic surgery has been performed, it should be assessed after at least 1 year. Success is indicated by the following:

- Absence of symptoms such as pain and swelling.
- No sinus tract.
- No loss of function.
- Satisfactory soft tissue healing.
- Radiographic evidence of bony infill at the surgical site.

Long-term follow-up is based on personal protocol after 1 year.

Surgical procedures

Incision and drainage

Incision and drainage are among the few surgical procedures that should be performed in the presence of acute inflammation. The main indication for incision and drainage is the presence of pus within the tissues that cannot be drained through the root canal. Anaesthesia is obtained with the use of surface analgesics, which can be supplemented with a few drops of local anaesthetic solution injected submucosally. An incision is made with a number 11 scalpel blade, a microbial swab is taken and drainage is effected. Alternatively, a wide-bore needle and sterile syringe can be used to aspirate the contents of the swelling, and culture and sensitivity testing can be carried out. Remember that in practical terms it will be days before the results of these tests are available. If there is no drainage, antibiotics such as a penicillin and/or metronidazole should be used. Significant infection (classically orbital cellulitis; see Chapter 10) beyond the confines of the dentoalveolar complex mandates aggressive antibiotic treatment (e.g. amoxycillin 500 mg and metronidazole 400 mg orally three times daily) and possibly referral.

Occasionally, a patient may present with severe pain resulting from exudate entrapped within the cortical bone. In this situation, anaesthesia is obtained and a mucoperiosteal flap is raised over the root apex. The cortical bone over the apex is penetrated with a hand or rotary instrument to release the exudate. This technique is known as *cortical trephination*.

Periradicular surgery

Numerous distinct stages are involved to effect apical surgery (apicectomy), and these include:

- Local analgesia.
- Raising a mucoperiosteal flap.
- Haemostasis.
- Identification of the root apex.
- Periapical curettage.
- Root end resection.
- Root end cavity preparation.
- Root end (retrograde) filling.

- Wound closure.
- Postsurgical care.

Local analgesia

Most surgical endodontic treatment can be performed using local anaesthesia (see Chapter 4). A careful technique at this stage ensures the patient's comfort throughout the procedure and does much to alleviate anxiety. A topical anaesthetic agent is applied to dry mucosa, followed by a slow supraperiosteal injection of 0.5 mL of the anaesthetic solution. Most of the discomfort resulting from the administration of local anaesthetic is caused by distension of the periosteum. Therefore, the remainder of the anaesthetic cartridge is given slowly at a rate of approximately 1 mL/minute. In the maxilla, infiltrations are almost exclusively used, whereas in the mandible nerve blocks should be supplemented with local infiltrations. This will help with haemostasis during surgery. Lidocaine with 1:80 000 adrenaline is commonly used in the United Kingdom, whereas in other countries lidocaine with 1:50 000 adrenaline is available and aids haemostatic control.

Flaps

A wide variety of flap designs has been used, but the six main types are:

- Semilunar (Figure 7.5).
- Triangular (Figure 7.6).
- Rectangular (Figure 7.7).
- Trapezoid (Figure 7.8).
- Vertical incision.
- Ochsenbein-Luebke flap (Figure 7.9) (this design is not very common in Germany, where the distinction is between marginal and paramarginal flaps).

Whichever design is chosen, there should be an unobstructed view of the operating area and good access for instrumentation. The triangular and rectangular flap designs are currently the most commonly used. Incision should allow a full-thickness mucoperiosteal flap to be raised

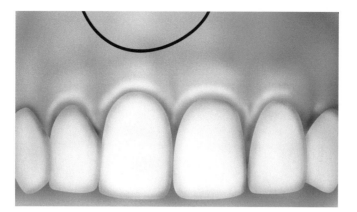

Figure 7.5 Semilunar flap.

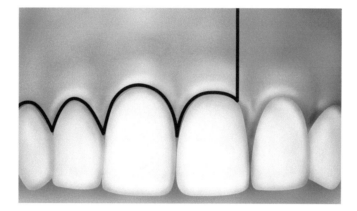

Figure 7.6 Triangular flap. Note that the vertical relieving incision does not bisect the dental papilla.

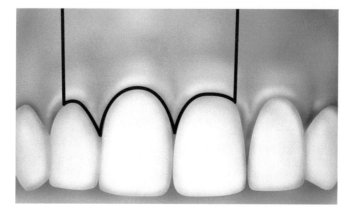

Figure 7.7 Rectangular flap.

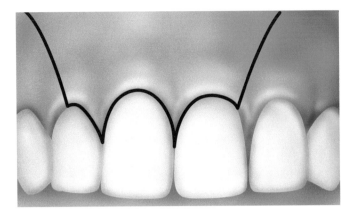

Figure 7.8 Trapezoidal flap.

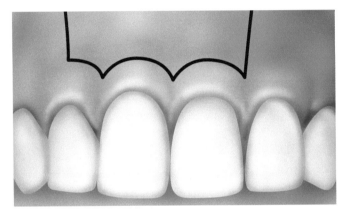

Figure 7.9 Ochsenbein-Luebke flap.

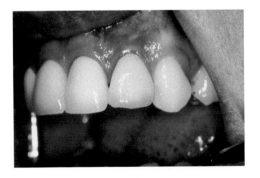

Figure 7.10 Appearance 1 year after periradicular surgery at UL2. Note the minimal gingival recession as a result of careful surgical technique.

cleanly from the bone. Any relieving incisions should be made vertically rather than at an angle, and they should avoid bulbous areas such as the canine prominence in the maxilla, where root dehiscences may prevent adequate healing of the flap margin. The flap is reflected from the crown toward the apex, starting in the sulcus, and it is kept moist and free of tension. This minimizes any postoperative gingival recession (Figure 7.10).

Haemostasis

Adequate haemostatic control is important during endodontic surgery to improve visualization of the surgical area and thus reduce surgical time and postoperative pain and swelling. It also allows the root end filling to be placed under favourable conditions. The adrenaline in local anaesthetic solutions can significantly reduce intraoperative haemorrhage by stimulating the alpha-receptors in gingival blood vessels and causing their vasoconstriction. Solutions with 1:50 000 adrenaline have been found to cause half the blood loss of those with 1:80 000, with no significant difference in systemic effects.

The design of the flap is also important when considering haemostatic control for endodontic surgery. The supraperiosteal blood vessels run parallel to the long axis of the tooth, and therefore vertical relieving incisions as opposed to angled incisions will decrease the number of blood vessels severed. Furthermore, reflection of a full-thickness periosteal flap that retains the microvasculature within the body of the flap also limits haemorrhage.

In addition to local anaesthetic solutions containing adrenaline and a careful surgical technique, various haemostatic agents are available to effect adequate moisture control. Although these agents are usually used after periapical curettage, they are considered here for convenience. Commonly used haemostatic agents include the following:

- Cotton/gauze with or without vasoconstrictor – these agents reduce haemorrhage by applying physical pressure and can be readily impregnated with a vasoconstrictor.
- Oxycellulose (e.g. Surgicel) – these agents provide a framework for clot formation. There have been reports of a foreign body reaction to the material together with delayed healing.
- Wax – this exerts a pressure or tamponade effect to aid with haemostasis, but histologically a foreign body reaction is also shown to be elicited. It can sometimes be difficult to remove all the wax from the bony crypt.
- Calcium alginate (e.g. Kaltostat) – this agent aids haemostasis by stimulating coagulation via the release of calcium.
- Calcium sulphate – this usually comes as a powder and a liquid that, when mixed together, form putty that can be placed into the cavity. This putty then exerts a tamponade effect and blocks the vascular channels.
- Ferric sulphate – this is particularly useful for arresting multiple small, bony bleeding points. However, it must be thoroughly rinsed out to prevent a foreign body reaction and abscess formation.
- Gelatin (e.g. Gelfoam and Spongostan) – this acts by stimulating the intrinsic clotting pathway.
- Collagen (e.g. CollaPlug) – this agent acts in a number of ways. In addition to having a mechanical tamponade effect, it also stimulates platelet adhesion and aggregation, activates factor VIII and releases serotonin, which in turn causes vasoconstriction.
- Tranexamic acid mouthwash given preoperatively and postoperatively – this is sometimes used to aid haemostasis by inhibiting fibrinolysis.

Identification of the root apex

If the lesion has perforated the cortical plate, identification of the apex is relatively simple. However, if this has not occurred, an estimation of the tooth length from a good preoperative radiograph is made. A small round burr, running in a slow handpiece with water irrigation, can then be used at this length with gentle pressure to explore the area and locate the lesion. Care is required to avoid damage to the roots of the adjacent teeth. The bone is gently pared away until the apex is located, and further bone is removed to provide good access.

Periapical curettage

Any soft tissue lesion is carefully curetted from around the apex with excavators and is sent for histopathology examination if appropriate. Where possible, the lesion should be excavated in one piece and any remnants curetted out with sharp instruments. Sometimes, the tissue is firmly adherent to the apex, in which case the apex is resected and removed together with the soft tissue lesion.

Root end resection

The aims of root end resection are to present the surface of the root so that the apical seal of the orthograde root filling can be examined and to provide access for preparation of the root end. Approximately 2 to 3 mm of the root end is resected at right angles to the long axis of the tooth. A bevelled resection is avoided where possible because a larger surface area of dentinal tubules is exposed, and this can lead to microleakage. Also, if the root end is bevelled, there is the possibility of leaving behind infected tooth tissue or of missing part or all of the root canal system (Figure 7.11).

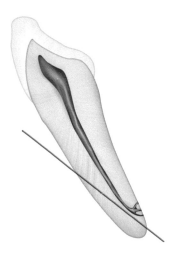

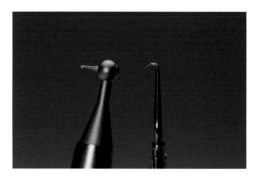

Figure 7.12 A comparison of the sizes of a micro-head handpiece and an ultrasonic tip.

Figure 7.11 A bevelled root end resection resulting in the canal being missed.

Root end resection is effectively an apicectomy, and although the term 'apicectomy' has been commonly used to describe apical surgery, that word describes only a small part of the whole procedure and is best avoided.

Root end cavity preparation

The ideal root end cavity preparation is defined as a class I preparation at least 3 mm into root dentine with walls parallel to and coincident with the anatomical outline of the pulpal space. A contra-angled slow-speed microhead handpiece with a small round burr has conventionally been used to prepare the cavity, but this does not relate to the anatomy of the pulp, and often the apical dentine is weakened by unnecessary overenlargement. There is also a considerable risk of perforating the root end. Therefore, specifically designed ultrasonic instruments have been developed to effect an accurate preparation, and their small tip size allows much greater access than even the micro-head handpiece (Figures 7.12 and 7.13). Ultrasonic instrumentation enables the isthmus running between some canals to be prepared and sealed. This isthmus is often a reservoir for bacteria that have not been removed during conventional RCT. In Germany and many developed countries the use of magnification and piezo (ultrasonic) instruments are the accepted standard.

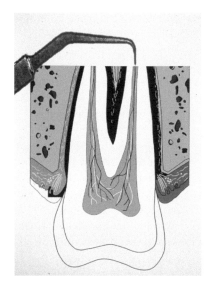

Figure 7.13 The contour and size of the ultrasonic tip allow better access to difficult areas of the mouth.

Root end (retrograde) filling

The purpose of the root end filling is to seal the apical section of the tooth and thus prevent any leakage between the oral environment and periradicular tissues. Before the root end filling is inserted, one of the haemostatic agents described in the section on haemostasis can be packed into the bony cavity to prevent contamination of the root end cavity.

In most situations a retrograde root filling is indicated, but when the source of irritants is removed by the resection and the rest of the canal is completely cleaned and obturated, it is acceptable

Table 7.1 Materials used for root end fillings

Commonly used materials	Less common materials
Amalgam	Gutta percha
Zinc oxide eugenol	Gold foil
Mineral trioxide aggregate	Teflon
Glass ionomer	Cyanoacrylate
Composite	Apatite cement
Zinc phosphate	Gallium alloy
Zinc polycarboxylate	

simply to burnish the apical gutta percha. When a root end filling is to be used, there is a wide variety of materials at the clinician's disposal (Table 7.1), although not all these materials have been commonly used.

Amalgam has been used for many years because it is cheap, easy to handle and not particularly moisture sensitive. However, there are problems with its dimensional stability and corrosion, and it can cause staining of the mucosa if it is carelessly placed. Furthermore, amalgam does not provide an ideal apical seal. It is no longer regarded as an acceptable root end material in Germany

The zinc oxide–eugenol–based materials such as ethoxybenzoic acid (Super EBA) and intermediate restorative material (IRM) have been used to good effect as retrograde filling materials. Leakage studies suggest less microleakage around these materials than amalgam, and because they are eugenol based there is some antibacterial activity.

Glass ionomer has been shown to give a better seal than amalgam by adhering to dentine, and it has antibacterial activity against some endodontic pathogens. As well as being placed in the root end cavity, a thin smear of glass ionomer can be used to seal the whole root end surface. Composite has also been used as a root end filling and, like glass ionomer, can be used to seal the root face. Both glass ionomer and composite materials are very moisture sensitive, which is a distinct disadvantage in apical surgery.

Mineral trioxide aggregate (MTA) consists of a fine powder of tricalcium silicate, tricalcium aluminate, tricalcium oxide and silicate oxide that sets in the presence of moisture. Hydration of the powder produces a colloidal gel with a pH of 12.5

that solidifies to hard cement. MTA has several reported advantages:

- Very good sealing ability.
- Low toxicity.
- Very low inflammatory reaction to the material.
- An inductive effect on osteoblasts and cementoblasts.
- No sensitivity to moisture.
- Low setting contraction.

The disadvantages of MTA are that it is relatively expensive and has a long setting time (4 hours) – although the initial set only takes several minutes. Despite this, current research is promising for the use of MTA in surgical endodontics, and it is the filling of choice for this purpose in Germany.

Wound closure

After placement of the root end material and débridement of the surgical area, the flap is reapproximated and compressed for 2 to 3 minutes before suturing. There is no evidence for the superiority of resorbable or nonresorbable sutures; 4-0 or 5-0 monofilament varieties have theoretical advantages. Cyanoacrylate adhesives and fibrin sealants have been used but are not widely adopted because of their unpredictable strength.

Postsurgical care

Patients are advised to use anti-inflammatory analgesics (see Chapter 4). Chlorhexidine mouthwash 10 mL rinsed twice daily is also prescribed. The use of prophylactic antibiotics is controversial. There is no current evidence base for this, although many still use this technique or even administer postoperative antibiotics, which have even less theoretical or evidence-based support. Ice packs, which are also commonly advised by some, have no real evidence base.

Sutures may resorb or be removed according to personal protocol. A radiograph is taken at 3 months. Further radiographs are taken as appropriate to each individual situation.

Treatment of specific areas of the mouth

Specific areas of the mouth pose various difficulties during apical surgery, and an understanding of the local anatomy is of immense importance when considering surgical treatment.

Upper anterior teeth

Reflection of the flap to provide adequate access to the apex of upper central incisor teeth can be compromised by a prominent and/or low anterior nasal spine. Extending the flap around more teeth and increasing the size of any relieving incisions often allow sufficient access to perform the surgery. The apices of upper lateral incisors can be deeply placed in the alveolar bone, which makes identification of the apex and access for apical surgery more difficult. The roots of upper canine teeth are occasionally very long, and access to the apex may be restricted by the buccal reflection. Adequate relieving incisions help overcome this.

Upper posterior teeth

The maxillary sinus is often in close relation to the apices of upper posterior teeth, but a careful surgical technique avoids damage to the sinus. It is advisable to burr down the root apex to the desired level, rather than resecting it, so that the resected tip cannot be displaced into the sinus or under its lining.

Apical surgery on upper first premolar teeth can be challenging for the operator because of the deeply placed palatal root. It may be necessary to resect a greater length of the buccal root than normal to provide sufficient access to the palatal root. The upper second premolar tooth is usually single rooted, but there may be two separate root canals or two canals joined by an isthmus. In these situations, it is important to seal both canals, together with any isthmus of tissue that may be present. Access to the palatal root of the upper molars is almost impossible, but fortunately the palatal root is readily treated by conventional endodontics. The buccal roots are normally fairly superficial but occasionally they are deeply placed beneath the zygomatic buttress.

Lower anterior teeth

The apices of the lower anterior teeth are usually deeply placed in the mandible, and this makes access extremely difficult. In addition, the mentalis and buccinator muscles are attached at a relatively high level, so that reflection of the flap to the level of the apices can be problematic. Therefore, a rectangular flap design with two relieving incisions is advised, and a *small* bevel of the root face may be necessary so that the canal or canals can be visualized. Local anaesthesia can also be surprisingly difficult, possibly because of sensory innervation by the nerve to mylohyoid.

Lower posterior teeth

The mental nerve usually emerges from the mental foramen below and between the lower premolar teeth. Therefore, vertical relieving incisions should be avoided in this area. Also, during root resection it may be desirable to resect the root at the desired level, rather than burring it down, to reduce the risk of damage to the mental nerve. Whether or not apical surgery is possible on lower molars depends on the degree to which the corner of the mouth can be retracted. If adequate retraction can be obtained and the attachment of the buccinator muscle is sufficiently low, surgery may be possible. A wide flap is usually required to enhance access, and it is often necessary to remove a considerable thickness of bone to gain access to the roots. Care is needed to avoid damage to the inferior alveolar nerve, and again it is advisable to resect the root rather than burring it down.

Corrective surgery

Corrective surgical endodontics includes:

- Perforation repair.
- Root resection.
- Tooth resection.

Many of the basic surgical principles outlined under apical surgery can be applied here (e.g. flap design, haemostasis, and root end filling materials), so the surgical procedures are not described in detail.

Perforation repair

Common causes of root perforations are endodontic instruments, posts and resorption cavities. If the prognosis of the tooth is acceptable, surgical access is gained to the site of the perforation, and the area is prepared and then filled with one of the materials mentioned earlier (e.g. IRM or MTA) (Figures 7.14, 7.15 and 7.16; note the apparent overbevelling is a consequence of this being a perforation repair and not a conventional apicectomy.)

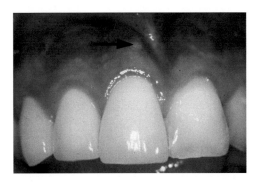

Figure 7.14 Labial swelling (arrow) related to a post perforation at UR1.

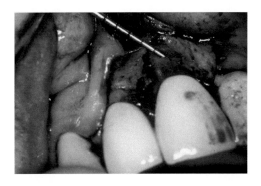

Figure 7.15 Flap raised and curettage of the surgical area effected. A periodontal probe was used to identify the defect.

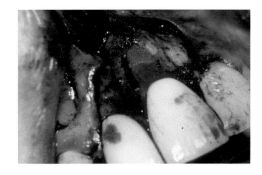

Figure 7.16 Defect repaired with mineral trioxide aggregate to reestablish the correct root contour.

Root resection

The objective of root resection is to remove an entire root or roots from a multirooted tooth, but without removing any portion of the crown. The main indications are when one root is affected by advanced periodontal disease but the rest of the periodontium is relatively unaffected or when it is impossible to carry out RCT in a root.

A suitable mucoperiosteal flap is reflected and the root is exposed by removing the overlying bone. The root is then resected from the tooth and is removed, and the portion of the crown adjacent to the resected root is recontoured to make the site easily cleanable. The flap is sutured, and postoperative instructions are issued.

Tooth resection (hemisection)

Here, the coronal tooth structure, as well as the root, is cut and the procedure is mainly performed on mandibular molar teeth with furcation involvement. The separated part of the tooth may either be removed or left *in situ* and restored. In the latter case, a molar is effectively converted into two premolar units.

Extraction with replantation

This procedure involves intentionally removing the tooth from its socket, carrying out the surgical endodontic procedure of choice (e.g. apical surgery, perforation repair) extraorally, and replanting the tooth. Although not commonly performed, extraction with replantation is useful when access for surgery *in situ* is impossible and the alternative would be loss of the tooth. The patient should be warned of the risk of damage to the tooth during the extraction process, which may preclude the procedure. (For the surgical technique for tooth transfer, see Chapter 9.)

Revision surgery

The cause of failure of surgery should be identified before considering revision surgical endodontics, and an assessment should be made of the likelihood of correcting this cause. Success rates for repeat apical surgery are in the region of 30% to 40%, which is much lower than for the initial procedure.

Root canals that have not been adequately sealed are the most common causes of failure of both conventional and surgical endodontic therapy. If surgical treatment has been performed in the absence of adequate cleansing and obturation of the root canal system, failure is to be expected. Repeat surgery will be successful in these situations only if the principles of conventional endodontic treatment are carried out first to ensure the best possible coronal seal. Failure caused by an inadequate apical seal can be rectified by ensuring that there is no contamination of the root end cavity at the time of surgery and by using an appropriate root end filling material.

Sometimes during apical surgery root canals are incompletely sealed surgically because an additional root has not been identified. This should be suspected if, at the time of repeat surgery, the apical seal in the treated root appears intact and the surrounding tissues have healed. Radiographs taken at different angles can be useful in identifying additional roots. Often it is the deeply placed palatal root that is missed, particularly of upper premolar teeth. An incomplete seal may also be present when there are two portals of exit of the root canal in the same root and only one has been treated. Alternatively, if both canals within a single root have been sealed but the intervening isthmus of tissue has remained untreated, treatment failure can ensue.

From a practical view point, revision surgery is more difficult for the operator, particularly when raising a flap that is scarred from previous surgery. The cause of the failure will determine which procedure is undertaken, but often the retrograde seal requires replacement. Care is needed when removing the old material to ensure that it does not scatter unnecessarily in the surgical field. Depending on which material is used, these small fragments can cause staining of the mucosa or a foreign body reaction in the tissues. Consideration also needs to be given to whether the root should be resected further at the time of second surgery. In most cases it is acceptable to reduce the root length a further 2 to 3 mm during revision surgery. However, in the presence of periodontal pocketing, resection of too great a length of root will reduce the distance between the epithelial attachment and the root end. Therefore, a small amount of further periodontal breakdown and migration of the epithelial attachment will result in a full-length pocket from the gingival crevice to the apical tissues.

Summary

There are a number of ways in which nonvital teeth may be preserved, but with the increasing body of evidence supporting the long-term viability of dental implants, it may be that atraumatic removal of these teeth with preservation of the maximum amount of healthy bone and immediate implant replacement may become the standard treatment for nonvital teeth that cannot be salvaged endodontically.

FURTHER READING

Barnes IE. *Surgical endodontics: colour manual.* Oxford: Wright, 1991, pp. 55–64, 95–102.

Chandler NP, Koshy S. The changing role of the apicectomy operation in dentistry. *J R Coll Surg Edinb* 2002;47:660–7.

Cohen S, Burns RC. *Pathways of the pulp*, 8th ed. St. Louis: Mosby, 2002, pp. 683–725.

Johnson BR. Considerations in the selection of a root-end filling material. *Oral Surg Oral Med Oral Pathol Oral Radiol Endod* 1999;87:398–404.

Kim S. Principles of endodontic microsurgery. *Dent Clin North America* 1997;4(3):481–597.

Nair UP, Yazdi MH, Nayar GM, Parry H, Katkar RA, Nair MK. Configuration of the inferior alveolar canal as detected by cone beam computed tomography. *J Conserv Dent* 2013;16:518–21.

Song M, Kim EA. prospective randomized controlled study of mineral trioxide aggregate and super ethoxy-benzoic acid as root-end filling materials in endodontic microsurgery. *J Endod* 2012;38:875–9.

Torabinejad M, Chivian N. Clinical applications of mineral trioxide aggregate. *J Endod* 1999;25:197–205.

Tsurumachi T. Current strategy for successful periradicular surgery. *J Oral Sci* 2013;55:267–73.

Von Arx T, Peñarrocha M, Jensen S. Prognostic factors in apical surgery with root-end filling: a meta-analysis. *J Endod* 2010;36:957–73.

Wälivaara DÅ, Abrahamsson P, Fogelin M, Isaksson S. Super-EBA and IRM as root-end fillings in periapical surgery with ultrasonic preparation: a prospective randomized clinical study of 206 consecutive teeth. *Oral Surg Oral Med Oral Pathol Oral Radiol Endod* 2011;112:258–63.

Wesselink PR. Consensus report of the European Society of Endodontology on quality guidelines for endodontic treatment. *Int Endod J* 1994;27:115–24.

8

Third molar surgery

Contents

Aims

- To understand third molar pathology and its treatment.
- The aims and objectives for undergraduates and postgraduates are similar and vary only in degree.

Learning outcomes

- To describe the indications and contraindications for third molar surgery.
- To identify those third molars for which surgical removal is appropriate or inappropriate.
- To identify those third molars that may be within your capability and those that need to be referred to a specialist.

- To be able to describe the techniques involved in removing third molars.
- To be able to discuss the management of postoperative sequelae.

Surgical removal of the third molar or 'wisdom' tooth is one of the most common procedures undertaken in oral and maxillofacial practice. It is also a common cause of litigation. In the United Kingdom, even the indications for removal of third molar teeth excited controversy, although this has now been addressed by guidelines developed both by the British Association of Oral and Maxillofacial Surgeons (BAOMS; www.baoms.org.uk) and the National Institute for Health and Care Excellence (NICE; www.nice.org.uk). UK guidelines are being reviewed in 2014. The 2013 guidelines of the German Society of Oral and Maxillofacial Surgeons

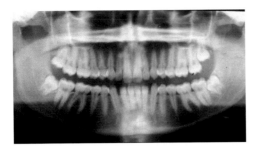

Figure 8.1 Dental panoramic radiograph showing mesioangular impacted third molars with lower incisor spacing.

are fairly similar. Many other countries have devised their own guidelines, and there is a lack of international consensus on when and when not to remove third molars; the American Association of Oral and Maxillofacial Surgeons views are quite different from those in the United Kingdom. The prevention of lower labial segment crowding is **not** an evidence-based indication (Figure 8.1). The safest way to remove wisdom teeth is a source of continual controversy – this relates particularly to how the lingual nerve is best protected.

The most common cause for failure of a tooth to erupt is lack of space into which it can pass. Other reasons include malposition of the follicle and congenital absence. Rarely other associated pathology such as cysts, odontomes or tumours will prevent eruption. Treatment is then directed at the primary pathology. Developmental conditions such as cleidocranial dysostosis or cleft lip and palate are associated with an increased incidence of unerupted third molars. In the presence of an obstruction (e.g. another tooth), the unerupted tooth is said to be 'impacted'. Third molars normally erupt between the ages of 17 and 21 years, although later eruption can occur. Because they are the last teeth to erupt, they have the least space available and therefore they commonly become impacted. Soft Western diets have also been implicated because the absence of attrition between the adjacent lower teeth does not provide any additional space for the teeth to erupt into. It is often possible to assess the potential for eruption by the age of 16 years on the basis of clinical examination and the use of radiographs, but 'prophylactic' removal of third molars is no longer considered justifiable in the United Kingdom, and the concept of lateral trepanation (removal of the third molar as a follicle) has passed into history. The

decision to remove third molars depends on a balance between symptoms or pathology and relative risks in removing them (e.g. injury to the inferior dental (ID) nerve and/or the lingual nerve, risk of fracture). If one third molar needs removing with the patient under general anaesthesia, it may be worth considering whether the opposite tooth should be removed at the same time. This is a balance between avoiding a second general anaesthetic regimen in the future and risking complications in otherwise asymptomatic teeth. This is an area of fine clinical judgement that is poorly addressed by the UK NICE guidelines.

Indications for removal of third molar teeth

- Pain, specific to the third molars (myofacial pain is not an indication).
- Pericoronitis or infection (Figure 8.2).
- Advanced caries.
- Periodontal disease.
- Periapical pathology.
- Disease of follicle, including cyst or tumour (Figure 8.3).
- Fractured tooth.
- Resorption of adjacent teeth.
- As part of an orthodontic or orthognathic treatment plan.
- Mandibular angle fracture (Figure 8.4).
- Prophylactic removal in the 'at risk' patient (e.g. bacterial endocarditis).
- As an aid to denture provision.

The most common indication is recurrent pericoronitis. Pericoronitis is inflammation and

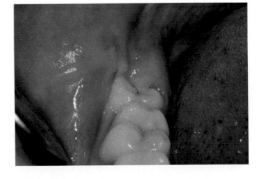

Figure 8.2 The pericoronal flap (operculum) over the lower third molar is the site of pericoronitis.

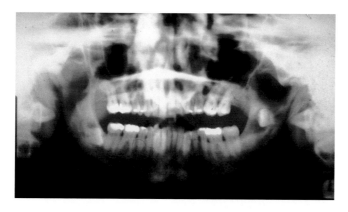

Figure 8.3 Radiograph of a third molar displaced by a dentigerous cyst.

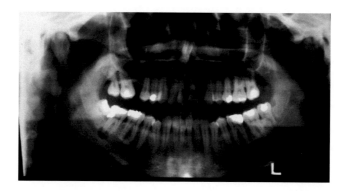

Figure 8.4 Radiograph of a fractured mandible through the lower left third molar. Note the apical area around the lower right 7. The patient was being managed medically for pyrexia of unknown origin.

infection of the mucosal flap (operculum) overlying a partially erupted tooth, usually the lower third molar. It may be acute or chronic. Treatment involves removal of the opposing third molar, irrigation under the operculum and topical application of silver nitrate or trichloroacetic acid (TCA) and glycerol. Systemic antibiotics (metronidazole 400 mg orally three times daily with or without amoxycillin 500 mg orally three times daily) and analgesics (ibuprofen 400 mg orally three times daily) are indicated in patients who present systemically unwell.

Contraindications to removal of third molars

- Patient's refusal.
- Active acute pericoronitis (although evidence disputing this exists).
- Absence of symptoms.
- High risk of injury to the ID nerve (relative contraindication).
- Uncontrolled clotting disorder.

Assessment

Before narrowing down to assessment of the individual tooth, think for a moment about the patient. Is there anything in the medical history that will contraindicate or modify your planned anaesthesia and surgery? (see Chapter 5). If the patient is physiologically healthy, is he or she psychologically able to cope with local anaesthesia (or in some instances, general anaesthesia)? If the patient's condition is otherwise straightforward, are there any local physical problems (e.g. limited mouth opening)?

Now you have an understanding of what sort of patient you are dealing with start to look at the third molar itself.

Assessment of the tooth is both clinical and radiographic. If a patient presents in pain, it is important to establish that this pain is coming from the third molar and not elsewhere. Pain is often vague, poorly localized and possibly referred from another tooth or as part of facial arthromyalgia (see Chapter 14). A dental panoramic radiograph is ideal because it helps to assess all the teeth at once. Another useful test is simply applying ethyl chloride to any suspect teeth. The health of the adjacent molars may influence the decision whether to remove the third molar. Large crowns or old restorations are all at risk of dislodgement during surgery, and this must be explained to the patient. It is also worth considering whether alternative treatment options are available. For instance pericoronitis resulting from an overerupted upper third molar may be dealt with by extracting that tooth only, with or without operculectomy. In the presence of other teeth with poor prognosis, will it be better in the long term to save the third molar, which may be used as a denture or bridge abutment?

Having established that the wisdom tooth needs to be removed, other points in the assessment include the following (Figures 8.5, 8.6, 8.7 and 8.8):

- Tooth position (vertical, mesioangular, distoangular, horizontal or across the arch) – a lower occlusal film may also be required if the last position is suspected.
- Depth and degree of impaction.
- Obstruction to eruption – what is the tooth impacted against?
- Root morphology – the curvature of the roots controls the path of withdrawal.

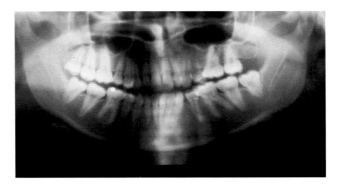

Figure 8.5 Radiograph showing vertically impacted lower third molars.

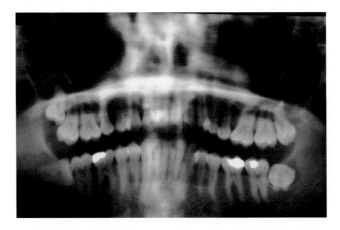

Figure 8.6 Radiograph showing horizontally and transversely impacted third molars.

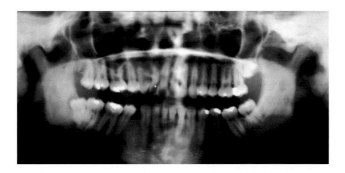

Figure 8.7 Radiograph showing distoangular impactions.

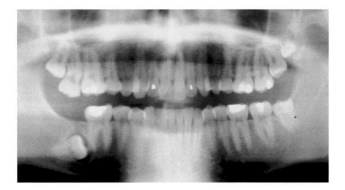

Figure 8.8 Radiograph showing an impacted upper *fourth* molar and a deep lower third molar.

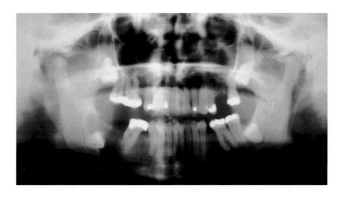

Figure 8.9 Radiograph showing a third molar with associated dentigerous cyst arising from the amelocemental junction (see Chapter 11).

- Relationship with the ID canal.
- Associated pathology (cysts; see Chapter 11) (Figure 8.9).
- Bone density.
- Status of second molar tooth – in selected cases where this tooth has a poor prognosis, it may be better to extract it and leave the third molar.

These points help to determine whether the tooth can be simply elevated or will need a surgical approach. If surgical removal is necessary, the surgeon needs to decide:

- The path of withdrawal.
- Obstructions to this path – do they need to be removed or left?

- The amount of bone that needs to be removed to allow application of an elevator.
- The direction of withdrawal (distoangular teeth are renowned for looking easy radiographically but being much more difficult to remove).
- Is the tooth best divided and removed in pieces?

With experience, many of these points are determined intuitively by careful examination of the radiograph. For novices, however, a structured system can be helpful – depth in bone of the maximal bulbosity of the crown, line of movement, point of elevation and impediments to movement. Removing the tooth is really removing the impediments and applying correctly orientated force (Figure 8.10).

'Buying time' – treating pericoronitis, temporizing

It is extremely important that you develop skills in temporizing, by using appropriate analgesics (particularly nonsteroidal anti-inflammatory drugs such as ibuprofen or diclofenac), antibiotics and TCA/glycerine techniques for recurrent pericoronitis and removal of upper third molars to alleviate the more significant symptoms while patients are waiting for definitive surgical treatment (Figure 8.11).

Taking consent – what can the patient expect?

The patient must be competent and understand the risks and benefits (see Chapter 2). The benefits are, fairly obviously, the removal of symptoms and (more difficult to convince people of) prevention of further disease.

All patients having third molars (particularly lower) removed **will** have:

- Some pain or discomfort.
- Swelling (widely variable), possibly with bruising.
- Stiffness of the jaws that makes eating difficult.

These symptoms last for about 7 days and gradually get better; if not, then the usual problem is wound infection, which can occur in 5% to 10% of patients even if prophylactic antibiotics have been used. Very rarely iatrogenic fracture of the mandible is the cause of worsening pain. From 5% to 10% of patients experience temporary altered sensation in the lingual or inferior alveolar nerve distribution. In 0.5% to 1% of cases this is permanent. Patients should take 2 to 5 days off work in most instances.

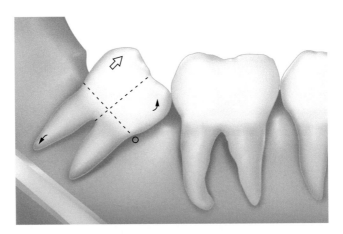

Figure 8.10 The dashed lines indicate efficient lines of tooth division. The circle indicates the usual point of application for the elevator. The solid arrows ↘ ↙ indicate movement if elevation alone is relied on; note the risk of driving the distal apex into the inferior alveolar nerve. The open arrow ⇧ indicates the 'natural' line of removal; anything that impedes this creates an 'impaction'. The aim is to remove impediments leading to impaction while causing the least trauma to the patient (i.e. cut up the tooth to be removed most, the surrounding bone as little as possible, and the adjacent teeth never).

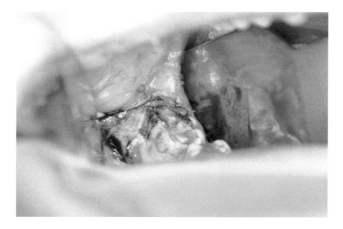

Figure 8.11 Occasionally, excision of the operculum relieves symptoms.

Surgical technique – lower third molars

Some aspects of this are controversial – Should we raise a lingual flap? Should we use burrs or chisels? Should antibiotics be prescribed? If so, for how long? Should steroids be prescribed? Given this is such a common operation it is astonishing there have not been adequately powered randomized controlled trials and a huge dataset for meta-analyses. For these, and many other points, there are no hard and fast rules. What seems to be emerging from the literature is that some techniques work well for some individuals and should therefore be encouraged. Only by supervised training and carefully conducted audit can these issues be answered and safe techniques developed for each surgeon. The various stages in the technique are as follows:

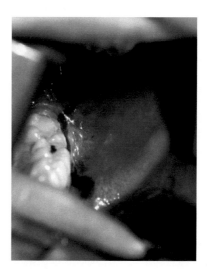

Figure 8.12 The markings for a buccal flap in third molar removal.

Anaesthesia – local anaesthesia helps haemostasis and postoperative pain relief even if the surgery is carried out using a general anaesthetic regimen. This involves local infiltration where the flap is to be raised; some surgeons augment this with a block even if the patient is receiving a general anaesthetic.

Buccal flap – a full-thickness mucoperiosteal flap is raised from the buccal surface of the wisdom tooth area. The choice of incision varies, but it commonly involves an incision along the external oblique ridge that passes forward either around the second molar tooth or out into the buccal sulcus (Figure 8.12). If little

or no bone is to be removed, a simple relieving incision may be all that is necessary. The important point is that dissection proceeds in a subperiosteal plane because this minimizes postoperative swelling and trismus (Figure 8.13).

Lingual flap – some authorities do not raise a lingual flap at all. The popularity of this approach was from the days when accurate very high-speed surgical drills were not available and the 'lingual split bone' technique was popular in the United Kingdom and in areas influenced by UK training. These experts argue that it is the process of actually raising

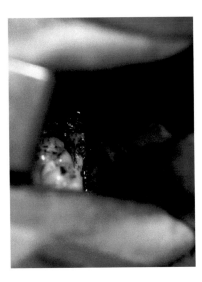

Figure 8.13 Buccal bone is exposed to identify how much needs to be removed to clear the bulbosity of the crown.

the flap that causes the injury to the lingual nerve. Conversely, it is argued that the nerve is at risk from direct trauma from the burr or chisel if it is not retracted. Again, if used, the flap is raised by subperiosteal dissection. Here it is important not to 'bow-string' the nerve over the retractor (usually Howarth's elevator), but to undermine the lingual periosteum widely to allow the tissues to lie passively and use a wide subperiosteally placed retractor. The elevation of a small cuff of distal attached

mucosa is designed for visibility, not for 'lingual nerve protection', and is not associated with an increase in morbidity (Figure 8.14).

Bone removal – this is usually done with either a burr or (rarely now) chisels. The piezoelectric saw has been used but much less commonly. How much needs to be removed depends on the position of the tooth. Care is required to ensure that enough bone remains to support the second molar tooth. If chisels are used, mesial and distal stop cuts need to be placed to prevent fracture propagation (Figure 8.15).

Tooth removal – in less impacted cases a point of application may be drilled into the tooth, which is then elevated out of the socket (Figure 8.16). Here it is important not to lever the tooth out because any resistance may change the fulcrum of elevation and cause the ID nerve to be crushed. If the tooth does not elevate it may be better to divide it and remove it in pieces. This is where the unprotected lingual nerve may be damaged if the burr is passed too deeply.

Coronectomy – there has been a reinvention of the concept of decoronation for third molars that are coronally symptomatic (causing pericoronitis or caries) but have significant risk of neurological damage associated with the operation to remove the tooth conventionally. In these cases some surgeons simply remove the crown through the amelodentinal junction, reduce the root surface to allow 2 mm of alveolar bone

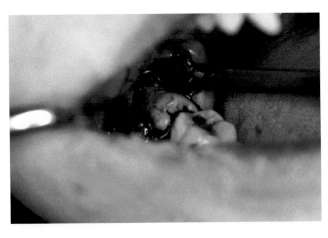

Figure 8.14 Elevation of a small distal lingual gingival flap for visualization – this is not the same as using Howarth's elevator for lingual nerve protection.

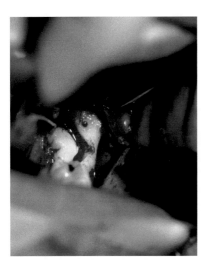

Figure 8.15 Bone removal. If bone is to be removed the burr must penetrate into cancellous bone; anything less is simply traumatic scratching.

above the resection line and either close the wound or place an antiseptic pack. This was a popular preprosthetic technique many years ago, in which the retained roots preserve alveolar bone (see Chapter 15). The obvious risk is of infection of the retained root at some time in the future. Clinical trials have suggested that coronectomy carries a lower risk of damage to the ID nerve, with no increase in symptoms related to the retained root, which sometimes migrates coronally, at least in short-term follow-up. Whether coronectomy becomes as

common as conventional third molar removal or cone beam computed tomography (CBCT) scans mandatory seems at least as likely to be influenced by funding issues as by rational science. Residual follicle is removed by curettage, working on the bone of the socket. Take care if the inferior alveolar nerve (IAN) is exposed in the base of the socket. Smooth bone spicules and wash bone dust from under the periosteal flap. Irrigation of the socket may be counterproductive if a healthy clot is forming. All last remnants must be irrigated out from under the periosteum (Figure 8.17).

Closure – free mucosa is sutured to fixed mucosa with one to two resorbable sutures only. A pressure pack is placed to create clot. Note that this is not first intention healing in most cases; the flap protects the clot and allows the socket to granulate (Figure 8.18). The root pattern (Figure 8.19) and relationship with the inferior alveolar nerve bundle, adjacent second molar and bone of the ascending ramus create problems with simple elevation of third molars. Sectioning the tooth is the safest technique to overcome this situation. Decoronation is performed by cutting through the amelocemental junction (about 80% through) and then fracturing off the crown with an elevator. If the tooth is still resistant to elevation, the roots are separated by cutting through the bifurcation and elevating them individually (Figure 8.20).

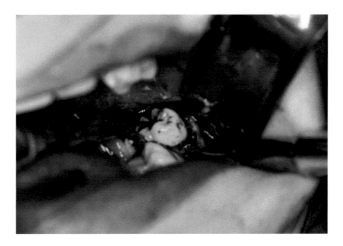

Figure 8.16 The third molar is elevated at the safest point of application.

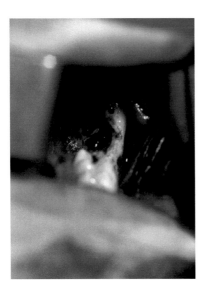

Figure 8.17 The socket is checked for retained fragments.

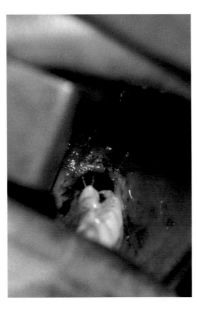

Figure 8.18 Closure should not be 'watertight' because the socket is being protected by the flap to allow a healthy clot, and a small amount of oozing is to be expected. Overly tight closure leads to haematoma.

Surgical technique – upper third molars

Here a buccal flap is raised with an incision either around the second molar or a 'slash' passing from the distobuccal cusp into the buccal sulcus (Figure 8.21). Bone can often be removed buccally with Coupland's elevator and the tooth then elevated with Warwick-James or Cryer's elevator. Deeply placed teeth rarely cause symptoms and are probably best left alone. Beware the fused, ankylosed or multirooted upper third molar (Figure 8.22).

Postoperative care

- Instructions.
- Medications.
- To review or not?

Complications

These include the following:

- Pain – if anticipated this can be minimized by the regular use of analgesics for the first 3 to 4 days. This is a painful procedure, and common humanity dictates we prescribe adequate rather than over-the-counter analgesia. Pain is more difficult to control once it is established.
- Swelling – steroids are often given when surgery is carried out using general anaesthesia; this is unusual in patients having an operation using local anaesthesia.
- Trismus – some muscle spasm may occur during the first few days. Gentle exercises are required after to prevent contracture. If there is still limitation in mouth opening at 3 weeks, some authorities elect to manipulate the mandible while the patient is under general anaesthesia.
- Bleeding (see Chapter 6).
- Fractured mandible (rare), maxillary tuberosity (uncommon) (Figure 8.23).
- Displacement of upper third molar into maxillary antrum or infratemporal fossa (Figure 8.24) – This is fortunately very rare (and scary!).
- Nerve injury (see later).
- Dry socket (see later).
- Infected haematoma.

Nerve injury

An important complication of mandibular third molar removal is injury to the lingual nerve – this

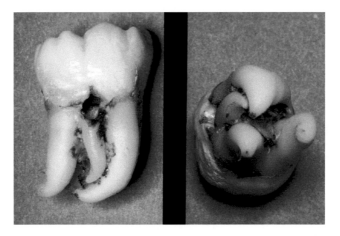

Figure 8.19 Multirooted third molars should be sectioned (the tooth is being removed and confers no additional morbidity; bone removal creates more patient morbidity).

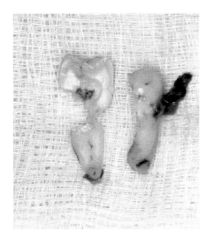

Figure 8.20 Example of a sectioned third molar.

is a common cause of medicolegal claims. The lingual nerve carries sensory fibres to the tongue and taste buds and secretomotor fibres to the submandibular and sublingual glands. Injury can therefore result in loss of sensation (including taste) on the side of the tongue. Most patients describe abnormal sensations, such as pins and needles, tingling, or itching although a few find these sensations painful (dysaesthesia).

The reported incidences of lingual nerve injury in the United Kingdom vary considerably from 0% to 15%. Of these patients, most make a full recovery within a few weeks, but it can take up to 12 months. However, a few (approximately 0.5%) patients are left with permanent sensory disturbance. Temporary disturbance of the lingual nerve

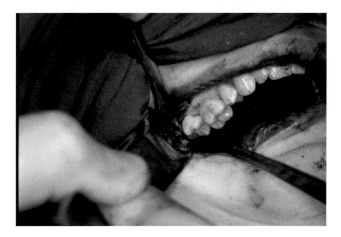

Figure 8.21 Exposing the upper third molar.

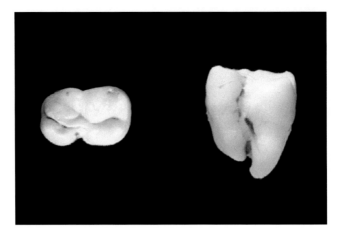

Figure 8.22 Potential problems – fused upper third molar.

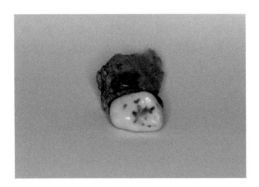

Figure 8.23 Potential problems – fractured tuberosity.

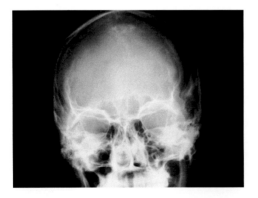

Figure 8.24 Potential problems – upper third molar displaced into the infratemporal fossa.

is often caused by retracting the mucoperiosteal flap during surgery. Permanent injuries often result from nerve division during burring.

Timing for referral

In selected cases, exploration of the nerve may be undertaken. Scar tissue is released (neurolysis) and if the nerve is found to be injured, the segment may be excised and the cut ends sutured together or grafted. Results vary considerably, but improvements have been noted in up to 75% of cases. Timing is crucial. It has been suggested that in the absence of any sensory recovery by 3 to 4 months following injury, exploration is indicated.

Injury to the ID nerve is less common but more difficult to manage. The nerve may be directly injured by the needle during the injection of local anaesthetic or crushed by the tooth root during elevation. Rarely the roots of the tooth may surround and encase the nerve so that elevation is unavoidable. Clues to this injury can be seen on the radiograph and when the tooth will not elevate easily (it actually feels as if it is attached by a rubber band).

Dry socket

Dry socket is localized inflammation of a socket following extraction, most commonly of the lower wisdom teeth (see Chapter 6). Typically the patient complains of severe dull, throbbing pain around 4 to 5 days after extraction and often has a bad taste in the mouth. Pain is often exquisite, with inflammation, exposed bone and halitosis. Treatment is described in Chapter 6.

Infected haematoma

An infected haematoma is a more significant problem than dry socket, mainly because the mass of haematoma can rapidly liquefy and become pus, which will create a large abscess. Try to avoid this by careful haemostasis before closing the wound (i.e. if it is continuing to bleed, do not just ignore it; identify the bleeding point and control before you close). If a patient has a large, tense swelling, start antibiotics immediately. Common regimens are amoxycillin 250 mg three times daily or ampicillin 250 mg four times daily and metronidazole 400 mg three times daily. Either clarithromycin or clindamycin is given to penicillin-allergic patients.

Does it need doing and when to refer

It must be abundantly obvious by now that not all third molars need to be removed simply because they are there. The concept of prophylactic removal of third molars has long been outmoded in the United Kingdom, although it remains a controversial point in some countries. It is therefore essential to ask yourself when a patient attends with vague aches and pains and impacted third molars on radiographs – Does this patient actually require surgery? The questions to ask yourself are as follows: Are the symptoms directly related to the third molars, and if they are, are they related to all the third molars, or can symptoms be ameliorated by removal of, say, a single standing overerupted upper third molar? If the third molars, particularly the lower third molars, do require to be removed, do you have the facilities and the experience to remove these third molars in a safe, straightforward and stress-free manner? Distoangular third molars are, generally speaking, to be avoided in a dental practice environment given that they are considerably more difficult to remove than they first appear. This is because the pathway of withdrawal is directly back into the ramus of the mandible, and the entire crown will almost certainly need to be removed to elevate them. Otherwise straightforward-appearing teeth such as vertical impactions that have square or rectangular-appearing roots on radiographs are often densely sclerosed and frequently will not move despite bone removal and appropriate use of an elevator. These are another group to beware.

Anxious patients who require bilateral third molar removal are probably not practice builders, and mesioangular and horizontally impacted third molars in close proximity to the inferior alveolar bundle may require fairly painstaking removal that is best avoided in practice. Once you have the knack of thinking through these particular problems, it makes it easier to select appropriate third molars for removal using local anaesthesia in a practice environment or removal using local anaesthesia in a hospital environment, as well as those third molars that require referral for either day case surgery or, even occasionally, inpatient surgery.

There is a threshold for referral, which varies widely depending on the facilities available in any individual region. If you are surrounded by specialists in oral surgery, there will be a much higher threshold for referral into the local hospital department. If you are not, then it is an unfortunate fact that many of these patients will have to be referred into the hospital service, and it is important to understand that it is difficult to see these patients on an urgent basis because many other high-priority clinical conditions take priority in the hospital oral and maxillofacial surgical service.

North America

In North America there is increasing availability of cone beam computed tomography (CBCT) in offices and clinics. CBCT can be useful in assessing lower third molars whose roots are in close proximity to the inferior alveolar nerve and in helping to determine the risk of neurosensory disturbance. If such cases are identified a decision may be made to remove the crown of the tooth only (coronectomy), as described earlier.

FURTHER READING

Dimitroulis G. *A synopsis of minor oral surgery.* London: Wright, 1997.
A bit 'book of lists' like but has a comprehensive approach to most of the dentoalveolar field.

McGowan DA. *An atlas of minor oral surgery; principles and practice.* London: Martin Dunitz, 1989.
A dated book now but gives a well-illustrated step-by-step guide.

Mitchell DA, Mitchell L. *Oxford handbook of clinical dentistry,* 6th ed. Oxford: Oxford University Press, 2014.
Never miss an opportunity!

National Institute for Clinical Excellence. *Guidance on the removal of wisdom teeth.* London: National Institute for Clinical Excellence, 2000.
The current UK rules being updated in 2014.

Piecuch JF, Arzadon J, Lieblich SE. Prophylactic antibiotics for third molar surgery. *J Oral Maxillofac Surg* 1995;53:53-60.
Part of the American journal's 'controversy' series summarizes most of the evidence base in this contentious area.

Specific literature includes the following:

Adde CA, Soares MS, Romano MM, Carnaval TG, Sampaio RM, Aldarvis FP, Federico LR. Clinical and surgical evaluation of the indication of postoperative antibiotic prescription in third molar surgery. *Oral Surg Oral Med Oral Pathol Oral Radiol* 2012;114(Suppl):S26–31.

Bezerra TP, Studart-Soares EC, Scaparo HC, Pita-Neto IC, Batista SH, Fonteles CS. Prophylaxis versus placebo treatment for infective and inflammatory complications of surgical third molar removal: a split-mouth, double-blind, controlled, clinical trial with amoxicillin (500 mg). *J Oral Maxillofac Surg* 2011;69:e333–9.

Briguglio F, Zenobio EG, Isola G, Briguglio R, Briguglio E, Farronato D, Shibli JA. Complications in surgical removal of impacted mandibular third molars in relation to flap design: clinical and statistical evaluations. *Quintessence Int* 2011;42:445–53.

Carvalho RW, do Egito Vasconcelos BC. Assessment of factors associated with surgical difficulty during removal of impacted lower third molars. *J Oral Maxillofac Surg* 2011;69:2714–21.

Kim DS, Lopes J, Higgins A, Lopes V. Influence of NICE guidelines on removal of third molars in a region of the UK. *Br J Oral Maxillofac Surg* 2006;44:504–6.

Macluskey M, Slevin M, Curran M, Nesbitt R. Indications for and anticipated difficulty of third molar surgery: a comparison between a dental hospital and a specialist high street practice. *Br Dent J* 2005;199:671–5.

Zeitler DL. Prophylactic antibiotics for third molar surgery: a dissenting opinion. *J Oral Maxillofac Surg* 1995;53:61–4.

9

Dentoalveolar surgery for orthodontic treatment

Contents

Aims for undergraduates and postgraduates

- To appreciate the range of dentoalveolar surgery procedures necessary as part of orthodontic treatment.
- To appreciate the broad principles of treatment for each procedure.

Learning outcomes

- To be able to outline the different options for treatment of impacted or ectopic teeth and describe the steps in operative treatment.
- To describe when a frenectomy is appropriate and the steps in the procedure.

- To be able to discuss the role of circumferential supracrestal fibrotomy in orthodontic treatment and the steps in the procedure.
- To be able to discuss the limited but important role of single tooth osteotomy and tooth transplantation.

Introduction

Orthodontic treatment is primarily concerned with the growth of the face, development of the dentition and the prevention and correction of malocclusion. As such, there is much that oral (and/or maxillofacial) surgeons and orthodontists can offer each other when treating patients, and very often a joint approach is necessary. Surgical

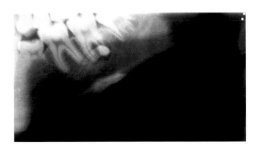

Figure 9.1 An extreme example of a migrating ectopic tooth; note LL5.

techniques that may help the orthodontist include the following:

- Removal of impacted or ectopic teeth (Figure 9.1).
- Treatment of impacted supernumerary teeth (Figure 9.2).
- Removal of infraoccluded teeth.
- Exposure of unerupted teeth.
- Tooth transplantation.
- Frenectomy.
- Pericision.
- Single tooth osteotomy.
- Orthognathic surgery (see Chapter 19).

General factors to be taken into account when orthodontic treatment is considered

The presence of a malocclusion does not *per se* indicate a need for treatment. In addition, there are often many different treatment options, and only by consideration of all factors can the most appropriate treatment be determined. These factors are:

- Patient's expectation, desire and cooperation.
- Patient's age.
- Oral hygiene and diet.
- Caries experience.
- Teeth of poor prognosis.
- Crowding.
- Hypodontia and microdontia.
- Other space requirements including levelling curves of Spee, centreline correction and expansion or constriction of the arches (including overjet reduction).

In determining the most appropriate treatment for a patient when a combination of dentoalveolar surgery and orthodontics may be required, it is imperative that the patient and those undertaking both the surgery and the orthodontic therapy all have a full understanding of the aims of treatment. This is best achieved by undertaking a joint consultation in which the risks and benefits of all options can be discussed and considered. Although the age at which treatment starts seems to vary from country to country, there seems to be little difference in clinical practice in our countries.

Impacted or ectopic teeth

Although any tooth may become impacted (i.e. its path of eruption is obstructed), those affected commonly are the lower third molars, upper canines, upper second premolars and upper incisors. These teeth may also be ectopically placed (i.e. the follicle develops in a remote position). Untreated, many impacted or ectopic teeth cause no problems and remain largely asymptomatic. However, a significant number may either develop complications or,

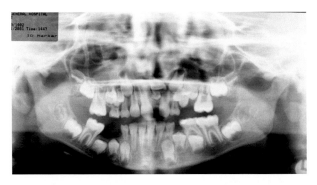

Figure 9.2 Supernumerary teeth preventing eruption of UL1.

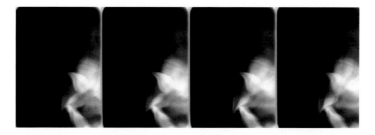

Figure 9.3 Tomograms of a dilacerated upper central incisor.

if an anterior tooth is affected, may cause aesthetic or functional problems.

If a decision is made not to undertake active intervention, the affected tooth must be kept under close observation, both clinically and, where appropriate, radiographically. Complications of impacted or ectopic teeth include:

- Prevention of eruption of adjacent tooth.
- Cystic change in associated follicle – a very rare occurrence.
- Resorption of adjacent teeth with loss of vitality – this most commonly occurs when upper canines resorb the roots of upper lateral and central incisors. Initiation of this process is, however, extremely rare after 15 years of age.

In view of these rare sequelae the value of routine radiographic screening of impacted or ectopic teeth is controversial, especially in view of more recent radiation exposure guidelines. Because complications are relatively rare, the healthcare benefit to the patient of repeated radiographs is limited. The decision therefore to radiograph these teeth regularly is a difficult one, especially if they have been quiescent and asymptomatic for a number of years.

If ectopic or impacted teeth are partially erupted, then they are at risk of the usual complications, particularly if their position prevents adequate oral hygiene measures:

- Advanced caries.
- Periodontal disease.

Failure of incisor eruption

Failure of eruption of upper incisors is relatively rare and can occur for many reasons including

previous trauma, root dilacerations (Figure 9.3), presence of a supernumerary, local failure of eruptive mechanisms or the presence of pathology. If an upper central incisor is noted to be delayed in its eruption, then a thorough clinical and radiographic examination is warranted. This would be the case if the tooth remains unerupted significantly after the expected time of eruption (6 to 7 years of age), if one incisor is unerupted more than 6 months after its contralateral partner has erupted or if it is unerupted after the eruption of the lateral incisors.

Clinical examination should note the status of the primary dentition and the position and angulation of adjacent teeth and should involve palpation of the buccal sulcus and palatal vault. Primary radiographic investigation of the area should identify the reason for failure of eruption, and an upper anterior occlusal view is a useful means to do this. Radiographs should be examined for evidence of supernumerary teeth and root dilaceration and to ensure an intact periodontal ligament. If failure of eruption results from dilaceration of the root, orthodontic alignment will be possible only if the degree of dilaceration is not severe. This is best determined using two views perpendicular to each other (e.g. an upper anterior occlusal view and a lateral cephalogram).

If failure of eruption results from severe dilaceration, ankylosis or resorption (internal or external), then the only option is to extract the tooth. This should be undertaken in the same manner as for any unerupted tooth, with accurate localization, adequate surgical exposure and careful removal. If the unerupted incisor appears of normal morphology with no obvious cause for the failure of eruption, then it should be exposed and given the opportunity to erupt.

Supernumerary teeth

Supernumerary teeth are relatively rare, with an incidence of 1% to 3% in the permanent dentition and 0.3% to 0.6% in the primary dentition. Most are located in the maxilla (90% to 98%), with most of these found in the premaxilla.

These teeth can be described by their morphology, being either rudimentary or supplemental. Supplemental supernumerary teeth tend to erupt and are then usually extracted to allow normal alignment of neighbouring teeth.

There are three types of rudimentary supernumerary teeth:

- Conical – these have normal root development and can be inverted. They are usually positioned between the upper incisors but can become palatally placed as the rest of the dentition develops forward and downward.
- Tuberculate – these are barrel-shaped teeth with little or no root formation.
- Complex/compound odontomes.

The decision whether treatment is required depends on the site of the supernumerary teeth and whether they will affect the eruption or development of adjacent teeth. To localize the position of the supernumerary teeth, the parallax technique should be used. Parallax is the apparent movement of an object relative to another object when the position of view is altered. As the position of view is shifted, the farthest object away moves in the same direction as that of the view.

Therefore, unerupted teeth can be localized using either vertical parallax, with an orthopantomogram (OPG) and one other view (either upper anterior occlusal or periapical), or horizontal parallax using two periapical views taken at different angulations. In orthodontic practice it is usual to use vertical parallax with an OPG and upper anterior occlusal view. In this situation the position of view has shifted vertically upward. If the object is palatal or lingual to the reference structure, then it will move in the same direction vertically. This is also known as the SLOB rule (i.e. same lingual opposite buccal). Conversely, if the object is buccal, then it will move in the opposite direction (i.e. downward) (Figure 9.4 (a) and (b)).

Conical supernumerary teeth often erupt and in these cases often have no effect on adjacent tooth

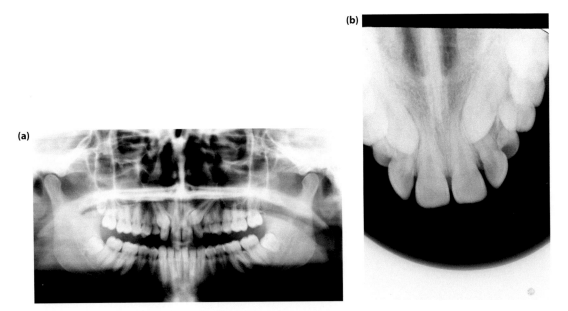

Figure 9.4 (a) and (b) Vertical parallax using an orthopantomogram and an upper anterior occlusal view allowing localization of ectopic canines. Note how the crowns of both canines move with the tube toward the apex of the incisors, thus revealing them to be palatally placed.

eruption but may affect tooth position. They can also be a rare cause of a median diastema. If they erupt, then they should be extracted. Inverted conical supernumerary teeth will not erupt and may, depending on their position, affect adjacent tooth development. If this is the case, then they should be surgically extracted. Tuberculate supernumerary teeth often develop in the cingulum area of the upper central incisors and are a common cause of their failure to erupt.

If a supernumerary tooth is present and preventing tooth eruption, it requires removal. The decision how and when to undertake treatment will involve thorough assessment of the severity of the problem and general patient-related factors including the patient's attitude to treatment and what other treatment may be required. Both immediate removal and delayed removal of supernumerary teeth have been advocated.

Immediate or early intervention for all supernumerary teeth has the advantage that it prevents or minimizes disturbance of development of surrounding teeth. However, it does place adjacent teeth at risk of damage and may not be necessary because no problems may ensue. Delayed treatment ensures there is less risk of damage to adjacent teeth, a significant risk in younger patients with incomplete root formation.

The decision whether to undertake immediate or delayed treatment has therefore caused much debate. Conical supernumerary teeth should be left under observation unless they are causing developmental disturbance. Tuberculate and inverted conical supernumerary teeth should be removed immediately if this can be achieved with no harm to adjacent teeth. If, however, the upper central incisors have erupted, treatment should be delayed until after the eruption of the lateral incisors because early treatment will not have any significant effect on tooth position.

Surgery is usually best undertaken using a general anaesthetic because treatment is often on relatively young patients and good access is required. If the unerupted incisor is relatively superficial, then an open eruption technique should be used. If the tooth is deep, then a closed eruption technique is probably better. In the past some have advocated simple removal of the supernumerary teeth alone to allow eruption of the incisor teeth, whereas others have advocated concurrent bonding of an attachment in case orthodontic traction is subsequently required.

There is evidence that a significant proportion of incisors will subsequently fail to erupt. In that case reoperation will be needed if supernumerary tooth removal alone has been undertaken to bond an attachment to allow orthodontic traction. Therefore, a decision to undertake supernumerary tooth removal alone may mean a further operation, and for some clinicians placing an attachment has become the 'default' position. This decision will be influenced by how ectopic the incisor is, the age of the patient, the relative stage of root development and the space available. If it is believed that there is a possibility that the tooth will not erupt, then it is appropriate to attach a bracket to the tooth or teeth to allow orthodontic traction at a later date if there is no evidence of subsequent spontaneous eruption.

A bracket and gold chain combination is usually the attachment of choice, and this allows orthodontic traction to be placed on the tooth either using a sectional fixed appliance or a removable appliance.

Surgery

A full-thickness mucoperiosteal flap is raised palatally. If possible the nasopalatine structures should be preserved, although there are few reported adverse consequences if for reasons of access they need to be transected. They do bleed, however, so have bone wax handy. The primary teeth and any overlying bone should be carefully removed to expose the supernumerary teeth. Only enough bone should be removed to expose the tooth adequately because excessive bone removal has no advantage and may lead to poor periodontal support. Care should be taken not to involve the exposed tooth below the cementoenamel junction because damage to this structure can lead to ankylosis. Care should also be taken not to disturb or damage the adjacent incisors. Before wound closure an attachment should be placed if clinically necessary (see later for technique).

Canines

The incidence of impaction of the maxillary canine is between 0.9% and 2.2%. It is twice as common in female patients as in male patients and is much more common palatally than buccally. The incidence of impacted lower canines is low. Many aetiological factors have been cited including generalized systemic causes, crowding, prolonged retention or early loss of the deciduous canine, ectopic development of the tooth bud, presence of an alveolar cleft, ankylosis, formation of cysts or neoplasms or dilacerations of the root. Palatal impaction is known to be more common in individuals with diminutive or absent lateral incisors. This has led to the theory that the lateral incisor root is important to guide the canine into position, although this theory is unproven and perhaps simplistic. Impacted upper canines, both palatal and buccal, are often causes of lateral incisor resorption and this tends to be initiated relatively early, before the age of 11 years (Figure 9.5 (a) and (b)).

Permanent upper canines normally erupt around 11 to 12 years of age. If they cannot be palpated in the buccal sulcus by 9 to 10 years of age, then a thorough clinical and radiographic investigation should be undertaken to locate them accurately. If the canine is buccally placed it can usually be palpated and the lateral incisor may appear proclined because its root has had to take up a relatively palatal position to accommodate the buccally placed root. If, however, the canine is palatally placed, then the lateral root is usually in a normal position. A bulge may be palpable palatally, although this is often present only when the canine is relatively superficial in older patients. Radiographic investigation by the parallax technique should again be used to localize the canines. Radiographs should also be used to assess the condition of the roots of adjacent teeth because a significant proportion of patients will suffer some root resorption, although this is rarely severe.

If ectopic canine development is identified at an early stage, interceptive treatment can be instigated to correct the canine's eruptive path. This involves the removal of the deciduous predecessor and has a good success rate, especially in less severe cases where there is no crowding.

If, however, the problem is not identified until later, then other treatment options are required, frequently involving both orthodontic treatment and surgery. Treatment planning again needs to take account of general patient-related factors including issues such as the patient's desire, expectation and cooperation (Figure 9.6).

Management options are protean and should be fully discussed with the patient and parents or carers before any definitive treatment planning decisions are made. Informed consent should be sought because what could be a routine although complex treatment for a patient during adolescence may become extremely difficult if it is delayed until later in life.

Options include those discussed in the following subsections:

Observation

Observation can be performed clinically, including vitality testing of adjacent teeth, and radiographically using a number of techniques. There are, however, a number of potential problems that need to be considered before it is decided to leave the canine under observation. An ectopic canine can occasionally cause severe root resorption of adjacent teeth, and this is often apparent only on radiographic investigation while being unsuspected clinically.

When the deciduous canine is retained, its long-term prognosis is uncertain. If it is lost, the patient

(a)

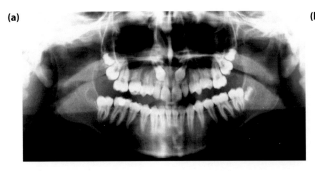

(b)

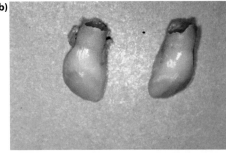

Figure 9.5 (a) An orthopantomogram shows severe resorption of both upper lateral incisors by ectopic canines. (b) Appearance of the upper lateral incisors after their removal.

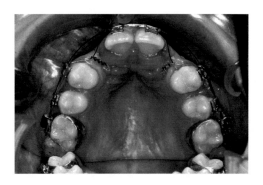

Figure 9.6 Fixed appliances used to align ectopic canines that have had gold chains attached.

either will be left with an unaesthetic gap or will require a complex restoration that will, in all probability, have to be replaced at regular intervals. The deciduous canine may also suffer significant attrition by the lower permanent canine if it is retained for an extended period, and this is concomitant with overeruption of the lower canine, potentially complicating any future restorative care because of the lack of vertical space in which to place a restoration.

In view of the potential long-term problems that can arise if no active treatment is undertaken, it is best to discuss all options carefully. Patients with ectopic canines often have acceptable aesthetics and function, unlike patients with other types of malocclusion. The benefits of treatment are consequently less obvious, and only later in life will a problem manifest, such as when the deciduous canine is lost.

Surgical removal

An ectopic canine should be removed only if it is resorbing adjacent teeth, if its follicle has undergone cystic change or if retention will prevent adoption of a comprehensive orthodontic approach. The decision to electively remove the permanent canine rather than any other tooth as part of comprehensive treatment is somewhat controversial. Aligning the canine is potentially advantageous for many reasons, including the fact that some clinicians believe that it is functionally important to establish canine guidance. In addition, because it has excellent longevity, the canine may be useful for future restorative care if required or preferred over the first premolar on aesthetic grounds. This view that the canines should always be retained is based

on a somewhat historical perspective and does not take into account changes in the pattern of dental disease. It is now accepted that as long as there is a mutually protected occlusion, canine guidance *per se* is not required. Prolonged treatment to align a canine is difficult to justify for aesthetic reasons or for future restorative considerations, especially as we can now expect most adults to retain the majority of their teeth in the long term.

There are risks associated with upper permanent canine removal, including not only those associated with general anaesthesia (which is normally required), but also iatrogenic damage to adjacent teeth and supporting structures. These risks often outweigh the benefits of removal in most cases.

The principles of surgical removal are no different from those described for removal of retained roots. Accurate localization is essential because this affects the approach to the tooth, especially for upper canines. Most are palatally positioned and therefore require a palatal flap for access. After the flap is raised, bone may have to be removed either with chisels or a burr and the tooth localized. It can be removed either *en bloc* or divided and removed in pieces. Extreme care should be taken not to damage adjacent roots. Occasionally the broken instrument technique can be applied, passing the elevator through the buccal cortex or the nasal floor.

Surgical exposure and alignment

Before the decision is made to expose and align the canine, the patient has to be aware that to achieve a satisfactory result, complex fixed appliance treatment will be required. This often takes in excess of 2 years and may include the need for dual arch fixed appliances to allow for the use of interarch elastics and to allow arch coordination.

Before surgery is undertaken, a decision has to be made between open or closed eruption. The aim of any exposure is to uncover enough of the crown either to place an attachment or to prevent recovering of the crown during the healing phase. The most important principle of surgery is to ensure the tooth will erupt through keratinized mucosa. If this does not happen, as can occur with buccally placed canines, then the post-treatment periodontal condition will be compromised. This can obviously affect gingival aesthetics and health.

Closed eruption

Closed eruption uses an attachment secured to the tooth to apply orthodontic traction and is useful in the treatment of markedly ectopic teeth in which it would be difficult to undertake an adequate open exposure. It is often used when the canine is palatally positioned. It can be used for the treatment of buccal canines, but the results can be disappointing if the attachment herniates through the thin buccal gingivae. To avoid this, the attachment should be placed either on the tip of the tooth or palatally. This is sometimes not possible because the crown position increases the risk of either excessive bone removal or iatrogenic damage to adjacent structures. It is, however, useful in the treatment of buccal canines if the crown overlies an adjacent tooth and it would be difficult to undertake an apically repositioned flap.

Surgery involves the same access as that for the removal of the tooth, except that great care must be taken not to damage the cementum of the root surface because this can lead to ankylosis of the tooth and subsequent failure of eruption. An adequate amount of the crown should be exposed to allow attachment of the bracket and chain. Before bonding the bracket to the tooth the area should be as uncontaminated as possible. Bleeding should be arrested as much as practicable with the use of local vasoconstrictors (as would be found in local anaesthetics) or the use of diathermy. Once the area is prepared the tooth surface should be washed with saline or water and then prepared for bonding either with acid etch or with self-etch priming agents. The latter agents offer the advantage that they do not need to be rinsed off, they need less time to prepare the tooth and they are to some extent hydrophilic.

Once the tooth surface has been prepared the bracket can be secured either with chemical or light cured composite. The bracket should be tested to ensure that it is securely in place before wound closure. The chain or ligature can exit either through the wound margin on the alveolar ridge or through a stab incision elsewhere if it is believed that this would give a better vector of traction to align the tooth.

With teeth that are significantly ectopic or are close to the roots of adjacent teeth it is sometimes useful for the orthodontist to be present at the time of surgery. This allows an assessment of the relationship of the canine with adjacent structures and to plan the vector of traction that will be most appropriate.

Open eruption

Open eruption is often the treatment of choice for both buccally and palatally ectopic teeth.

> Buccally placed teeth – the most important principle of surgery is to ensure that the tooth erupts through keratinized gingivae, and this means that care has to be taken with flap design. This can effectively be achieved if an apically repositioned flap technique is used. A flap is raised either from the keratinized gingivae of the alveolar ridge if the area the tooth is to erupt into is edentulous or from the gingival cuff of the deciduous predecessor, which should be extracted at the same time as the surgery is undertaken. The design and direction of the relieving incisions allow the tooth to be exposed and the flap to be sutured into position, thus exposing an adequate amount of the crown of the canine (Figure 9.7 (a) and (b)).

(a)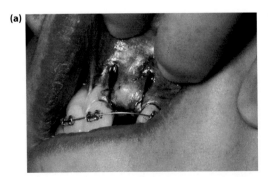
(b)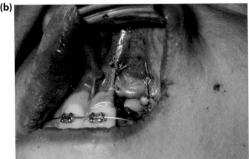

Figure 9.7 (a) Incision for apically repositioned flap UL3. (b) Apically repositioned flap complete.

Palatally placed canines – open eruption can also be used in the treatment of palatally ectopic canines, especially when they are relatively superficial. Because the palatal mucosa is all keratinized the problem of ensuring that the tooth erupts through keratinized gingivae is less relevant. The most important principle of surgery is to ensure that adequate crown is exposed to guarantee that there is no chance that the crown will be covered again during the healing phase. If necessary a bracket can be attached at the time of surgery in the same manner as for closed eruption. Again, care must be taken to ensure that the cementum is not damaged during surgery and that keratinized mucosa is left overlying the cementoenamel junction. Interestingly, even if large areas of bone are left denuded, postoperative healing is usually excellent and uneventful. Packs can be placed over the exposed tooth to aid haemostasis, to promote the patient's comfort and prevent the tooth from becoming covered again. This has historically involved the placing of ribbon gauze soaked in Whitehead's varnish secured in place with mattress-type sutures. Periodontal dressings, such as Coe-Pack, can also be used. This pack should be removed after 7 to 14 days, after which vigorous oral hygiene measures should be instigated by the patient to encourage healing, prevent gingival overgrowth and promote eruption (Figures 9.8 and 9.9).

Surgical repositioning

With the development of fixed appliance therapy and its relative acceptance by patients, the need

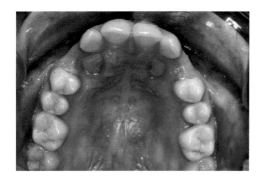

Figure 9.8 Exposed ectopic canines 3 months postoperatively.

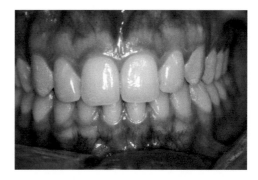

Figure 9.9 Exposed canines following comprehensive orthodontic treatment.

for surgical repositioning has become relatively rare. The most common indication is in a patient who is unwilling to accept fixed appliance therapy, who has sufficient space for the tooth to be repositioned and in whom it is believed possible to remove the tooth surgically without damaging it or adjacent teeth. This procedure is synonymous with tooth transplantation and the technique is covered later. If space needs to be created for the tooth before implantation, then it can be 'parked' by placing it underneath the mucosa in the buccal sulcus until it is required. This maintains the vitality of the cells of the cementum and periodontal ligament.

Other ectopic teeth

The same principles used in the treatment of ectopic canines can be applied to other ectopic or impacted teeth. The underlying principle to consider is whether it is possible, desirable and necessary to align the tooth. If greater harm or little benefit will accrue, then it is probable that another course of action should be undertaken.

Infraoccluded primary teeth

Infraocclusion of primary teeth is relatively common and is caused by a focal area of ankylosis preventing normal eruption during dentoalveolar development. It is often self-limiting, with the tooth either re-erupting or being exfoliated before the eruption of its permanent successor.

Occasionally, severe infraocclusion occurs, and this is defined as when the marginal ridge of the primary tooth is below the level of the gingival margin. In these situations the tooth should be extracted. These extractions are usually uneventful, and the area of ankylosis does not cause any significant problem. Occasionally, when the infraocclusion occurs early, the deciduous tooth totally submerges and not only prevents eruption of its successor but may also cause adjacent teeth to tip toward the infraoccluded tooth, restrict development of the dentoalveolus (leading to lateral open bites) or, because of its continued communication with the oral cavity, may lead to decay, periodontal disease or periapical pathology. In these cases it is appropriate to remove the tooth, and the technique employed depends on accurate localization of the tooth by clinical and radiographic examination (Figures 9.10 and 9.11).

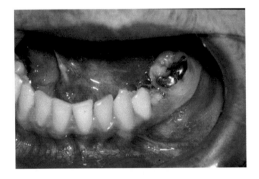

Figure 9.10 Infraoccluded LLE.

Tooth transplantation

Tooth transplantation is a useful technique in a small number of clinical situations. For example, transplantation has been advocated to reposition ectopic canines, to replace developmentally absent teeth or to replace a tooth lost following trauma or pathology. In most of these situations there are other more appropriate treatments, but in recent years there has been renewed interest in tooth transplantation to replace upper incisors lost following trauma. The most commonly affected are the upper anterior segment incisors, lost from root fracture, periapical infection, ankylosis or external or internal root resorption (Figure 9.12 (a)). It is usually possible to undertake premolar transplantation only to replace lost central incisors because lateral incisors, unless they are extremely large, do not have adequate mesiodistal width for this to be a good aesthetic alternative. This is an especially useful treatment choice if the patient has crowded dentition and would require premolar extractions as part of a course of comprehensive orthodontic treatment.

The technique can be used for any ectopic teeth, such as canines, in which a decision has been made to undertake transplantation rather than orthodontic alignment. Teeth should be transplanted just before or on completion of root formation, ideally when there is still an open apex. In these situations there is the possibility of revascularization and possibly reinnervation of the transplanted tooth.

Preoperatively space is created orthodontically (Figure 9.12 (b)). A socket is prepared to accept

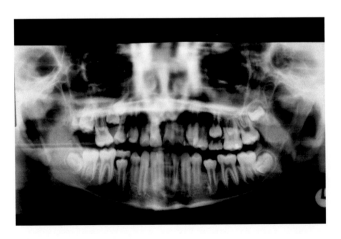

Figure 9.11 Severely infraoccluded URE preventing eruption of UR5.

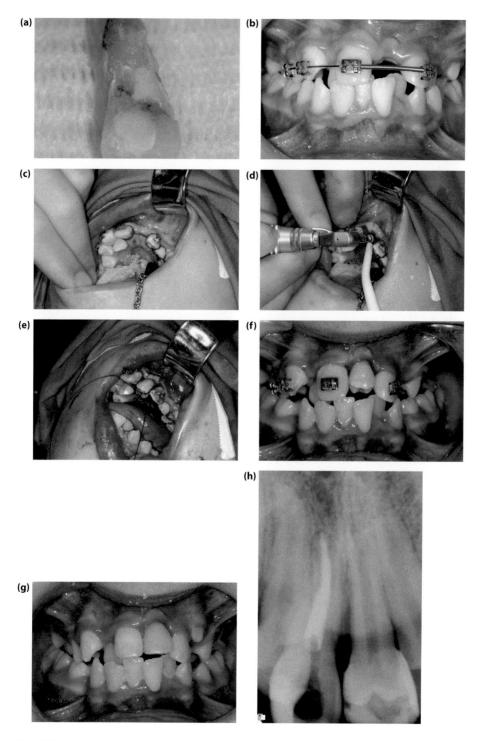

Figure 9.12 (a) Extracted UL1 previously traumatized and suffering root fracture. (b) Space created for premolar transplant by using fixed appliances. (c) Incision for premolar transplant. (d) Donor site created with trephine. (e) Transplanted tooth held in place with mattress suture. (f) Postoperative appearance of transplanted lower first premolar. (g) Transplanted premolar following placement of composite veneer. (h) Radiograph showing good periapical healing. Note root-filled UR1 traumatized at the same time as lost UL1.

the tooth by using burrs with water irrigation to prevent bone overheating and subsequent necrosis (Figure 9.12 (c) and (d)). If further future eruption would be beneficial (e.g. in a growing patient), then again, care should be taken to prevent damage to the cementum; otherwise, ankylosis may occur that would prevent further eruption.

Once the tooth has been transplanted it should be splinted for 7 to 14 days. This may be with a preformed splint cemented with a luting material or even with appropriately placed sutures (Figure 9.12 (e)). The patient should be warned not to disturb the area during the healing phase to allow optimal healing of the periodontal ligament.

If the apex of the tooth was closed before transplantation, then a root filling should be placed immediately. If, however, the apex was open at transplantation, then there is still the possibility of revascularization of the pulpal tissue. In this situation the tooth should be reviewed using the same protocol as would be used for an avulsed incisor. This involves assessment of the tooth's colour, colour when viewed with transillumination, pulpal vitality (response to electrical or thermal testing) and radiographic appearance. Obviously if there is evidence of pulpal necrosis, then the pulpal tissue should be extirpated and root canal therapy instigated (Figure 9.12 (f)). Once good healing of the periodontal ligament has occurred and the tooth is quiescent, then appropriate restorative treatment can be undertaken to improve aesthetics.

The long-term success of tooth transplantation appears excellent in experienced hands, and it is definitely an option to be considered in certain appropriately selected cases. There does, however, need to be good multidisciplinary support from other specialties, such as paediatric and restorative dentistry, in order that optimal results can be achieved (Figure 9.12 (g) and (h)).

Frenectomy

A prominent labial frenum is often thought to be the most common cause of a midline diastema, and resection of the frenum has therefore been advocated as a cure. Unfortunately, the frenum is rarely implicated in the aetiology of midline diastemas, which usually have other causes such as generalized spacing, microdont laterals, the stage of dental development (the so-called ugly duckling stage), the presence of pathology or the presence of a midline supernumerary tooth.

Even if the frenum is thought to be implicated in the presence of the diastema, its resection will not guarantee the stability of closure, and permanent retention will be required. Early intervention should be avoided because spontaneous closure may occur with continued dental development. The decision whether resection is necessary should therefore be delayed until the patient is established in the adult dentition.

Assessment of whether the frenum is a primary aetiological factor in the presence of a midline diastema is difficult. If, on gentle pulling of the upper lip to place pressure on the frenum, there is blanching of the palatal mucosa in the area of the incisive papilla, then this may indicate that fibres are passing through the diastema into the palatal tissues and there will therefore be little chance of spontaneous closure (Figure 9.13). If radiographs reveal a notch in the midpalatal suture, it is believed to indicate that fibres are passing through the diastema. However, both these tests are open to criticism regarding their accuracy and validity.

Therefore, a labial frenum should be removed only if it is causing problems with aesthetics or is preventing adequate oral hygiene procedures to be undertaken. Some clinicians still believe that resection is beneficial, even though neither spontaneous closure nor stability of orthodontic closure is guaranteed.

If resection is undertaken, then its timing is also controversial. Some authorities advocate labial frenectomy before orthodontic treatment, whereas others advocate it to be undertaken just

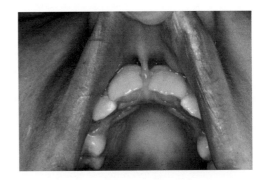

Figure 9.13 Prominent labial frenum showing blanching of the incisive papilla on gentle tension.

before or on completion of space closure so that the scar tissue formed will prevent reopening of the diastema. Neither method has any evidence of efficacy that recommends it over the other. Also as previously stated, to guarantee stability, long-term retention will still be required, and so the reason for the resection has to be brought into question.

Lingual frenectomy

This is not a procedure directly related to orthodontics, but release of the lingual frenum (tongue tie) is a relatively common operation. It may be requested at a range of ages. Neonates are sometimes referred for and in some services offered simple resection of a tight frenum. The child is wrapped in a blanket, and the frenum is cut with scissors. This is not a technique we advocate because it is impossible to visualize the submandibular ducts and it is painful to the neonate. Other children are referred by paediatric speech and language therapists when the children are between 6 and 12 months old and sometimes later with a concern over speech development. Although it may well be reasonable to carry out frenectomy, it is essential to ensure that the parent and the practitioners involved understand that release of the tongue tip may or may not improve aspects of speech.

Older children may request lingual frenectomy at the ice cream licking stage, and teenagers and adults may request it for other reasons related to tongue tip mobility.

Technique

The simplest effective technique is, after appropriate anaesthesia, to put the tongue tip on traction and incise the tightest part of the frenum. This allows the tongue to lengthen, and a diamond-shaped wound opens up that can be simply closed with a few interrupted resorbable sutures. Z-plasty has been described but runs a higher risk of damaging the submandibular ducts for no discernible advantage.

Circumferential supracrestal fibrotomy

Circumferential supracrestal fibrotomy or pericision is a technique used to prevent or reduce relapse

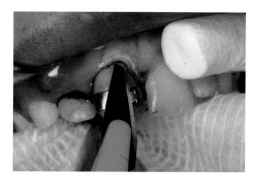

Figure 9.14 The incision for pericision.

of rotated or severely ectopic teeth. Following orthodontic treatment, most fibres in the periodontal ligament rearrange within 4 to 6 months. The supracrestal fibres, however, do not and remain displaced in the long term. The exact mechanism of how these fibres cause relapse is poorly understood. Collagen fibres have no contractile properties, and this could explain the relapse of tooth position toward the pretreatment position, although fibres are seen to be stretched following tooth movement, and it may be that the recovery of these fibres to their normal length is responsible for the relapse seen.

Pericision involves the sectioning of these fibres in order that they reattach to the tooth in its new position. Unfortunately, many studies have shown that there is not complete prevention of relapse and therefore other adjunctive retention techniques are still required if alignment is to be maintained.

The sectioning of the fibres should be undertaken using local anaesthesia. A scalpel blade is passed down the periodontal ligament to the alveolar crest around the whole circumference of the tooth (Figure 9.14). In the lower incisor region where the gingivae are thinner and more friable, if complete circumferential supracrestal fibrotomy is undertaken, then there is the danger of gingival recession labially. In these areas, therefore, sectioning of the interdental papilla alone should be undertaken. This involves passing of a scalpel blade directly through the interdental papillae to the alveolar crest.

Single tooth osteotomy

Very occasionally it is necessary to undertake a localized osteotomy to reposition a single tooth

(a) 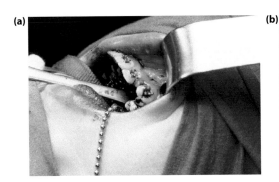 (b)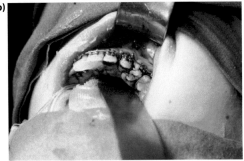

Figure 9.15 (a) Single tooth osteotomy, tooth and bone segment osteotomized. (b) Canine repositioned with supporting bone and immobilized with arch wire.

that has, for whatever reason, been impossible to align orthodontically. This is usually a treatment of last resort, and the condition may be the result of ankylosis (secondary to trauma, infection, replacement, resorption) or primary failure of eruption. Before the osteotomy is undertaken, adequate space must be available to allow correct tooth positioning. It also has to be realized that there will be no further tooth movement or development following surgery, and so if there is significant further growth expected, then there will be relative recurrence of the problem after treatment. In addition, minimal further orthodontic tooth movement will be achievable.

A palatal flap is raised to allow mesial and distal cuts to be undertaken through to the buccal cortex. A superior cut is also made, although because of the angle of access this cut will not pass through to the buccal side. This cut is completed via a vertical incision in the buccal sulcus above the attached keratinized mucosa. This ensures that the keratinized mucosa on the buccal side is not disrupted and the blood supply to the osteotomized segment is maintained (Figure 9.15 (a)). Osteotomy is made simpler by piezosurgery, which minimizes bone removal. Once the segment has been gently mobilized it is possible either to reposition it immediately and immobilize it using an arch wire (Figure 9.15 (b)) or to undertake gentle alignment of the segment orthodontically over a period of days and weeks in a manner analogous to distraction osteogenesis. This second method

is useful if the tooth is a significant distance from its desired position.

FURTHER READING

Becker A. *The orthodontic treatment of impacted teeth,* 3rd ed. Oxford: Wiley-Blackwell, 2012.
A detailed look at this subject.
Faculty of Dental Surgery, Royal College of Surgeons of England. *National clinical guidelines, 1997.* London: Royal College of Surgeons of England, 1997.
Because if we are going to have guidelines you should know what they are!
Isaacson KG, Thom AR, Horner K, Whaites E. *Orthodontic radiographs: guidelines,* 3rd ed. London: British Orthodontic Society, 2008.
See above.
Lindhe J, Lang NP, Karring T. *Clinical periodontology and implant dentistry,* 3rd ed. Copenhagen: Munksgaard, 2003, Chapter 25.
A definitive guide to this area from one of the much published masters of international periodontology.
Mitchell L. *An introduction to orthodontics,* 4th ed. Oxford: Oxford University Press, 2013.
Self-evident really, it contains a good overview of the surgical-orthodontic interface.
Tsukiboshi M. *Autotransplantation of teeth.* Chicago: Quintessence, 2001.
Beautiful pictures.

10

Orofacial infections

Contents

Aim

- To appreciate the importance of infectious processes in oral and maxillofacial surgery.

Learning outcomes for undergraduates and postgraduates

- To be able to describe how microorganisms may cause infections of the maxillofacial region.
- To be able to discuss how infections remote from the maxillofacial region may complicate treatment of the oral and maxillofacial surgery patient.
- To be able to describe how these infections may be prevented and treated.

- To understand the role of infection in the prevention and treatment of bisphosphonate-related osteonecrosis of the jaws.

The oral and maxillofacial microbial flora

The oral and maxillofacial region is the major interface between the individual and the external environment. As a result it is constantly exposed to microorganisms that may give rise to infection.

Three areas, each with their own specific microflora, are of importance to the oral and maxillofacial surgeon:

- The cutaneous regions of the face.
- The oral cavity.
- The nasal cavity and paranasal air sinuses.

A basic knowledge of the microflora of these areas is important when planning prophylaxis or empirical treatment of infection.

Skin flora

- Staphylococci.
- Streptococci of the viridans group.
- Gram-positive and gram-negative diphtheroids.
- *Candida albicans.*
- *Malassezia furfur.*

Mouth flora

- Alpha-haemolytic streptococci.
- Nonhaemolytic streptococci.
- Gram-negative cocci.
- *Actinomyces* species.
- *Actinobacillus actinomycetemcomitans.*
- Gram-negative anaerobic rods.
- Spirochaetes.
- *Candida* species.

Nasal cavity and paranasal sinuses

- Gram-positive rods.
- Gram-positive cocci.
- Gram-negative cocci (e.g. *Neisseria*).

Host defence mechanisms

Specific and nonspecific host defence mechanisms exist to prevent microbial infection. These are well developed in the head and neck region. These mechanisms include the following: an intact epithelial surface; and nasal mucus, saliva and tears, all of which have antimicrobial properties. The mixed microbial flora that is present also acts as an important nonspecific defence mechanism (commensal microflora). If this flora is altered, overgrowth of certain organisms can occur, leading to symptomatic infection (opportunistic infection). This is exemplified by the frequency with which candidal infection occurs following broad-spectrum antibiotic therapy.

Diagnosis of infections

Accurate diagnosis of infection is important both for treatment and for public health management. Prompt identification of the organism causing infection enables the antimicrobial therapy to be specifically directed, which may allow rapid resolution of symptoms and minimizes the opportunity for the development of resistant strains of bacteria. This approach requires careful collection of specimens, accurate labelling and the provision of adequate clinical details to allow the clinical microbiologist to carry out the appropriate culture and sensitivity testing. It is important to be aware that the specimen can be contaminated by normal flora, and where possible the sample should be obtained by aspiration, rather than by swabbing the area or collecting a 'pure' pus sample from a drained abscess. If anaerobic or specific infections (e.g. tuberculosis) are suspected, then designated containers should be used. Samples should be sent to the laboratory without delay to ensure that culture of any organisms is possible. Warn the laboratory if a biohazard specimen such as tuberculosis is suspected.

Serology can be useful, particularly in the case of viral and mycoplasmal infections. It may be possible to identify viral antigens in serum, but it is more common to measure serum antibodies. This can allow the demonstration of a rising antibody titre over several days. It can also allow for identification of previous exposure.

Prophylaxis

It is not possible to sterilize the oral cavity before intraoral surgery, and bacteraemia is inevitable. What is not known is the significance of this bacteraemia.

This is also the case in traumatic wounds to the facial skin. The bacteraemia may be mild and readily dealt with by a patient with an intact host defence system. However, in the presence of underlying systemic disease, host defences may be overwhelmed. This may give rise to wound infection or more generalized sepsis. If the patient has a foreign body in place (e.g. a prosthetic joint or a structural lesion of a heart valve), then infection may develop at these sites following the bacteraemia. Examples of at-risk patients include the following categories:

- Advanced age.
- Prolonged surgery – longer than 3 hours.
- Prosthetic material placed (e.g. implants including plates and screws).
- Impaired host defences – malignancy, malnutrition, uncompensated metabolic disease (e.g. diabetes, patients on steroids or other immunosuppressants).
- Patients with cardiac valve lesions (e.g. after rheumatic fever, endocarditis; patients with prosthetic valves). This illustrates well the capacity for international controversy – the current UK National Institute for Health and Care Excellence (NICE) guidelines do not require clinicians to provide antibiotic cover for patients at risk of infective endocarditis (CG64). However, similar national bodies in many other countries recommend the exact opposite.

The principles of prophylaxis are as follows:

1. The procedure must carry a significant risk of postoperative infection or the consequence of infection must be significant.
2. The correct antibiotic should be used (i.e. one that the relevant bacteria are sensitive to and the patient is not allergic to).
3. The antibiotic should be administered in the correct manner at the correct time (i.e. just before the bacteraemia, to ensure a microbicidal level of antibiotic is in the tissue that will be contaminated).

Acute bacterial infections

Pericoronitis

The lower third molars are the most commonly affected in pericoronitis (see also Chapter 8). During eruption the tooth is covered by a flap of gingival tissue, the operculum. This can result in the formation of a pocket, which may act as a food trap and provide a favourable environment for anaerobic bacteria. This flap can be traumatized by the opposing tooth and become inflamed. The most common symptom is pain associated with a partially erupted tooth. The operculum is inflamed, and it may be possible to express pus or food debris from beneath the flap. The degree of systemic upset is variable. There may be trismus, lymphadenopathy and spread of infection to the adjacent fascial spaces.

Treatment

Débridement of the infected area may be all that is required in uncomplicated cases if the tooth is to be retained. Any abscess should be drained. If there is obvious trauma from an opposing tooth that is otherwise nonfunctional, then removal of this tooth may allow resolution of the symptoms. The affected tooth can be reviewed and arrangements made for its removal, if indicated.

Alveolar osteitis

Dry socket occurs when there is loss of the clot formed at the time of tooth extraction (see also Chapter 6). This results in local osteitis of the extraction socket. It is characterized by a distinctive pain (often described as a toothache getting worse after the tooth has been removed) and an offensive smell.

Treatment

Treatment consists of irrigation of the socket and placement of an obtundent dressing. This may be supplemented with metronidazole 200–400 mg three times a day for 3 days to eradicate any secondary anaerobic infection that is present.

Acute periodontal disease

This is much less common than chronic periodontal disease, which is universal. It is being seen much more frequently in patients with impaired host mechanisms such as those with human immunodeficiency virus (HIV) infection. It tends to be an exacerbation of underlying chronic periodontal disease. Treatment of the underlying condition must be considered when planning management of these patients.

Necrotizing ulcerative gingivitis

This is a painful and unpleasant condition. It is most commonly seen in patients who smoke and have poor oral hygiene. It may be more common at times of severe stress. Pain is a prominent feature and may prevent the patient from achieving adequate food and fluid intake. There is usually an offensive odour from the mouth and bleeding from the gingivae following minimal pressure. The interdental papillae are initially affected, with the rest of the gingivae subsequently becoming involved (Figure 10.1). There may be marked loss of periodontal support. Cancrum oris (noma) is an extreme form with marked soft tissue and bony destruction. It is thought that a mixed spirochaete and fusiform bacterial infection is the cause. It is particularly common in the horn of Africa (e.g. Ethiopia), where malnutrition and lack of access to simple antibiotics such as metronidazole are an everyday problem.

Treatment

Adequate analgesia is vital to allow adequate fluid intake and débridement of the affected tissue. Good oral hygiene is essential. This is supplemented with antibiotic therapy. Metronidazole 200–400 mg three times a day is the initial drug of choice. Noma presents a chronic problem created by extreme, often absolute, trismus resulting from destruction of facial tissue that requires division and reconstruction with robust vascularized tissue – the submental flap works well for this.

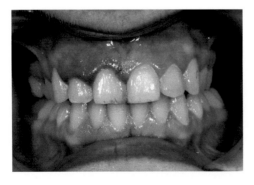

Figure 10.1 Necrotizing ulcerative gingivitis. (Courtesy of Mr R.F. Crosher.)

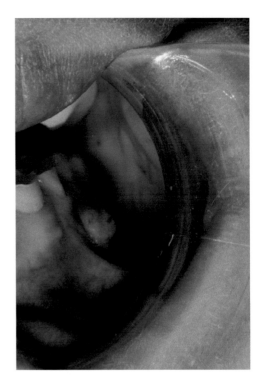

Figure 10.2 Dental abscess pointing intraorally.

Dentoalveolar abscess

Oral microorganisms can reach the periapical tissues via the root canal system or via the periodontal ligament. If the bacteria are sufficiently virulent and/or the host defences compromised, then the infection may give rise to a dentoalveolar abscess. The complex attachment of facial fascia determines how these infections spread. The abscess may remain localized and drain via a small intraoral sinus (Figure 10.2), or it may spread, giving rise to severe cellulitis involving multiple tissue spaces (Figures 10.3, 10.4, 10.5 and 10.6). Various organisms are involved in these infections. There is an increasing recognition of the role of anaerobic bacteria, especially streptococci, in these infections. The specific signs and symptoms depend on which tissue spaces are involved. The symptoms may include pain, swelling, discharge, tenderness to percussion of involved teeth, trismus and dysphagia. Trismus or dysphagia, particularly for fluids (ask whether the patient can swallow his or her own

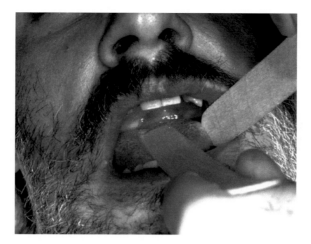

Figure 10.3 Submandibular and lateral pharyngeal abscess showing compromise of the airway.

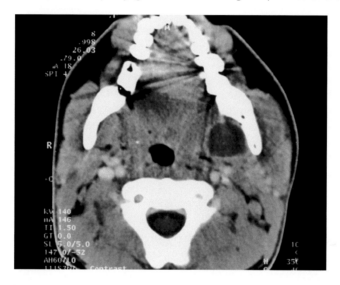

Figure 10.4 Computed tomography scan demonstrating submandibular and submasseteric space collections.

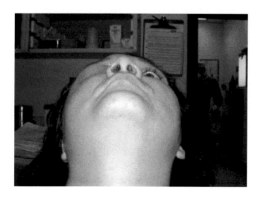

Figure 10.5 Temporal space abscess.

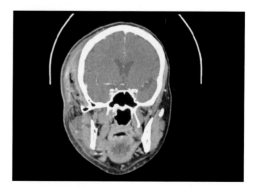

Figure 10.6 Computed tomography scan showing a temporal space abscess.

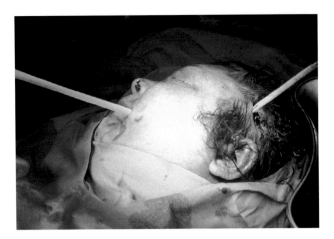

Figure 10.7 Postoperative incision and drainage of a temporal space abscess. Note the through and through drainage.

saliva), warns you that the airway may be at risk. Systemic upset is variable, but it may manifest as pyrexia, tachycardia and hypotension. Infections of the anterior maxilla may, rarely, give rise to cavernous sinus thrombosis, a condition that still has a mortality of 30% in spite of antibiotic therapy. The signs of cavernous sinus thrombosis include proptosis, chemosis, impaired eye movements (ophthalmoplegia) and marked systemic upset.

Treatment

Early assessment and control of the airway are essential in significant cervicofacial infection. Clinicians in secondary care must get used to the standard misconceptions in play with other specialties in relation to 'dental abscess'. Minor collections (true dental abscess sometimes known in lay terms as a 'gumboil') are manageable by simple incision and drainage using topical or conventional local anaesthesia. This has nothing in common with the potentially lethal severe cervicofacial infections seen in the hospital environment in which early involvement with anaesthesia in relation to securing early airway security (often combined with adequate drainage after awake flexible fibreoptic intubation) is mandatory.

The source of the infection should be eliminated by extraction or, if the tooth is believed to be salvageable, root canal or periodontal therapy (possible in minor infections but highly unlikely in the

significant infections requiring admission). Any pus present must be drained and samples cultured. All the involved tissue spaces should be explored (Figure 10.7). Monitoring the airway and hydration of the patient are very important. Antibiotics are an essential adjunct to drainage and should not be used in isolation.

Ludwig's angina

This is a feared condition in which there is bilateral involvement of the sublingual and submandibular spaces. This disorder results in elevation of the floor of the mouth and tongue and marked oedema of the soft tissues of the neck. Ludwig's angina is most commonly the consequence of dental sepsis but may complicate submandibular gland infection or infection of a mandibular fracture or of an intraoral wound. Patients have marked systemic upset and boardlike swelling of the neck and floor of mouth. Inability to swallow their own saliva is a major indicator of deterioration. The airway is at definite risk. Various oral commensal bacteria have been implicated.

Treatment

The airway must be maintained and secured at an early stage. This requires intubation to allow drainage of the compressed infected region usually by fibreoptic intubation. Tracheostomy or cricothyroidotomy should be procedures of last choice

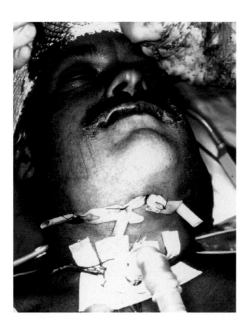

Figure 10.8 Ludwig's angina postoperatively. Note the multiple drains in place and the placement of a tracheostomy to secure the airway. Some clinicians claim a 50% mortality when tracheostomy is performed in this situation.

because a surgical airway under these conditions creates a high risk of mediastinitis and an approximate 50% mortality rate. The involved spaces should be decompressed, even though frequently little pus is obtained (Figure 10.8). High-dose intravenous antibiotics should be given to complement surgical decompression. Any infective focus should be removed.

Necrotizing fasciitis

This uncommon, but life-threatening, condition may affect the head and neck and be rapidly fulminant. The mortality approaches 40%. The term necrotizing soft tissue infection is preferred by some. This is because it is believed that this alternate term more accurately reflects the process, given that the fascial boundaries are frequently transgressed by the infection. It also overcomes arguments about whether 'deep fascial components' in the face are involved because in reality it is more frequently a necrosis of muscle, fat and skin in the head and neck, with necrotic muscle causing the classic undermining skin infection.

It is a frequently polymicrobial infection, with group A streptococci most commonly isolated (*Streptococcus milleri* is frequently found). This condition is believed to be more common in patients with some form of immunocompromise. The initial site of infection may be so trivial as to be unnoticed by the patient. The subsequent systemic upset and tissue destruction are disproportionate to the initial infection. The soft tissue destruction is characterized by liquefaction of the subcutaneous fat and connective tissue. Small vessel thrombosis gives rise to a mottled appearance of the affected skin. A rapidly progressive systemic inflammatory response syndrome (SIRS) with multiorgan failure is frequent.

Treatment

These patients require aggressive resuscitation and débridement. The initial surgery should be supported by broad-spectrum antibiotics (e.g. megadose penicillin, gentamycin and metronidazole). Second look surgery at 24 to 48 hours should be planned with further débridement as required. Hyperbaric oxygen therapy may be helpful for these patients to eradicate the infection and provide a favourable environment for subsequent healing and reconstruction, although there are few areas in the world where this is possible in the acute phase.

Osteomyelitis

This term describes inflammation of bone of infective origin. It starts in the medullary space of the involved bone and progresses as inflammatory changes in the nutrient vessels render the bone ischaemic. Any pus formed can compress the vessels further. The bone becomes necrotic and behaves as a foreign body, known as a sequestrum. This gives rise to a chronic inflammatory reaction as the body tries to eliminate it. Attempts at repair may cause the sequestrum to become encased in osteoid material, known as an involucrum.

Osteomyelitis can be divided into suppurative or nonsuppurative forms, although these may overlap considerably. There is frequently a predisposing factor for the development of osteomyelitis. This may be underlying systemic disease or local bony factors. Local bony factors include primary

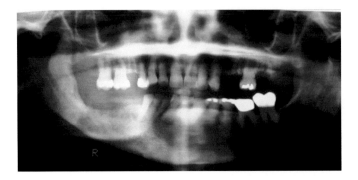

Figure 10.9 Chronic osteomyelitis of the right mandible. Note the loss of the right condyle and the diffuse radiopacity of the right body of the mandible.

diseases of bone (e.g. fibrous dysplasia, Paget's disease or osteopetrosis). It may be secondary to bone damage from trauma or foreign bodies in the bone (e.g. bone plates).

Previously irradiated bone may undergo osteoradionecrosis because radiation-damaged DNA breaks down when required to undergo replication. This necrotic bone is very susceptible to secondary infection. Bone rendered incapable of normal physiological healing such as by bisphosphonates or anti–rank ligand antibody in which the osteoclasts are effectively paralyzed is also very prone to superinfection to which it cannot respond and gives rise to a specific clinical osteomyelitis – bisphosphonate-related osteonecrosis of the jaws (BRON or BRONJ or, more recently antiresorptive-associated osteonecrosis of the jaws [ARAONJ], changed to recognize that other antiresorptives such as anti–rank ligand antibody can produce the same condition).

In the maxillofacial region osteomyelitis is most commonly seen in the mandible and is secondary to infection of the medullary space from an odontogenic infection. Rarely, in infants, there may be an acute infection of the maxilla. This is more correctly known as osteitis because the medullary space is negligible. The infection is thought to reach the maxilla by a haematogenous route. The infection is most commonly polymicrobial, with staphylococci predominating. *Salmonella* is commonly implicated in cases of osteomyelitis occurring in patients with sickle cell disease.

The typical signs and symptoms are pain, swelling, erythema of overlying skin and systemic upset. In suppurative osteomyelitis sinus tracts may

develop. Long-standing cases may undergo malignant transformation (Marjolin ulcers). Paraesthesia of local nerves may occur. Pathological fracture may also occur, and teeth become loose.

Imaging may be difficult because the radiographic findings lag behind the clinical stage. The first sign may be radiopacity (Figure 10.9), which represents the sequestrum that has lost its nonmineralized component. Bone scans show osteomyelitis as areas of increased bone turnover ('hot spots').

Treatment

General management, including the correction of any underlying systemic factors, is vital. Routine investigations should include:

- Full blood count.
- Routine biochemistry, including blood glucose.
- C-reactive protein with or without erythrocyte sedimentation rate.
- Blood cultures.

If the patient is systemically unwell, intravenous antibiotics should be started. Penicillin and flucloxacillin are a good best guess, with clindamycin used in patients with penicillin allergy. If necessary the antibiotics can be changed when culture results are available.

Surgical treatment includes the drainage of pus and the removal of any focus of infection (tooth, foreign body). In established cases, saucerization and decortication may be necessary to allow coverage of the medullary space by well-vascularized soft tissue. Measurement of C-reactive protein helps to monitor the response to treatment.

Resection of any bone sequestrum or clinically ischaemic bone is particularly important in radiation-related or bisphosphonate-damaged osteomyelitis; this may be helped by packing the defect with gentamycin-impregnated collagen 'fleece'. The remaining bone must be covered with sealed healthy vascularized tissue whenever possible. In pathological fractures associated with osteomyelitis, rigid fixation is shown to improve healing, and in those involving radiation or bisphosphonate damage, fresh vascularized bone and soft tissue to create watertight seals around healing bone are generally advocated.

Bite wounds

The oral cavities of all animals, including humans, are full of bacteria. Any bite therefore results in inoculating the wound with significant numbers of bacteria. This predisposes to infection, particularly if there is a significant injury (see also Chapter 17).

The infecting organisms depend on the source of the bite. The most common isolates from infected dog and cat bites are *Pasteurella* species, streptococci, staphylococci, *Moraxella*, *Neisseria,* and anaerobes such as *Fusobacterium* and *Bacteroides*.

The most common isolates from human bites are *Staphylococcus aureus, Eikenella, Haemophilus influenzae* and beta-lactamase–producing oral anaerobes.

Treatment

Irrigation and débridement of the wound are mandatory. Antibiotic treatment is based on the likely infecting organisms. For animal and human bites, amoxycillin-clavulinic acid is the drug of choice. A clarithromycin and metronidazole combination is used for penicillin-allergic patients. The patient's tetanus immunization status is reviewed.

Acute salivary gland infections

See also Chapter 21.

Acute parotitis

Less frequently seen nowadays thanks to better fluid management, acute parotitis is most commonly encountered in debilitated, dehydrated postoperative patients or in those adults with known chronic subacute obstructive sialadenitis. Decreased salivary flow creates a risk from ascending infection. *S. aureus* is, surprisingly, the most common infecting organism. Acute parotitis may occur secondary to duct obstruction by a mucus plug or, more rarely, a stone (Figure 10.10). The gland is typically swollen and tender. The overlying soft tissue may be oedematous. It may be possible to see pus discharged from the affected parotid duct. Abscess formation may occur and in subacute cases may mimic a parotid mass (Figures 10.11 and 10.12). Recurrent parotitis may be seen in children,

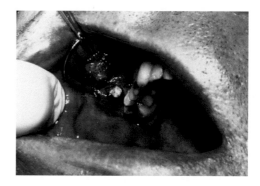

Figure 10.10 Parotid duct stone giving rise to acute parotitis.

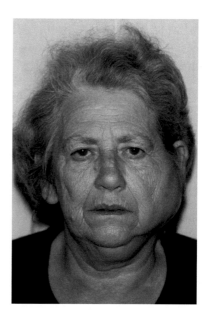

Figure 10.11 Parotid abscess.

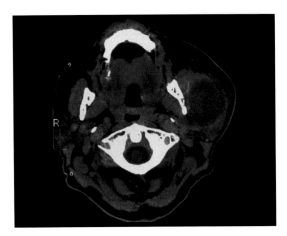

Figure 10.12 Computed tomography scan demonstrating abscess formation within the parotid gland.

usually in a gland that has been damaged by previous viral infection. This disorder has a tendency to burn out over several years, but it may leave the gland scarred and requiring removal.

Treatment

Treatment consists of fluid rehydration, analgesia, optimizing oral hygiene and intravenous antibiotics. The antibiotics should have antistaphylococcal activity. Any pus expressible from the ducts should be cultured to guide antibiotic therapy. The removal of any duct obstruction will help the drainage of infected secretions. If abscess formation occurs (true parotid abscess is comparatively rare), then incision and drainage of the abscess are required. Dissection through the gland, if absolutely essential, should be carried out parallel to the facial nerve fibres.

Submandibular sialadenitis

This disorder is usually secondary to gland obstruction. A calculus is the most common cause, but the obstruction may result from stricture of the duct. *S. aureus* is, again surprisingly, the most common infecting organism. There is frequently a history of intermittent swelling of the gland, associated with meal times. Acute presentation with a hot, tender submandibular swelling with systemic upset is not uncommon. Spread into the adjacent fascial spaces may lead to the development of Ludwig's angina.

A lower occlusal radiograph frequently shows the calculus causing the obstruction. In more chronic cases, where there is stricture of the duct, sialography may be diagnostic and therapeutic.

Treatment

In acute presentations the airway must be assessed. Fluid resuscitation and antibiotics are required. If there is abscess formation, then incision and drainage of the abscess will be required, followed by interval removal of the gland. In uncomplicated cases any obstruction that is present should be removed. This may require dilation of the duct if it is strictured and the removal of any associated calculus by a transoral open procedure, by interventional radiology using basket retrieval or sialoendoscopically. If the gland is scarred or the calculus is in the substance of the gland, then removal of the gland may be required.

Acute viral infections

Mumps

This condition is caused by a RNA paramyxovirus. It is most commonly seen in childhood. It is characterized by a painful swelling of the salivary glands, particularly the parotid. It is usually bilateral, and the patient frequently has trismus and halitosis. Although mumps is usually self-limiting, complications can occur, especially in adults. These include orchitis, meningoencephalitis, myocarditis and nephritis.

Acute skin infections

Impetigo

This spreading infection of the superficial layers of the epidermis is usually caused by beta haemolytic streptococci or coagulase-positive staphylococci. It frequently follows minor tissue trauma such as scratching of the skin. Initially there are thin-walled pustules, which spread rapidly circumferentially and burst, leaving a crusting wound. Treatment is with antibiotics, typically penicillin and flucloxacillin. In penicillin-sensitive patients an antibiotic with antistaphylococcal activity should be chosen.

Erysipelas

Erysipelas is a superficial cellulitis involving the dermis and is most commonly caused by beta-haemolytic streptococci. The lesions spread rapidly and systemic upset is common. Desquamation of the skin following resolution of the infection may occur. Treatment is with penicillins or cephalosporins or with equivalent drugs in allergic patients.

Furuncles and carbuncles

Staphylococcal infections of hair follicles give rise to a variety of conditions. Localized superficial infection of a hair follicle is known as folliculitis. If abscess formation occurs this is known as a furuncle or boil. These are very painful and may require drainage if they do not spontaneously discharge. Multiple adjacent follicles can be involved, and if these coalesce this is known as a carbuncle. A furuncle localized to an eyelash is known as stye. These infections frequently recur because of a reservoir of *S. aureus* in the nares, and eradication of this reservoir is important. Sebaceous cysts and acne cysts may become similarly infected.

Treatment

Any abscess present should be drained. Antistaphylococcal antibiotics should be prescribed and face hygiene optimized. Naseptin (chlorhexidine and neomycin) or mupirocin cream to the nares helps reduce staphylococcal carriage. When quiescent, any affected cyst should be excised.

Cat scratch disease

Bartonella henselae, formerly called *Rochalimaea henselae,* is the agent of cat scratch disease. The infection is usually self-limiting, but it may last weeks to months. *Afipia felis* has also appeared to be involved in causation.

Regional or solitary lymphadenitis is seen at or near the site of the injury, sometimes with an erythematous skin papule. Fever, malaise and other constitutional symptoms may also occur. In immunocompromised patients the infection can disseminate and cause a serious systemic illness.

A few patients report a cat scratch, and it is likely that the identical illness can be caused by other animals and even by splinters and thorns bearing the causative organisms. Cats are really the carrier.

No specific therapy is usually needed. The culpable organisms, however, have shown sensitivity to numerous antibiotics *in vitro*.

Appropriate serology testing may aid in the diagnosis and management of the underlying infection. There are case reports in which ciprofloxacin and azithromycin have been effective.

Acute fungal infections

Candidiasis

Candida is a yeast-like fungus and is commonly found in the oral cavity. *Candida albicans* is most commonly cultured and associated with disease. It is more commonly isolated in smokers, patients with xerostomia and those taking broad-spectrum antibiotics or steroids, particularly inhaled steroids. Underlying systemic disease such as diabetes can predispose patients to systemic candidiasis. Candidiasis is often known as the disease of the diseased.

Symptoms include the following: discomfort, often described as burning; altered taste and altered smell. Dysphagia may be present in patients with oral candidiasis. Pseudomembrane formation is common (Figure 10.13), and it is characterized by the fact that the plaque can be removed by rubbing, thus leaving a bleeding site. An erythematous form may be seen in which painful red areas are present in the absence of plaques. A hyperplastic form may be seen in denture wearers, as may angular

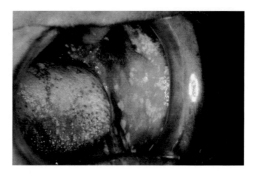

Figure 10.13 Candidiasis secondary to oral steroid inhaler use.

cheilitis, in which an associated *S. aureus* infection may be present. The hyperplastic form may give rise to possibly premalignant leukoplakia.

Diagnosis is largely clinical. Culture alone cannot be relied on because *Candida* is a common commensal. Biopsy confirmation may be required in cases of hyperplastic candidiasis.

Treatment

Any underlying factors should be dealt with (e.g. optimizing control of diabetes, stopping smoking). In patients whose candidiasis is associated with steroid inhalers, consideration should be given to the use of a spacer. Denture hygiene must be maintained at a high level. Antifungal therapy may be topical or systemic, and the decision to use systemic antifungal agents will be based on the severity and duration of symptoms in addition to the underlying systemic disease.

Azole antifungals are the mainstay of systemic therapy, with fluconazole the best tolerated (50 to 100 mg daily for 10 days to 3 weeks). Miconazole is used in gel (mouth) and cream (angular cheilitis) form as the topical agent of choice. Combining the two in recalcitrant cases may help because fluconazole-resistant (and itraconazole-resistant) cases have emerged. Voriconazole is an expensive reserve.

Chronic infections

Chronic osteomyelitis

Infection persisting for more than 1 month is viewed as chronic. There are a number of types described, and this can cause confusion. In broad terms, these conditions may be viewed as suppurative or nonsuppurative.

Chronic suppurative osteomyelitis is most commonly the result of inadequately treated acute osteomyelitis, and the treatment is the same. All correctable host factors should be addressed. Hyperbaric oxygen therapy may be of value in refractory cases, particularly those associated with previous radiotherapy.

Garré's sclerosing osteomyelitis

This is an unusual condition, most often reported in children and young adults. It typically manifests as a nontender bony swelling of the mandible associated with a carious first molar. Systemic upset is unusual. It is thought that low-grade chronic infection stimulates the active periosteum to lay down bone. The subperiosteal bone deposition often has a laminated appearance and needs to be distinguished from osteosarcoma and Ewing's sarcoma. In the absence of an obvious dental cause, early biopsy is required.

Treatment

Any source of infection should be removed, and sometimes this has to be surprisingly radical. Antibiotics are not helpful. Remodelling of the bone is the rule, but surgical recontouring may be needed.

Chronic sclerosing osteomyelitis

This disorder may be focal or diffuse. It is thought to be an inflammatory response to bacterial infection in which there is bone deposition rather than resorption. No specific organism has been identified. Intermittent refractory pain is a feature. It is more frequent in the mandible. The symptoms include pain swelling, paraesthesia, pressure and trismus. The symptoms may persist for years. Radiographs show mixed sclerosis and osteolysis, with the sclerotic component becoming more prominent over time.

Treatment

Treatment can be problematic. Long-term antibiotic therapy has been reported as being of benefit if given early in the course of the disease. In more refractory cases a course of corticosteroids and decortication may be of benefit. Hyperbaric oxygen therapy can be used to supplement surgery, although the evidence base is conflicting. Bisphosphonates have been advocated for chronic pain but have obvious conflicting risks.

Actinomycosis

Actinomyces israelii is a common oral commensal that can cause disease if it is inoculated into deeper tissues. It may be inoculated during trauma such as tooth extraction or fracture of the mandible. The infection rarely manifests as acute soft tissue swelling, similar to a dental

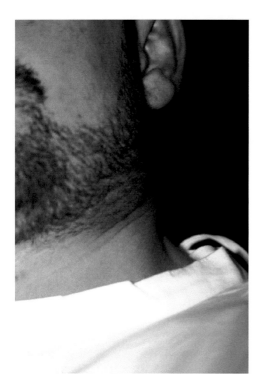

Figure 10.14 Clinical presentation of actinomycosis.

abscess. Pain may be less of a feature than in a simple odontogenic infection. Actinomycosis more frequently manifests as a slowly progressive mass, which may not be painful (Figure 10.14). Suppuration can occur via multiple tracts. These may resolve only to recur later. Bone involvement is characterized by deep-seated pain, low-grade pyrexia and paraesthesia. Serial radiographs may show variable areas of destruction with variable amounts of bone deposition.

Diagnosis is by culture of any pus present or biopsy of the involved tissue. *Actinomyces* is a fastidious anaerobe, and if this infection is suspected, it should be marked on the microbiological request form so that careful, prolonged, anaerobic culture can be carried out. The US literature shows increasing recognition of the association of actinomycosis and ARAONJ.

Treatment

Prolonged, high-dose antibiotics are required. Depending on response this treatment may even need to be continued for 12 months. Penicillin is the drug of choice; erythromycin or clindamycin is used in patients with penicillin allergy. If there is significant bone involvement, then resection of the involved bone and saucerization of the involved bone will be required. Older texts and some microbiologists advocate prolonged (6 weeks) intravenous amoxycillin. Although this regimen can be achieved in some communities with highly developed outreach services, a high-dose oral equivalent has regularly been effective.

Mycobacterial infections

Mycobacterial infections, both tuberculosis and atypical mycobacterial infection, have become more prevalent in recent years. They are seen in homeless, chronically malnourished and immunocompromised patients, particularly those with HIV infection and acquired immunodeficiency syndrome (AIDS). Atypical mycobacterial cervical lymphadenitis is seen regularly in otherwise healthy children. The maxillofacial manifestations of tuberculosis include the following: cervical lymphadenopathy, in which the lymph nodes may coalesce and give rise to a discharging sinus; chronic oral ulcers, typically of the tongue (Figure 10.15); and rarely

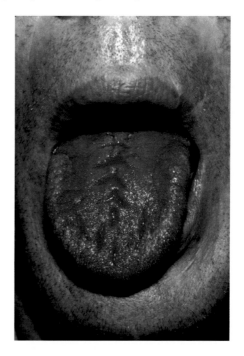

Figure 10.15 Fissured, ulcerated tongue in a patient with tuberculosis.

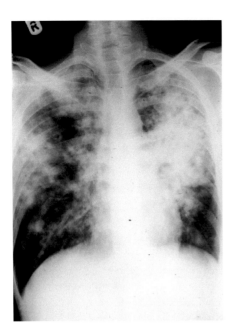

Figure 10.16 Chest X-ray of the patient in Figure 10.15 showing classic appearances of pulmonary tuberculosis.

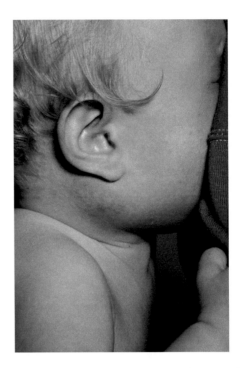

Figure 10.17 Cervical lymphadenopathy in a child that is caused by atypical *Mycobacterium* infection. (Sometimes called 'scrofula' or 'the king's evil', it was believed in the Middle Ages that the condition could be cured by the touch of the king.)

osteomyelitis. Diagnosis can be difficult and may require multiple cultures, skin testing, chest radiography and occasionally biopsy. If active pulmonary tuberculosis is present, national reporting and isolation nursing will be required (Figure 10.16.)

It is of immense importance not to confuse the quite common cervical lymphadenopathy of atypical mycobacteria (*Mycobacterium avium-intracellulare* complex, *Mycobacterium kansasii*, *Mycobacterium marinum*) with tuberculosis. These infections with atypical mycobacteria do not respond to antituberculous therapy, do not need national reporting, rarely show any of the other manifestations of tuberculosis and are treated quite differently.

Treatment

Treatment is entirely dependent on the infecting organism. *Mycobacterium tuberculosis* responds to complex chemotherapy but atypical mycobacteria rarely do. Chemotherapy for tuberculosis is prolonged and involves optimizing host factors and long-term combination chemotherapy. Currently used drugs include isoniazid, rifampicin, pyrazinamide and ethambutol. Treatment should be carried out in consultation with infectious disease specialists because of the increasing problem with

drug resistance secondary to poor compliance with treatment.

Atypical mycobacteria, such as *M. avium-intracellulare* (and many others), may give rise to an isolated, occasionally discharging cervical mass in children (a scrofula) (Figure 10.17). Diagnosis is by culture and microscopy. Treatment is by excision of the affected glands. Antituberculous therapy is not particularly helpful, but long-term clarithromycin may improve resolution of nondischarging cervical lymph nodes.

Syphilis

This sexually transmitted infection may have oral manifestations at any point in its natural history. It is caused by the spirochaete *Treponema pallidum*.

In primary syphilis there is a painless ulcer, known as a chancre, at the site of entry of the infection. This may be at an intraoral site, with the lip, tongue and gingivae the most common areas.

Chancres are highly infectious and may persist for up to a month. Approximately 6 weeks later secondary syphilis may manifest intraorally as 'snail-track' ulcers of the mucous membrane. The infection may become latent for 5 to 10 years. The classic lesion of tertiary syphilis is the gumma, which may affect the palate, lips and tongue. Considerable destruction may occur. There can be associated glossitis, which may be premalignant.

Infection *in utero* causes congenital syphilis. There may be hypoplasia of the permanent teeth giving rise to notched, peg-shaped incisors (Hutchinson's incisors) and rounded first permanent molars (mulberry molars). Gumma formation may cause collapse of the nasal complex and a 'saddle nose' deformity. Diagnosis is by serology.

Treatment

Penicillin is the drug of choice. Contact tracing may be required. The possibility of other sexually transmitted disease, including HIV infection, should be considered.

Viral infections

Herpesvirus infections

These DNA viruses are all characterized by their capacity for latent infection and subsequent reactivation, particularly at times of stress or immunocompromise.

The herpesvirus family (human herpesvirus [HHV]) include: herpes simplex, varicella-zoster, Epstein-Barr, cytomegalovirus and Kaposi's sarcoma virus (HHV-8).

Herpes simplex

Herpes simplex is the most common HHV infection; most people are exposed to it by puberty. Most initial exposures are symptomatic. Primary infection can manifest as gingivostomatitis, with vesicles, ulcers and oropharyngeal pain (Figure 10.18). This is often misnamed as 'teething' in children. Primary infection tends to be more troublesome if it occurs in adult life. Treatment of the initial infection is symptomatic. Following the initial infection the virus travels to the regional ganglia. From here reactivation is common. In the maxillofacial region these reactivations are seen as

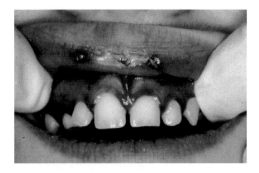

Figure 10.18 Herpetic gingivostomatitis.

mucosal and labial infections (cold sores, canker sores). A prodrome of tingling is common. These lesions are uncomfortable, unsightly and highly contagious. Diagnosis is usually clinical, although viral culture and cytology are possible. The infection is transferable to the genitals and *vice versa*.

Treatment

Systemic and topical antiviral agents, such as aciclovir and famciclovir, are available and may, if given early in the course of reactivation (first 2 to 3 days), shorten the course of the infection. Labial secondary herpes (type 1 usually) is commonly managed topically, whereas genital herpes (type 2 usually) is more often managed with systemic aciclovir and is an increasing problem as a sexually transmitted disease. There is a crossover between the two viruses and sites. Supportive measures are important, and adequate fluid intake must be ensured in young and debilitated patients.

Varicella-zoster

Primary varicella-zoster infection gives rise to chickenpox. This is a common contagious disease of children. The symptoms are fever, malaise and a rash, which spreads rapidly from the trunk to the head, neck and extremities. The rash gives way to vesicles and papules. These can involve the oral cavity and make eating and drinking difficult. The infection tends to be self-limiting, and complications such as pneumonia and encephalitis are uncommon.

The virus remains latent in the sensory ganglia and may reactivate in later life or if the patient is immunocompromised. This is known as herpes zoster or shingles. Following a painful prodromal period, vesicles appear that typically have a dermatomal distribution along the divisions of

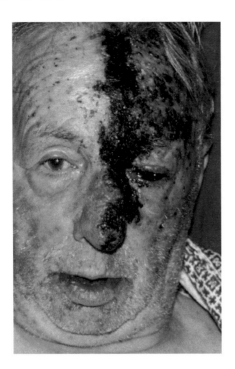

Figure 10.19 Herpes zoster infection showing dermatome distribution.

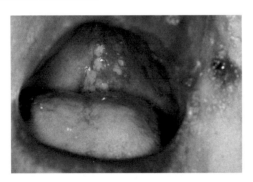

Figure 10.20 Intraoral herpes zoster infection.

the trigeminal nerve (Figures 10.19 and 10.20). The vesicles typically heal over a 3-week period. Preherpetic, periherpetic and postherpetic neuralgic pain is common and troublesome.

Diagnosis is usually clinical.

Treatment

Treatment of chickenpox is symptomatic, with attention paid to adequate fluid intake. In cases of shingles high doses of antiviral agents, such as aciclovir and famciclovir, are given early in the course of the disease. Some patients can develop a distressing postherpetic neuralgia. The cautious, early use of corticosteroids with the antiviral therapy may minimize the occurrence of this complication. If established, the neuralgia may require treatment with regular analgesia and coanalgesics such as tricyclic antidepressants, gabapentin or pregabalin.

Epstein-Barr virus

Epstein-Barr virus infection most commonly manifests as infectious mononucleosis (glandular fever). It is transmitted by contaminated saliva. It is also associated with nasopharyngeal carcinoma, lymphoma and hairy leukoplakia (Figure 10.21). Infectious mononucleosis is most commonly seen in adolescents and young adults and manifests as malaise, sore throat and cervical lymphadenopathy. There may be associated hepatosplenomegaly. Intraoral examination may show multiple petechiae. Treatment is supportive and the condition is self-limiting. In Germany it is sometimes referred to as Pfeiffer's disease or kissing disease because of the mode of transmission.

Cytomegalovirus

These infections may manifest as mucosal ulceration or salivary gland swelling in patients who are immunocompromised. Diagnosis may require biopsy of the affected tissue and special staining. Treatment is with aciclovir or ganciclovir.

Other infections of surgical importance

Hepatitis B virus

Hepatitis B is one of several viral infections that can complicate surgical treatment. Hepatitis B virus

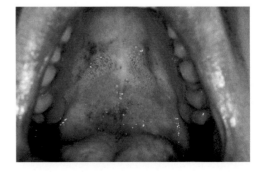

Figure 10.21 Palatal petechiae in infectious mononucleosis.

(HBV) is a DNA virus that can be spread by sexual contact or inoculation, particularly in association with intravenous drug abuse. It can be present in saliva as well as all in other bodily fluids. There is a long incubation period, so unwitting infection as a result of inoculation during surgical treatment can occur. This is why the use of universal precautions is so important. Signs and symptoms include malaise, abdominal discomfort, anorexia and jaundice. Liver function tests show elevation of the enzymes of the transaminase series. Diagnosis is by serology, with detection of the surface antigen (HbsAg) indicating current infection. Treatment of acute infection is largely supportive, although the use of alpha-interferon or the nucleoside lamivudine (3TC) may help with eradication of the virus. Chronic infection with persistence of the infectious state occurs in approximately 5% of cases. The development of cirrhosis and hepatocellular carcinoma can complicate infection. A vaccine against HBV is available, and all healthcare workers should avail themselves of it.

Hepatitis C virus

Hepatitis C virus (HCV) infection is an increasing public health problem. Transmission is similar to that of HBV, although HCV is arguably even more easily transmissible, with the highest rate of infection among intravenous drug abusers. There is no vaccine currently available. Approximately 20% of infected patients will develop cirrhosis and may require liver transplantation.

Human immunodeficiency virus

There are approximately 34 million people worldwide living with HIV, an RNA virus. Infection is bloodborne and spread by sexual contact or by inoculation with infected blood or blood products. HIV infection can complicate oral and maxillosurgical treatment both because of the cross-infection risk and because of the oral manifestations, some of which may be the first signs of the condition and may lead to the diagnosis. There is a 2- to 6-week incubation period followed by an episode of flu-like illness. There is then usually a period of persistent generalized lymphadenopathy before the disease enters its latent phase, which may last several years. During the

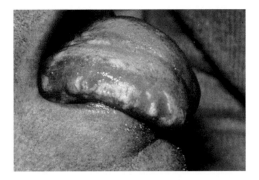

Figure 10.22 Clinical example of hairy leukoplakia in a man infected with human immunodeficiency virus.

latent phase there is an increase in the viral load and a reduction of the CD4 lymphocyte count. Eventually the lymphocyte reduction will give rise to symptoms and the development of AIDS.

Oral conditions associated with HIV/AIDS include oropharyngeal candidiasis, hairy leukoplakia (Figure 10.22), Kaposi's sarcoma, necrotizing gingivitis/periodontitis and the development of carcinomas or lymphomas (usually non-Hodgkin's) and parotid enlargement.

Treatment

Although there is no effective vaccine currently available and there is no cure for HIV infection, reverse transcriptase inhibitors and protease inhibitors can block viral replication. Combinations of these drugs, termed highly active antiretroviral therapy (HAART), allow the majority of HIV-infected individuals who have access to this treatment to live a normal life span. Immediate postexposure prophylaxis using these drugs may prevent the survival of HIV in a contaminated individual and may thus prevent the infected state.

Infected patients who have reached a stage of significant immunocompromise (much rarer nowadays in the developed world) may present with severe dentofacial sepsis. The removal of the source of infection may be difficult but is essential. High-dose antibiotics are required, and specialist advice about the possible need for granulocyte colony-stimulating factors should be sought.

Patients with HIV/AIDS are at risk of bacterial infection during treatment. Prophylactic antibiotics should be used. Patients with HIV infection but entirely controlled CD4/viral titres using HAART can be managed essentially as normal.

Universal precautions should be used to prevent transmission of infection, but this is hardly unique to HIV.

Bisphosphonate-related osteonecrosis of the jaws

There are many protocols, guidelines and suggestions on the management of this disorder, with little or no evidence to support one strategy over another. Better-quality trials are needed.

For most patients a conservative approach with minimal local intervention seems to be most sensible. On occasion, extensive débridement of necrotic bone with radical resection of bone and reconstruction are required when other interventions fail or pathological fracture develops.

CLINICAL STAGING OF BISPHOSPHONATE-RELATED OSTEONECROSIS OF THE JAWS

- **At risk category** – no apparent exposed or necrotic bone in patients who have been treated with either oral or intravenous bisphosphonates.
- **Stage 1** – exposed or necrotic bone in patients who are asymptomatic and have no evidence of infection.
- **Stage 2** – exposed or necrotic bone associated with infection as evidenced by pain and erythema in the region of the exposed bone with or without purulent drainage.
- **Stage 3** – exposed or necrotic bone in patients with pain, infection and one or more of the following: pathological fracture, extraoral fistula or osteolysis extending to the inferior border.

FURTHER READING

Bagan J, Scully C, Sabater V, Jimenez Y. Osteonecrosis of the jaws in patients treated with intravenous bisphosphonates (BRONJ): a concise update. *Oral Oncol* 2009;45:551–4.

Epstein MS, Wicknick FW, Epstein JB, Berenson JR, Gorsky M. Management of bisphosphonate-associated osteonecrosis: pentoxifylline and tocopherol in addition to antimicrobial therapy. An initial case series. *Oral Surg Oral Med Oral Pathol Oral Radiol Endodontol* 2010;110:593–5.

Flynn TR. Surgical management of orofacial infections. *Atlas Oral Maxillofac Surg Clin North Am* 2000;8(1):77–100.

Jones JL, Candelaria LM. Head and neck infections. In Fonseca RI, editor. *Oral and maxillofacial surgery*, vol. 5. Philadelphia: Saunders, 2000.

Laskin DM, Strauss RA. Current concepts in the management of maxillofacial infections. *Oral Maxillofac Surg Clin North Am* 2003;15:xi–xii.

Lindeboom JA, Kuijper EJ, Bruijnesteijn van Coppenraet ES, Lindeboom R, Prins JM. Surgical excision versus antibiotic treatment for nontuberculous mycobacterial cervicofacial lymphadenitis in children: a multicenter, randomized, controlled trial. *Clin Infect Dis* 2007;44:1057–64.

Lindeboom JA, Lindeboom R, Bruijnesteijn van Coppenraet ES, Kuijper EJ, Tuk J, Prins JM. Esthetic outcome of surgical excision versus antibiotic therapy for nontuberculous mycobacterial cervicofacial lymphadenitis in children. *Pediatr Infect Dis J* 2009;28:1028–30.

McLeod NMH, Patel V, Kusanale A, Rogers SN, Brennan PA. Bisphosphonate osteonecrosis of the jaw: a literature review of UK policies versus international policies on the management of bisphosphonate osteonecrosis of the jaw. *Br J Oral Maxillofac Surg* 2011;49:335–42.

Ruggiero SL. Guidelines for the diagnosis of bisphosphonate-related osteonecrosis of the jaw (BRONJ). *Clin Cases Miner Bone Metab* 2007;4:37–42.

Rui-feng C, Li-song H, Ji-bo Z, Li-qiu W. Emergency treatment on facial laceration of dog bite wounds with immediate primary closure: a prospective randomized trial study. *BMC Emerg Med* 2013;13(Suppl 1):S2.

Topazian RG, Goldberg MH, Hupp JR, editors. *Oral and maxillofacial infections,* 4th ed. Philadelphia: Saunders, 2002.

11

Cysts of the jaws

Contents

Aims for undergraduates and postgraduates

- To appreciate the nature of various cysts and how they behave clinically.
- To understand the importance of different types of cysts in relation to their management.

Learning outcomes

- To be able to describe how cysts are classified according to the epithelium of origin.
- To demonstrate the use of basic history and examination in the diagnosis of cystic lesions.
- To be able to request and interpret specific investigations in aiding diagnosis.
- To be able to plan treatment and take informed consent for the procedure.
- To be able to describe surgical management of the majority of cysts of the head and neck.

Classification of cysts of the jaws

Cysts can be broadly categorized into epithelial or nonepithelial. The epithelial cysts are further divided into their epithelium of origin, which is either odontogenic or nonodontogenic.

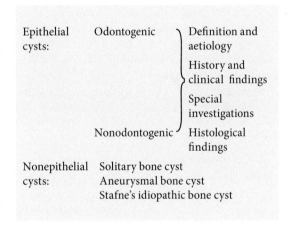

Epithelial cysts

The most common cause of chronic swelling of the jaws is a cyst.

A cyst is defined as a pathological cavity filled with fluid and lined by epithelium. This epithelium can originate either from the tooth-forming organ (odontogenic) or from other sources such as areas of inclusion of epithelium when the embryonic processes of the face fuse (nonodontogenic). Odontogenic cysts account for the large majority (90%) of jaw cysts.

Theories of epithelial cyst formation

There are several theories proposed for the formation of epithelial cysts:

- **Hydrostatic theory** – central epithelial necrosis results in a high osmotic pressure causing fluid to move into the cavity. The consequent increase in hydrostatic pressure leads to expansion of bone.
- **Proliferation of lining theory** – degeneration and liquefaction necrosis of granulation tissue result from toxic products of necrotic pulp or bacteria. The epithelium then proliferates to surround the area.
- **Prostaglandin theory** – epithelial cells within the lining produce prostaglandin release in response to some stimulus. The prostaglandins cause bone resorption, thus resulting in expansion of the cavity.

Epithelium within the tooth-forming organ gives rise to these 'odontogenic' cysts. The three different types of epithelium and the cysts they give rise to are shown in Table 11.1. In Table 11.1, radicular cysts are inflammatory, whereas the others are developmental.

Nonodontogenic cysts include nasopalatine (incisive canal), globulomaxillary, median and

Table 11.1 Types of epithelial cysts

Type of odontogenic epithelium	Cyst
Epithelial rests (glands of Serres)	Odontogenic keratocyst/keratocystic odontogenic tumour (KCOT/KOT)
	Lateral periodontal and gingival
Reduced enamel epithelium (enamel organ)	Dentigerous (follicular)
Eruption	
Epithelial rests of Malassez (root sheath of Hertwig)	Radicular

Table 11.2 Relative frequency of jaw cysts

Type of cyst	Frequency (%)
Radicular	65–70
Dentigerous	15–18
Nasopalatine	5–10
Keratocyst/KCOT/KOT	3–5
Lateral periodontal	<1

nasolabial. The relative frequency of these epithelial cysts is shown in Table 11.2. The percentages given in Table 11.2 can vary a little; for example, the keratocystic odontogenic tumour (KOT) seems twice as common in German-speaking countries as in the United Kingdom. The main issue is to obtain a correct diagnosis and treat the condition.

History and examination

A good history can yield a great deal of information about the likely nature of the problem. Signs and symptoms of the various types of cysts are frequently similar. They usually manifest either as an incidental radiographic finding or as a chronic, painless swelling. Pain becomes a feature when the cyst becomes infected or is so extensive that it causes a pathological fracture, most commonly of the mandible.

Common physical signs include:

- Swelling (intraoral or extraoral).
- Displaced teeth.
- Mobile teeth.
- Eggshell crackling (crepitus).
- Fluctuation.

Other signs that may be more specific to particular cysts are included here:

Odontogenic cysts
Radicular cyst

In a nonvital tooth, this cyst appears as a rounded periapical radiolucency with loss of lamina dura and a sclerotic margin if it is a long-standing lesion (Figure 11.1).

Residual cyst

A radicular cyst is left behind after tooth removal and continues to grow (Figure 11.2).

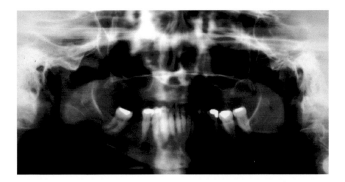

Figure 11.1 A dental panoramic tomogram showing a typical large radicular cyst in the body of the mandible associated with a lower canine and premolar.

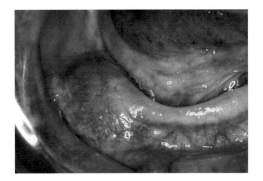

Figure 11.2 The distended mucosa over a residual cyst.

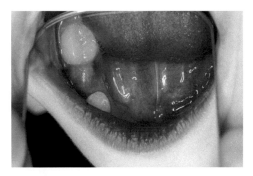

Figure 11.3 Typical blue appearance of an eruption cyst.

Dentigerous cyst

This cyst is found as an incidental finding on radiographs. The cyst envelopes the crown of a tooth. Lower third molars are most frequently affected, followed by upper canines and lower premolars.

Eruption cysts

These cysts are soft tissue analogues of dentigerous cysts and usually overlie unerupted teeth. They tend to affect children and involve deciduous teeth. They appear as a soft, translucent, bluish swelling (Figure 11.3).

Keratocyst/keratocystic odontogenic tumour
This cyst is thought to replace a missing tooth (may be a supernumerary). It is associated with unerupted teeth in 40% of cases. It appears radiographically as a uniloculated or multiloculated radiolucency with a well-defined sclerotic margin. These cysts tend to grow in an anteroposterior direction and therefore do not always cause bony expansion (Figure 11.4).

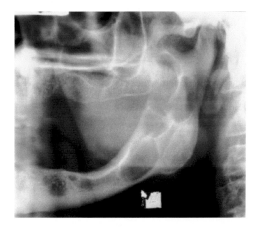

Figure 11.4 A dental panoramic tomogram of a multilocular odontogenic keratocyst (KOC).

The lesion formerly known as the odontogenic keratocyst was redesignated by the World Health Organization as the keratocystic odontogenic tumour (KCOT or KOT) in 2005. This change was based on the aggressive nature, histology and genetics of the lesion. Although this seems to be of interest to pathologists, it makes little difference to clinical management and certainly does not justify treating these cysts as 'malignancy'.

Multiple KOTs are a feature of 'naevoid basal cell carcinoma' syndrome (Gorlin's syndrome – multiple basal cell carcinomas, calcified falx cerebri, rib anomalies). This syndrome is characterized by new cysts appearing throughout the jaws over the lifetime of the patient (as opposed to locally recurring after treatment). The cysts do not need to be managed particularly radically; indeed, given that the cysts often start young, overaggressive surgical treatment can be a great disservice to the patient.

Nonodontogenic cysts

Nasopalatine cyst

Palatal swelling with pain and salty discharge is commonly associated with tooth displacement and loss of vitality (Figure 11.5). Suspect radiographically when the incisive canal is greater than 6 mm in diameter.

Nasolabial cyst

Soft tissue swelling obliterates the nasolabial fold.

Special investigations

These are specific tests carried out to help reach a diagnosis.

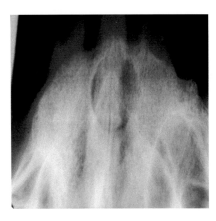

Figure 11.5 Anterior occlusal view of a nasopalatine cyst.

Radiography

This is an essential investigation for establishing the outline and extent of the lesion. It also shows the relationship of teeth and associated anatomical structures such as the inferior dental nerve. Cone beam CT can provide a more detailed picture to aid diagnosis or associated structures in relevant cases.

Aspiration

This can be helpful in establishing a diagnosis.

- Cheesy white material suggests a keratocyst/ KOT.
- Solid mass suggests a possible tumour or a very thick keratin mass.
- Pus indicates an infected cyst or abscess (also foul smell).
- Blood can suggest either an aneurysmal bone cyst or, more importantly, a vascular malformation.
- Air indicates that the needle is within the maxillary antrum or it indicates a solitary bone cyst.

Various tests can be carried out on the aspirate:

- Culture and sensitivity – this is performed if infection is suspected.
- Stain for keratin – keratinized squames are suggestive of a KOT.
- Soluble protein content – KOTs have low protein content because the cyst is filled with keratin, which is mostly insoluble protein. The aspirate therefore contains less than 4 g/dl soluble protein. Cysts and tumours generally have soluble protein concentrations greater than 5 g/dl.
- Electrophoresis – this is not often used now but the protein bands are compared with normal serum as a control. The procedure can distinguish KOTs because the keratin has little soluble protein compared with serum.

Incisional biopsy

If a lesion is very large or there is suspicion that it is more than a simple cyst (e.g. KOT or ameloblastoma), then a biopsy is indicated.

Histological features

Histological features of odontogenic cysts
Radicular cysts (inflammatory)

These cysts develop within a periapical granuloma. The epithelial lining is nonkeratinized squamous epithelium, and it is hyperplastic with occasional mucous metaplasia. Rushton bodies may be found in about 10% of odontogenic cysts, and they occur in odontogenic cysts because the material is secreted only by reduced enamel epithelium. Cholesterol clefts are often present in inflammatory cysts but are not diagnostic. A mixed inflammatory infiltrate of neutrophils, lymphocytes and plasma cells is present.

Dentigerous cysts (developmental)

These cysts are attached to the unerupted tooth at the amelocemental junction, and although this cannot be seen radiographically, it can be seen at operation. The epithelial lining, which is derived from the reduced enamel epithelium, has a flat basement membrane and is a feature of developmental cysts (i.e. dentigerous and KOT). If the cyst is infected there will be an inflammatory response, similar to a radicular cyst.

Keratocystic odontogenic tumours (developmental)

The epithelial lining in KOTs is very friable and therefore difficult to remove completely. Microscopic 'satellite' cysts can be left behind at operation, and this creates the problem of recurrence. The epithelium is keratinized and the keratin is shed into the lumen of the cyst, thus producing the characteristic cheesy contents (Figure 11.6). The basement membrane is flat as in a dentigerous cyst with palisaded columnar basal cells.

Histological features of nonodontogenic cysts
Nasopalatine duct cysts (developmental)

The epithelial lining of these cysts is variable among respiratory, columnar, cuboidal and squamous epithelia as it approaches the oral cavity. The specimen may contain the neurovascular bundle.

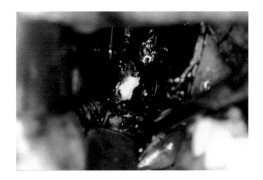

Figure 11.6 An unfortunate rupture of a keratocyst (KOT) lining demonstrates the cheesy, sebaceous-like contents.

Management of cysts

After history, examination and specific investigations, a provisional diagnosis is reached. The likely nature of the condition is explained to the patient. It should be understood that the final diagnosis would be made after a complete histological examination. The proposed surgical treatment, which in the case of epithelial cysts is either enucleation or marsupialization, is discussed with the patient. The major questions are: When is biopsy appropriate, and when is it unnecessary? Preoperative histological diagnosis is an advantage in most cases; the problem is that even if it is performed using local anaesthesia, this subjects the patient to an unpleasant and potentially unnecessary second procedure. Clinically and radiologically unicystic lesions in which the level of certainty of diagnosis is high can quite reasonably be treated primarily and the diagnosis confirmed postoperatively, as long as it is accepted that very rarely a surprise diagnosis of KOT, ameloblastoma or even squamous cell carcinoma will occur. Equally, if there is a level of uncertainty with the diagnosis with which you or the patient feel uncomfortable, then predefinitive treatment biopsy is the sensible option.

Local anaesthetic versus general anaesthetic

If the lesion is limited to the region of a single tooth, then treatment using a local anaesthetic is usually adequate. Lesions in the posterior mandible and those spanning more than two or three teeth are often better treated with the patient under general anaesthesia. These are only approximate guidelines, and the treatment plan should be tailored to the individual case, taking all other factors such as medical history, size and potential definitive diagnosis into account.

Warnings and potential complications

Informed consent is obtained from the patient (see Chapter 2). Serious and commonly occurring complications should also be discussed. Complications can be categorized as follows:

- Intraoperative – bleeding, fractured mandible in cases of mandibular cysts, oral antral fistula (Figures 11.7 and 11.8), damage to adjacent teeth and nerve damage (temporary and permanent).
- Early postoperative – pain, swelling, bruising, bleeding and infection.

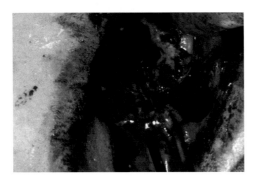

Figure 11.7 Enucleation of maxillary cysts often results in involvement of the antral lining.

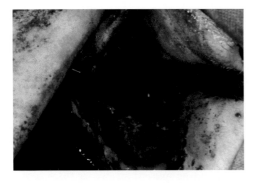

Figure 11.8 Oral antral communications should be closed primarily.

- Late postoperative – recurrence (particularly KOTs).

Postoperative course

Patients will want to know how long they will be in hospital in the case of inpatient procedures using general anaesthesia. If patients are having a local anaesthetic, then they will often ask how long the procedure will take. Postoperative recovery should be discussed, as well as time off work. In cases of large cysts where there is a risk of fracture postoperatively, a soft diet and avoidance of contact sports should be recommended.

Review

The patient will need to be reviewed to discuss the histopathology and to check the operative site. Further review will depend on the nature of the disease. In particular, KOTs will require longer-term follow-up in view of the risk of recurrence that can occur after many years, although the practicality of this follow-up varies with the available resources. Rarely, these lesions can undergo malignant transformation into squamous cell carcinoma.

Surgical treatment

Enucleation (termed cystectomy or Partsch II operation in Germany)

Most cysts are managed by enucleation. This involves stripping away the cyst lining from the resorbed bony cavity; the result is a clean 'hole' in the bone. This deficit is filled by blood, which organizes into osteoid and then into new bone. A step by step illustration of the procedure is shown in Figures 11.9 through 11.14.

Marsupialization (termed cystostomy or Partsch I operation in Germany)

Large cysts in which enucleation may result in extensive local damage or patients who are unfit for more extensive surgery can be managed by marsupialization. This involves exposing the cyst lining and removing a small window from the lining. This is then sutured to the mucosa. The cavity can be packed with an antiseptic dressing (a thermoplastic obturating material called KERR in Germany) and regularly changed as the cavity heals from underneath (Figures 11.15, 11.16 and 11.17).

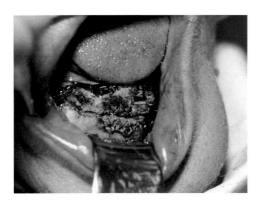

Figure 11.9 Subperiosteal flap to expose bone expanded by the underlying cyst.

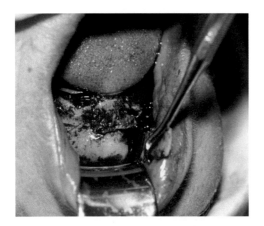

Figure 11.10 Buccal cortex is removed to create a bone 'window' for enucleation of the cyst.

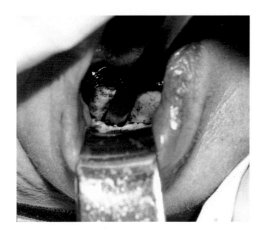

Figure 11.11 The plane between the cyst lining and the bone cavity is bluntly dissected with a periosteal elevator.

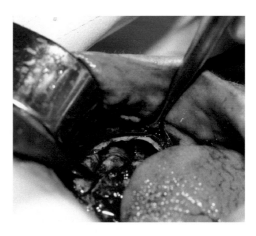

Figure 11.12 Teasing the cyst by direct traction and dissection with a periosteal elevator delivers the cyst.

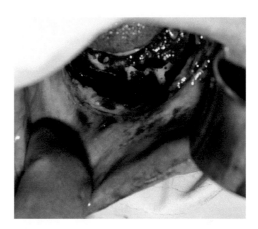

Figure 11.13 The empty bone cavity after removal of the cyst.

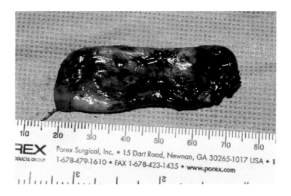

Figure 11.14 The removed specimen.

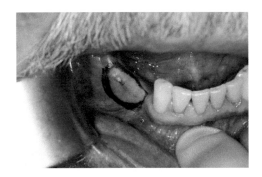

Figure 11.15 Marsupialization of a cyst that is in contact with the overlying alveolar mucosa in an infirm patient. The area of mucosa to be excised is marked out.

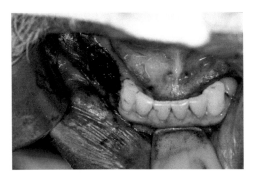

Figure 11.16 Cyst lining is retained and in continuity with oral epithelium 'externalizing' the cyst.

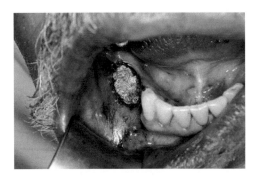

Figure 11.17 The defect is packed with iodoform gauze. This allows gradual resolution of the defect as new bone displaces the cavity lining toward the alveolus.

Decompression with oral 'grommets' has been used in extremely frail patients. This procedure removes little or none of the cyst lining and places a small 'ventilation tube' that seems to delay growth or even reduce the overall size of the cyst. This procedure is essentially palliative because no formal diagnosis is reached and the bone defect remains. The term 'marsupialization' in German means only suturing of the cyst lining to peripheral mucosa to achieve something similar.

Limited resection

Keratocysts/KOTs, aneurysmal bone cysts and cyst-like tumours (e.g. myxoma, unicystic ameloblastoma) need more aggressive forms of removal. A rim resection or modified enucleation removing bone in contact with the lining or treatment with Carnoy's solution or cryotherapy can be used. Resection with a reinforcing reconstruction plate is shown in Figures 11.18, 11.19, 11.20, 11.21, 11.22 and 11.23.

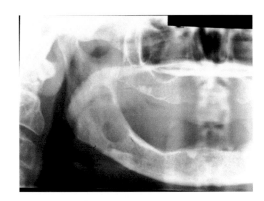

Figure 11.18 Large keratocysts (KOT), or benign cystic tumours, may require more radical excision.

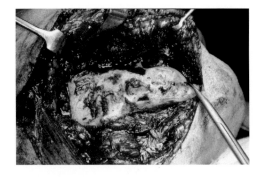

Figure 11.19 A cervical approach to a large recurrent keratocyst (KOT) that has grossly distorted the buccal cortex.

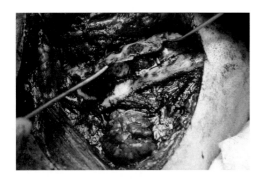

Figure 11.20 The involved bone is removed, thus exposing the cyst.

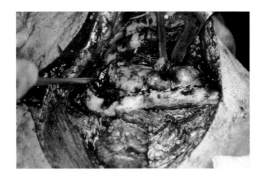

Figure 11.21 The thick-walled cyst is removed and the surrounding bone is excised.

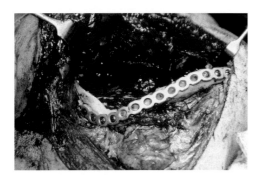

Figure 11.22 The hollow lower border and the lingual cortex are plated with a reconstruction plate. If a pathological fracture occurs, the bone will be held in its anatomical position while it heals.

Nonepithelial cysts

These cysts are sometimes referred to as 'pseudo-cysts' because they do not have an epithelial lining. They are fluid-filled cavities within the bone and can be broadly divided into three types:

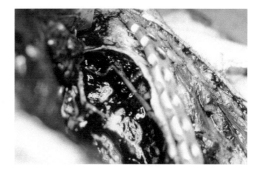

Figure 11.23 The inferior alveolar nerve branching into mental and incisive branches with a bicortical screw passing beneath the main bundle.

- Aneurysmal bone cyst.
- Solitary bone cyst.
- Stafne's idiopathic bone 'cyst'.

Aneurysmal bone cyst

These cysts are benign intraosseous lesions characterized by blood-filled spaces. They are most commonly found in the long bones (98.5%). They are rare in the facial bones and when they do occur they are usually seen in the mandible.

The aetiology is unknown. The lesions can be divided into two categories – primary (70%) and secondary (30%). Primary aneurysmal bone cysts have no associated previous lesions, and these cysts can be congenital (i.e. no history of trauma) or traumatic. Patients with secondary aneurismal bone cysts have a history of previous lesions such as fibrous dysplasia or dentigerous cyst.

Clinically, they manifest as firm, painless swellings that expand slowly. Sudden expansion and pain are usually indicative of sudden bleeding inside the cyst, often following minor trauma. Although the teeth generally remain vital, the patient may present with malocclusions or root resorption.

Radiographically the cysts form unilocular or multilocular radiolucencies, which can be mistaken for ameloblastoma or KOT.

Histologically, multiple blood-filled spaces are seen and are separated by fibrous septa with scattered multinucleate giant cells.

Simple curettage is usually all that is required, although some cases are complicated by severe bleeding. In these situations, limited resection is needed and curative.

Solitary bone cyst

These cysts are often seen in the humerus and femur. They rarely occur in the head and neck region, and when they do they are almost always in the mandible.

The aetiology is unknown, but it is thought to be related to a haemodynamic imbalance within the bone. It has been suggested that these cysts may be associated with a history of trauma, although the link is not strong and the history of trauma may range from months to years before the appearance of the cyst.

Clinically, these cysts are usually asymptomatic, but there is occasionally bone expansion and radiographically there is an irregular radiolucency with well-defined scalloping between the roots of the teeth. Histological examination shows a thin layer of loose vascular fibrous tissue but no epithelial lining and no cyst fluid.

The cysts often resolve spontaneously; however, the cavity is usually opened if only to confirm a diagnosis. Theoretically it could be healed by injecting the patient's own blood into the cyst to allow organization of clot into new bone.

Stafne's idiopathic bone cavity

This is thought to be a developmental defect on the lingual aspect of the mandible that contains a portion of normal submandibular salivary gland (or sublingual gland when seen in the anterior mandible).

Clinically, these cavities are asymptomatic and are usually discovered as incidental findings on radiographs, where they appear as a well-circumscribed area in the body of the mandible with a sclerotic margin. Their location and lack of symptoms are often diagnostic; however, further investigation (e.g. sialography, computed tomography scans or magnetic resonance imaging) can confirm the diagnosis. No treatment is required.

FURTHER READING

Chapelle KAOM, Stoelinga PJW, De Wild PCM, Brouns JJA, Voorsmit RACA. Rational approach to diagnosis and treatment of ameloblastomas and odontogenic keratocysts. *Br J Oral Maxillofac Surg* 2004;42:381–90.

Shear M, Speight P. *Cysts of the oral regions*, 4th ed. Bristol, UK: John Wright & Sons, 2007. *Remains one of the few textbooks on oral and jaw cysts.*

Soames JV, Southam JC. *Oral pathology*, 4th ed. Oxford: Oxford University Press, 2005. *Readable and up to date account of the pathological appearance and behaviour of jaw cysts.*

Stoelinga PJW. The treatment of odontogenic keratocysts by excision of the overlying, attached mucosa, enucleation, and treatment of the bony defect with Carnoy solution. *J Oral Maxillofac Surg* 2005;63:1662–6.

World Health Organization (WHO), International Agency for Research on Cancer Screening Group. WHO histological classification of odontogenic tumours. http://screening.iarc.fr/atlasoralclassifwho2.php *If you really feel the need to know why it's now called KOT.*

12

Benign surgical conditions of the mouth, jaws and neck

Contents

Aim for the undergraduate and postgraduate

- To develop a broad recognition of benign oral and maxillofacial lumps and their investigation and treatment.

Learning outcomes

For undergraduates:

- To be able to describe the majority of benign conditions that manifest as soft tissue swelling in the mouth, face, neck and jaw.
- To be able to describe the usual investigations indicated for these lumps.
- To be able to outline the general treatment of these lumps.

For postgraduates:

- To be able to recognize the surgical soft tissue swellings of the mouth, jaws, face and neck.

- To be able to describe appropriate investigations and treatment of these swellings.
- To be able to list those conditions that require urgent or routine referral.
- To be able to describe the surgical treatment of the common benign oral and maxillofacial lumps.

Introduction

The benign conditions that manifest as soft tissue swellings, particularly those appropriate for surgical management in the mouth, jaws, skin of the face and the neck, overlap with many of the other conditions outlined in other chapters (e.g. Chapters 11 and 21). It is important to recognize that many of the swellings detected on examination of the head and neck are entirely innocent and can be identified as being so by clinical examination, distinct history and some fairly simple diagnostic tests. Each condition is outlined with its appropriate treatment.

Soft tissue lumps of the mouth

Brown tumour of hyperparathyroidism

This is a giant cell lesion that can look extremely florid and mandates early biopsy for diagnosis. It occurs secondarily to hyperparathyroidism, but this diagnosis is usually made only after biopsy, either incisional or excisional, when the findings of giant cells in a fibrous stroma mandate an assessment of bone biochemistry and measurement of parathyroid hormone levels.

Treatment

After diagnosis by incisional biopsy, treatment consists of local excision and curettage of bone and periosteum if the lesion does not regress spontaneously after treatment of the hyperparathyroidism.

Congenital epulis

This is a sessile or pedunculated nodule containing granular cells on histological examination. Present at birth, the lesion is usually excised only once the child is 1 year old unless it significantly interferes with normal function.

Treatment

Local excision in a subperiosteal plane is curative.

Dermoid cyst

This developmental cyst is found in the midline of the neck, above the mylohyoid, where it causes swelling in the floor of the mouth. If it appears as an intraoral swelling, it can be confused with a ranula. Oral dermoids tend to manifest in young adults. There is a male-to-female ratio of 1:1.

There are three general variants:

1. The common epidermoid cyst, which tends to contain keratinous material similar to that seen in keratocystic odontogenic tumours.
2. The true dermoid cyst, which is lined by squamous epithelium and contains skin appendages.

3. The very rare keratoid cyst, which may contain other external derivatives.

The 'angular dermoid' is an epidermal cyst arising above the lateral canthus of the eye at the zygomaticofrontal suture. It manifests in childhood and may have an intracranial extension. This diagnosis should be excluded by computed tomography (CT) before excision.

Treatment

Treatment is by complete local excision. The approach depends on the size and location of the dermoid.

Epulis

This is any gingival lump that has nonspecific features.

Treatment

The lesion is classified from clinical or imaging features and is managed accordingly.

Fibroepithelial polyp

This is a benign but excessive response to low-grade recurrent trauma. These lesions may be sessile or pedunculated and can range from very small lumps looking like a genuine polyp in the cheek to lesions that can cover the entire palate ('leaf fibroma') (Figure 12.1). Histology will show very dense collagenous fibrous tissue lined by keratinized stratified squamous epithelium.

Treatment

These lesions, once diagnosed either on a clinical basis or by incisional biopsy, should be excised, including their base. The pedunculated lesion often has a very vascular stalk that requires local control with diathermy or sutures.

Granuloma

Granulomata are swellings that show a characteristic histological appearance and may be caused by orofacial granulomatosis (Figure 12.2), sarcoidosis, or implanted foreign bodies.

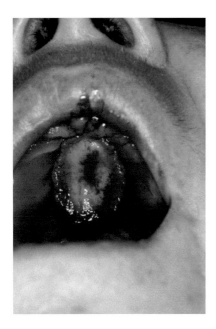

Figure 12.1 An example of 'leaf fibroma'.

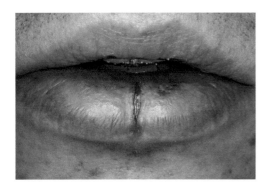

Figure 12.2 Orofacial granulomatosis may manifest with 'cobblestone' mucosal lumps, lip swelling and midline fissuring.

Treatment

Local granulomata are usually treated by simple local excision, although in the case of orofacial granulomatosis and sarcoidosis, intralesional steroids may help. Patients with orofacial granulomatosis, in particular, should undergo patch testing for allergic-type responses to cinnamates often found in toothpastes. Elimination diets to exclude a dietary cause can be both diagnostic and therapeutic and may prevent serious facial distortion later (Figure 12.3).

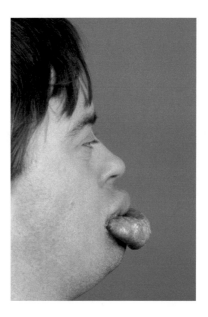

Figure 12.3 Early treatment of orofacial granulomatosis can prevent gross labial distortion.

Giant cell granuloma (giant cell epulis)

This is a very vascular gingival swelling and is probably caused by chronic irritation (Figure 12.4). Histological examination demonstrates multinucleate giant cells in a vascular stroma.

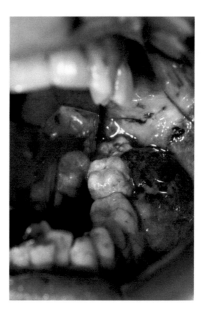

Figure 12.4 Granuloma can mimic malignant disease.

Treatment

Excision should include the underlying periosteum.

Gingival fibromatosis

This condition can be hereditary or, more often, drug induced. Phenytoin, Cyclosporin A and calcium channel blockers are the main causes (Figure 12.5).

Treatment

Treatment consists of excision by gingivectomy unless drugs can be changed and this change induces an involution of the swelling.

Hyperplasia

Particularly notable is irritation hyperplasia, which is a hyperplastic response to repeated trauma following denture-induced ulceration (see Chapter 15). Rolls of hyperplastic tissue that may be quite erythematous and resemble malignant disease are seen, particularly in the buccal sulci (Figure 12.6). This condition is more common in the lower jaw than the upper. Histology is very similar to that of fibroepithelial polyp.

Treatment

Treatment consists of removing the offending denture to see whether there is any spontaneous resolution. If so, then it may be possible to manage this condition nonsurgically; if not, the area should be excised and allowed to heal, and then new dentures

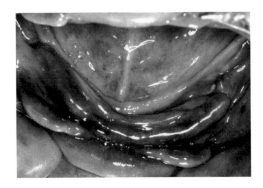

Figure 12.6 Irritation hyperplasia caused by an ill-fitting full lower denture.

should be provided. Simple preprosthetic measures may also be needed.

Haemangioma

Haemangiomata are developmental lesions of blood vessels. They are usually congenital (i.e. present at birth) and tend to grow with the child. Most (up to 80%) of these lesions regress spontaneously.

Treatment

Haemangioma can be identified by blanching under pressure (classically by using a glass slide) (Figure 12.7). Some haemangiomata respond to the use of steroids or propanolol to promote resolution. Localized cryotherapy and laser therapy can also resolve these lesions. However, it should be remembered that 80% will resolve spontaneously. These are quite different from vascular malformations.

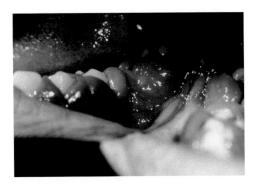

Figure 12.5 Drug-induced gingival fibromatosis.

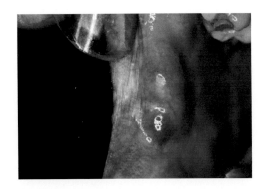

Figure 12.7 Low-flow venous vascular malformation of the buccal mucosa.

Lipoma

Lipomata are benign tumours of fat cells found anywhere in the body including the mouth (Figure 12.8).

Treatment

Treatment consists of excision with primary repair.

Lymphangioma

Lymphangiomata are rare developmental abnormalities of lymphatics. Most are simple, thin-walled, capillary-sized lymphatic channels, although some can be larger, termed cavernous lymphangioma, containing dilated lymphatic spaces. The rarest variant is called cystic hygroma, which creates a cystic malformation containing multiple cysts of various sizes. Cystic hygroma arises mainly in the neck where it can encroach and spread between surrounding tissues. Intraoral lymphangioma can cause significant enlargement of the tongue, lips and cheek. The male-to-female ratio is 1:1, and more than 90% of these lesions are present by the second birthday (Figure 12.9).

Treatment

Treatment of cystic hygroma and lymphangioma is usually by excision, although Picibanil a (a streptococcal antigen) injections have demonstrated value in some of the variants of cystic hygroma. Surgery is extremely difficult for microcystic lesions but comparatively simple for large, solitary macrocystic lymphangioma (which perversely is the easiest

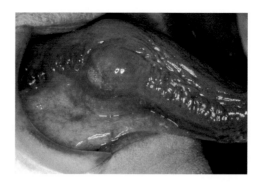

Figure 12.9 Lymphangioma of the tongue.

to sclerose with Picibanil). Microcystic lymphangioma may require multiple excisions over many years, and it is essential to have the child's parents fully cognizant of this. Recurrence rate is up to 15%, although this shows a preponderance toward the microcystic variant.

Mucocele

Mucoceles are mucous extravasation cysts in which saliva leaks from traumatized minor salivary ducts and pools of usually mucinous saliva create a connective tissue capsule. They almost always affect the lower lip, and treatment is by excision (see Chapter 21) (Figure 12.10).

Papilloma

Squamous cell papillomas are multiple papillated pink and white asymptomatic lumps; they

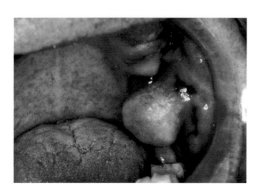

Figure 12.8 Intraoral lipoma.

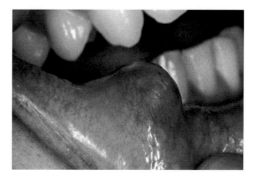

Figure 12.10 Mucocele of the lower lip (most common site).

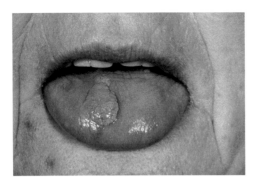

Figure 12.11 Squamous papilloma of the tongue tip.

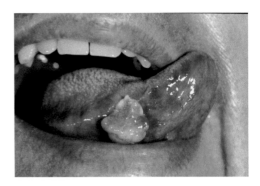

Figure 12.12 Large pyogenic granuloma of the tongue.

look like and are very similar to warts in skin. These lesions should be readily identifiable as such (Figure 12.11). The main aetiological factor is the human papilloma virus (HPV), and there is an increase in patients with sexually transmitted diseases. Most oral papillomata are of no real significance and are not related to oral infection with HPV-16 or HPV-18, which is a transient infection affecting up to 10% of the population (occurring more in male than in female patients) and is cleared within a year. This virus type (HPV-16 and HPV-18) is, however, clearly associated with HPV-driven oropharyngeal squamous cell carcinoma (see Chapter 22), which has a much better prognosis in nonsmokers. The relationships among virus type, transient infection and virally driven cancer in specific anatomical sites in the head and neck remains unclear, but prevention of infection by vaccination, changing safe sex practices or some as yet unenvisioned intervention to remove an identified cause of head and neck cancer is a vital area of further research.

Treatment
Excision biopsy is performed.

Pyogenic granuloma

Pyogenic granuloma is an inflammatory response to chronic irritation. Lesions are found in a variety of intraoral sites, depending on aetiology. Puberty and pregnancy 'epulides' are hormonally sensitive examples.

Treatment
Excision, usually in a deep plane, is performed if the patient is symptomatic (Figure 12.12).

Ranula

Ranulas are mucoceles of the floor of the mouth, usually arising from the sublingual gland or the duct of the sublingual glands. Simple marsupialization tends to cause recurrence because the underlying damaged duct has not been dealt with. Plunging ranulas cross the mylohyoid and can appear in the neck (see the later section on neck swelling). Treatment is by excision of the cyst and the associated sublingual gland. This is performed transorally for simple ranula and externally via the neck for plunging ranula (see Chapter 21).

Vascular malformation

These malformations are divided into arteriovenous fistulae, high-flow venous malformations and low-flow venous malformations.

Treatment
Treatment is conventionally by interventional radiology, either embolization or sclerosant injection coupled with surgical excision and reconstruction where indicated. As the move toward minimal intervention by embolization techniques has progressed, it is important to recognize that these malformations tend to recur without synchronized excision.

Hard tissue lumps of the mouth and jaws

Ameloblastoma

This is the most common tumour of dental epithelial origin. It is found particularly in the posterior mandible in African male patients. It is benign and has three clinical and histological variants – unicystic, follicular/plexiform and peripheral.

Unicystic ameloblastoma

Unicystic ameloblastoma is a cystic swelling distinguished by resorbing adjacent tooth roots and the lamina propria on radiographs. According to Ackermann there are three histological groups of **unicystic ameloblastomas** – groups 1 and 2 (tumour confined to the epithelium of the cyst) and group 3 (tumour present in the connective tissue wall of the cyst).

Although this lesion is an ameloblastoma histologically, it has predominantly fluid contents (Figure 12.13).

Treatment

Treatment consists of 'radical' enucleation, in which a margin of the surrounding bone is resected or otherwise treated (cryosurgery, Carnoy's solution). This is similar to the approach to recurrent keratocystic odontogenic tumours.

Follicular/plexiform ameloblastoma

This solid tumour, again found in the mandible, is more aggressive in its clinical behaviour and resembles a solid tumour histologically (Figure 12.14).

Treatment

Conventional bone resection is performed with a small (0.5 cm) margin, preserving vital structures when possible. Segmental resection may be needed (Figure 12.15).

Peripheral ameloblastoma

Peripheral ameloblastoma is an extraosseous soft tissue version of ameloblastoma. It is rare and is more often seen in the maxilla.

Treatment

Subperiosteal soft tissue excision is performed with a 0.5-cm margin of normal tissue.

An ameloblastoma in German textbooks is commonly specified as a benign hard tissue tumour. However, an ameloblastoma is said to behave like a basal cell carcinoma (BCC) in principle (i.e. usually no metastases) and therefore is nicknamed the BCC of the bone.

Running through all these varying interpretations are essential useful clinical behaviours; ameloblastoma has a range of pathological behaviours based on local destructiveness and a propensity for recurrence. These tumours do not metastasize but do need wide local excision and sometimes reconstruction.

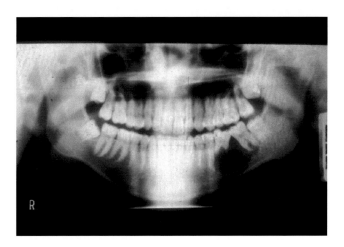

Figure 12.13 'Unicystic' ameloblastoma resorbing tooth roots.

BENIGN TUMOURS

Odontogenic epithelium with mature, fibrous stroma without odontogenic ectomesenchyme

Ameloblastoma, solid/multicystic
type 9310/0
Ameloblastoma, extraosseous/
peripheral type 9310/0
Amcloblastoma, desmoplastic
type 9310/0
Ameloblastoma, unicystic
type 9310/0

Ameloblastic carcinoma is a malignant version of the ameloblastoma and is managed as any intraosseous malignancy of the head and neck.

Other odontogenic tumours are extremely rare. They are all managed by conservative excision:

- Adenoameloblastoma, most common in the anterior mandible of female patients.
- Calcifying epithelial odontogenic tumour, radiographically distinguished as a cyst with flecks of calcification.
- Myxoma, which affects young adults and is radiographically a multilocular radiolucency.
- Ameloblastic fibroma, which is radiographically a unilocular radiolucency but is more prone to recurrence after excision.

Brown tumour

See the earlier section on brown tumour of hyperparathyroidism.

Cherubism

Cherubism is a hereditary variant of fibrous dysplasia that manifests between 2 and 4 years of age. It appears bilaterally and tends to burn out in a similar fashion to fibrous dysplasia.

Treatment

Skeletal resculpting is performed.

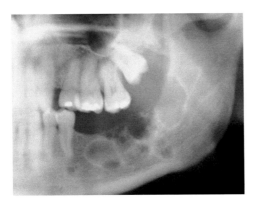

Figure 12.14 Sectional dental panoramic tomogram of the 'soap bubble' appearance of the solid variety of ameloblastoma.

Fibrous dysplasia

This is characteristically a disease of young adults in which areas of bone are replaced by fibrous tissue. Onset is in childhood, and the disease tends to stabilize with age. Jaw involvement usually manifests as a hard, painless swelling, with a characteristic radiographic appearance of 'ground glass' (Figure 12.16). Histology shows fibrous replacement of bone with osseous trabeculae that look like irregular Chinese characters.

Treatment

Treatment should wait until completion of growth because this is a hamartomatous problem that can be resculpted after growth is completed.

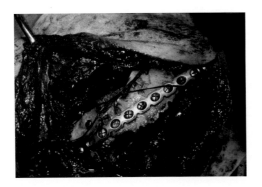

Figure 12.15 Bone and nerve grafting supported by a reconstruction plate to repair the mandibular discontinuity after segmental mandibular resection.

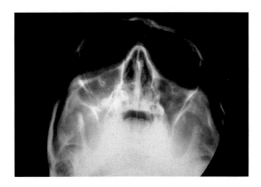

Figure 12.16 Radiographic appearance of fibrous dysplasia of the maxilla.

The ossifying fibroma, thought to be a localized tumour, may be a variant of this condition.

Giant cell granuloma

Giant cell granuloma can manifest as an intrabony swelling treated in the same way as the soft tissue version (see earlier). In the United States there are some clinicians who manage these lesions medically with intralesional steroid, calcitonin or interferon.

Ossifying fibroma

This is probably a localized variant of fibrous dysplasia that appears clinically as a bony hard mass in the jaws that is capable of enlarging both bony cortices. It appears well circumscribed radiologically.

Treatment

This lesion can usually be safely enucleated within a fibrous envelope (Figure 12.17). Significant bone resection is not necessary.

Osteoma

Osteoma is a benign tumour of bone. It may appear singly (Figure 12.18) or as multiple small bony protuberances characteristic of Gardner's syndrome (multiple familial polyposis coli). Always enquire about gastrointestinal symptoms in these patients and refer for gastrointestinal and genetic investigations.

Treatment

Local excision is performed (Figure 12.19).

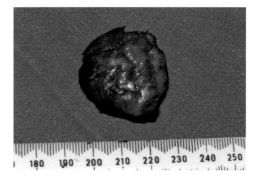

Figure 12.17 Postexcision specimen of an ossifying fibroma showing how it can be 'shelled out' from the surrounding bone (no recurrence after 17 years).

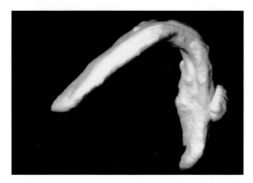

Figure 12.18 Three-dimensional computed tomography reformat of a single large mandibular osteoma.

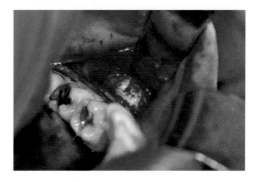

Figure 12.19 Transoral resections of mandibular osteoma showing the subperiosteal plane common to most jaw surgery.

Paget's disease of the bone

This multisystem condition affects the skull, pelvis and long bones as well as the jaws. It is relatively common after the age of 55 years. Respiratory syncytial and measles viruses have been indicated

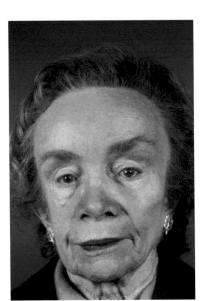

Figure 12.20 Clinical example of distortion of the left zygoma and skull in Paget's disease.

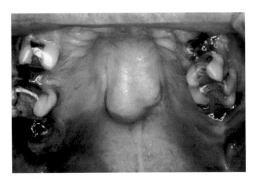

Figure 12.21 The appearance of torus palatinus.

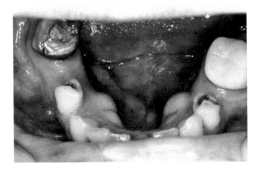

Figure 12.22 Torus mandibularis. Both torus palatinus and torus mandibularis are benign and require no treatment.

in its aetiology although this correlation is still unclear. The maxilla is more frequently affected than the mandible, and of particular note is that the bones are prone to hypercementosis, which makes extractions difficult (Figure 12.20). There is a replacement of normal remodelling by a chaotic alternation of resorption and deposition, with resorption dominating in the early stages and deposition later. Bone pain and cranial neuropathies can occur, and patients may present with altered sensation of the face associated with bony swelling. Plain radiographs show a cotton wool appearance, and biochemistry shows elevations in alkaline phosphatase and urinary hydroxyproline.

Treatment

Treatment is complex, but bisphosphonates and calcitonin may be used. However, because this is a multisystem disease, localized lesions may be diagnosed on bone biopsy, and referral would be indicated. The risk of bisphosphonate-related osteonecrosis of the jaw in patients with Paget's disease treated by bisphosphonates is of obvious relevance.

Torus

Tori are bony exostoses found in both jaws. Torus palatinus occurs in the centre of the hard palate (see Chapter 15) (Figure 12.21), and torus mandibularis occurs in the lingual premolar or molar region of the mandible (Figure 12.22). These lesions are entirely benign and require removal only if the patient is very concerned about them or for preprosthetic reasons. Multiple bony exostoses as found in Gardner's syndrome or significant isolated exostoses may require excision both for diagnostic and symptomatic purposes.

Neck lumps

Traditionally and for practical reasons, these lesions can be divided into those commonly manifesting in children and those commonly manifesting in adults. There are fundamental differences in the underlying pathology of neck lumps in the two groups.

Neck masses in children

It is important to remember that head and neck neoplasia is a very rare cause of neck swellings in children. In children, neck swellings are usually either congenital or inflammatory.

Congenital conditions
Branchial sinus

These sinuses arise either from the branchial cleft or arches (usually the first and second branchial arches) or from the thyroglossal tract.

Branchial derivatives – These are preauricular sinuses and remnants of notochord just in front of the ear. Many of these preauricular sinuses and cartilaginous remnants are probably **not** specifically of branchial origin. True branchial sinuses arising from the first branchial arch have openings usually just below the angle of the mandible or along the uppermost border of the sternomastoid. They usually manifest as a discharging sinus with an epithelial lined tract. It is thought that the internal openings of the sinuses are related to the arch of origin. Sinuses of first arch origin tend to open near the bony and cartilaginous external auditory meatus. The second arch opens into the tonsillar fossa, whereas sinuses of third or fourth arch origins would arise lower down in the pharynx.

Treatment Treatment is by excision of the entire sinus by using multiple small cervical incisions in a stepwise fashion, sometimes coupled with an open approach (Figure 12.23). A modified

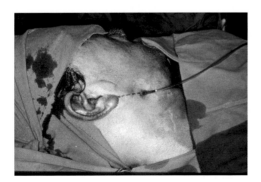

Figure 12.23 Preoperative photograph of a sinus probe in a branchial sinus before excision.

parotidectomy may be needed for some first arch sinuses.

Branchial cyst

These cysts have two theories of origin:

1. The branchial cyst is a remnant of the second branchial arch, but this fails to explain why most branchial cysts manifest in adolescence or adulthood.
2. The branchial cyst is actually an epithelial inclusion within cervical lymph nodes. This theory is supported by the findings that branchial cysts have no internal opening and most branchial cysts do include lymphoid tissue in their wall.

Other theories exist based on the embryonic development theory. There is no agreement on which theory is the more favourable, although in terms of popularity, origin from the branchial apparatus is probably the leader.

Clinical findings Two thirds of these cysts lie anterior to the anterior border of the upper third of the sternomastoid muscle, one third will lie lower than this. These cysts usually manifest as a persistent swelling, although pain can be a presenting feature if the cyst is infected. They are more frequent in male than in female patients and are more common on the left than on the right side; approximately 2% are said to be bilateral.

Investigations These lesions should be diagnosed clinically; specific imaging either with ultrasound or CT may confirm the clinical impression of an isolated cyst in a classical position. Fine needle aspiration cytology may demonstrate cholesterol crystals but is otherwise unhelpful.

Treatment Treatment is by excision, preserving the great auricular nerve wherever possible (Figures 12.24 and 12.25).

Thyroglossal derivatives – thyroglossal cyst

The thyroid develops from the tuberculum impar at the junction of the posterior and anterior two thirds of the tongue, which descends during fetal life to the neck. In some instances no migration

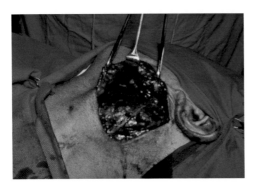

Figure 12.24 Skin flap elevated to show the distortion of sternomastoid caused by a branchial cyst and the preserved great auricular nerve.

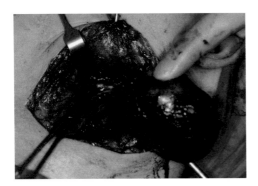

Figure 12.25 The dissected branchial cyst being removed from beneath sternomastoid. Note the bipolar burns – small vessels usually lie deep to these cysts.

occurs, and the thyroid gland can develop as a lingual thyroid. On rare occasions this may be the only functioning thyroid, but more commonly the tract of descent is the source of pathology, usually in the form of a thyroglossal duct cyst. It is important to remember that the persisting thyroglossal duct runs from behind the thyroid gland, through, around or in front of the hyoid bone and ends at the foramen caecum in the tongue. Thyroglossal fistulae may occur when an infected thyroglossal cyst discharges spontaneously onto the skin or when inadequate surgery has been attempted to excise a thyroglossal cyst.

Clinical features These cysts most frequently manifest in young children, although the age range is wide; most of these lesions lie in the midline of the neck (90%). These are mostly painless central

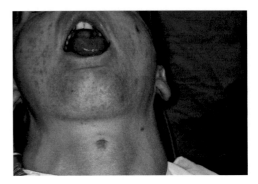

Figure 12.26 Sinus from a thyroglossal duct cyst moving up on tongue elevation.

neck masses that move on swallowing and elevate on protruding the tongue (Figure 12.26).

Investigations These cysts can be transilluminated but are usually easy to diagnose on a clinical basis. If the patient is euthyroid with a normal thyroid-stimulating hormone value, no further investigations are needed, although many clinicians recommend ultrasound of the neck to image the usual position of the thyroid.

Treatment Treatment is by the operation described by Sistrunk that includes removal of the cyst and the central portion of the hyoid bone to allow complete excision of the length of the duct (Figure 12.27).

Lymphangioma

Cystic hygroma manifests more commonly in the neck than in the mouth and appears as a cystic mass that infiltrates through tissue planes and will not spontaneously resolve. Because of the problems associated with completely resecting this nonmalignant mass, various sclerosant agents have been used. Picibanil, a form of inactivated streptococcal antigen, and bleomycin are examples of these agents. The easiest and most effectively sclerosed lymphangiomata are also those that could be most easily and safely excised (the macrocystic variants). This means that treatment should be the patient's, rather than the practitioner's, choice.

Sternomastoid tumour

This is probably a combination of spasm and small haematoma within the fibres of sternomastoid that

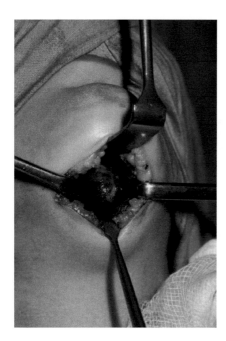

Figure 12.27 The Sistrunk approach to excision of a thyroglossal cyst includes the tract and central portion of the hyoid bone.

creates the physical appearance of a mass. This can result in torticollis, which can itself result in asymmetrical development of the head and face (postural plagiocephaly).

Treatment Direct physiotherapy and manipulation are performed, if at all possible. If this lesion has been missed as a child and manifests in later life, formal excision (cranial and caudal ends of the sternomastoid with or without Z-plasty) may be necessary because areas of extremely tight fibrosis and sometimes ossification can occur.

Cervical lymphadenopathy

It is important to realize that children develop cervical lymphadenopathy very easily indeed, and persisting cervical lymphadenopathy in children, unlike in adults, is more frequently the result of transient reactive lymphadenopathy than anything else. There are, however, specific infective and inflammatory conditions that cause lymphadenitis. These include cat scratch fever (see Chapter 10), which causes generalized lymphadenopathy, but particularly cervical lymphadenopathy. Many other bacterial infections including dental infections cause cervical lymphadenitis

(see Chapter 10). Of particular importance is mycobacterial lymphadenitis, usually caused by atypical mycobacteria. There is a balance needed between surgical treatment of atypical mycobacterial lymphadenitis (which remains the most effective modality) and watching and waiting with long-term clarithromycin therapy (which may avoid operation but can take a very long time and sometimes leaves scars worse than those of surgery).

Adult neck masses

Unlike in children, the finding of a soft tissue mass in the neck of an adult is more often indicative of serious pathology. These neck masses can be divided into congenital, acquired, infective and tumours.

Congenital neck masses

Lymphangioma

Lymphangiomas have already been discussed and usually manifest in childhood.

Dermoid

Intra oral dermoids have already been discussed; however, it is important to realize that of all craniofacial dermoids the most common site of origin is between the outer angle of the eye and the hairline. These lesions can also occur on the nasal bridge, submentally without manifesting in the mouth and very low in the neck, just below the sternoclavicular notch. Dermoids arise at lines of fusion where exodermal tissue can become submerged in the development and fusion of the facial processes. These later secrete sebaceous material and appear as cystic swellings that are called dermoids.

Investigation There is seldom any need for a specific investigation. However, if there is any suspicion, particularly of an angular dermoid of the lateral border of the eye fixed to the underlying tissues, it should be investigated by CT scan because on rare occasions dumbbell phenomena can occur in which two dermoids, one intracranial and one extracranial, are connected.

Treatment Treatment is generally by simple excision of the cyst.

Thyroglossal duct cyst

See the earlier section on neck masses in children.

Branchial cyst

See the earlier section on neck masses in children.

Branchial fistula

See the earlier section on neck masses in children.

Haemangioma

See the earlier section on neck masses in children.

Acquired neck masses

Ranula

Ranula has already been mentioned within the mouth and is covered in Chapter 21.

Laryngocele

Laryngoceles arise within the circle of the laryngeal ventricle. They are more common in men than in women and usually occur in patients in their 60s. Most are unilateral, and 1% will contain malignant disease.

Clinical findings   Clinical findings include neck lump, hoarseness, sore throat and sometimes stridor, and 10% of patients will present with infection of the laryngocele. Because of the association with the larynx these patients are much more likely to present to an otolaryngologist.

Pharyngeal pouch

This is a diverticulum of the pharyngeal mucosa, usually of the median posterior wall passing through Killian's dehiscence. It is more common in men than in women and is usually a condition found in patients who are more than 70 years old. Most patients present with difficulty in swallowing, although halitosis and regurgitation of undigested food can also be found. Some may present with cough, recurrent chest infection, hoarseness or a neck mass.

Investigation   These patients require a barium swallow and pharyngeal oesophagoscopy and again are much more likely to present to an otolaryngologist.

Treatment   There is a range of endoscopic and open procedures for the excision of pharyngeal pouches. The profusion of different treatments would suggest that no one is ideal, but most of these diverticula are now managed endoscopically.

Infective neck masses

These masses tend to be either manifestations of cervical lymphadenopathy or abscesses of the cervical fascial spaces (see Chapter 10).

Benign tumours of the neck

Benign tumours of salivary gland origin are most common (see Chapter 21).

Schwannoma, neurofibroma and malignant tumours such as neurosarcoma account for approximately 25% of primary neck tumours, and the paragangliomas account for approximately 15%. Miscellaneous lumps such as lipoma (Figure 12.28) and rhabdomyoma are comparatively rare in the neck.

Neurogenic tumours

These tumours can arise from any of the major nerves of the neck and are either schwannomas (neurolemmoma) or neurofibromas. The most common nerve of origin is the vagus.

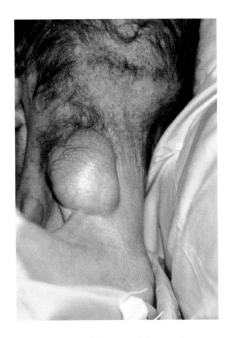

Figure 12.28 A rare lipoma of the neck.

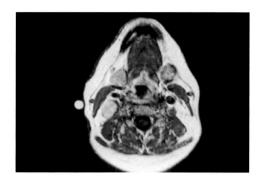

Figure 12.29 Computed tomography scan of a C5 schwannoma.

Neurofibromas These may be part of von Recklinghausen's neurofibromatosis or they may be solitary. If part of von Recklinghausen's syndrome, they are associated with multiple neurofibromas and café au lait spots over the skin. The association between neurofibromatosis and multiple neuroendocrine syndromes needs to be borne in mind. Isolated neurofibromas can be excised, although generally speaking the nerve will be irrevocably damaged by the excision and will require primary nerve repair. Schwannomas, conversely, tend to stretch the surrounding nerve sheath and can often be excised while maintaining the integrity of the nerve of origin (Figure 12.29).

Paragangliomas

Glomus vagale tumours are vagal paragangliomas arising from the mass of paraganglionic tissue within the perineurium of the vagus nerve just below the skull base. These may extend through the jugular foramen. This is a slow-growing mass in the upper neck, and symptoms are relatively late – pulsatile tinnitus, vertigo, deafness and pharyngeal pain. These tumours need to be investigated by magnetic resonance imaging (MRI) or CT scanning and should be excised because they are at risk of spreading into the cranial cavity. These are extremely vascular tumours, and because most of them are crossed by the internal carotid artery, there is a high level of risk of vascular injury.

Carotid body tumours The carotid body tumour (glomus tumour) is the most common paraganglioma in the head and neck. These are uncommon tumours representing 0.6% of head and neck neoplasms and approximately 0.03% of all neoplasms. These tumours arise from the chemoreceptor bodies at the bifurcation of the carotid artery. Carotid body tumours can be distinguished on imaging from glomus vagale and glomus jugulare tumours because they tend to splay the internal and external carotid arteries, whereas the other two tend to displace the internal carotid artery anteriorly. Patients give a clinical history of a slowly enlarging painless lump in the middle of the neck that may be pulsatile. The tumour feels firm and rubbery, and it is classically described as being mobile from side to side, but not up and down, although this is not a particularly useful clinical sign in reality. The higher prevalence of carotid body tumours has been related to chronic hypoxemia from chronic obstructive pulmonary disease and high altitudes. The sporadic form of carotid body paraganglioma is more common than the inherited variety and tends to occur more often in women. Familial tumours account for about 10% of all carotid body tumours and have an autosomal dominant mode with variable penetrance and higher incidence of bilateral tumours (exclude with ultrasound scanning).

Investigations: These are extremely vascular tumours, and biopsies should not be attempted. They are characteristic on CT, MRI or magnetic resonance angiography (MRA). Contrast CT and MRI and carotid angiography may demonstrate widening (classical contrast and angiographic finding) of the carotid bifurcation (lyre sign). Most of these tumours are benign, although it is impossible to distinguish benign and malignant carotid body tumours on the basis of histology alone. The tumour is typically mobile in the lateral plane, but its mobility is restricted in the cephalocaudal direction (Fontaine's sign). Occasionally the tumour may transmit the carotid pulse or demonstrate a bruit or thrill. Because of its close proximity to carotid vessels and cranial nerves X to XII, enlargement of the tumour may cause progressive neurological symptoms such as dysphagia, odynophagia or hoarseness.

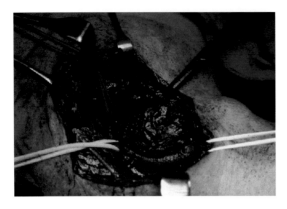

Figure 12.30 Perioperative view of resection of a carotid body tumour; the coloured silicon bands control the common, internal and external carotid arteries.

Patients with carotid body tumours may give a history of symptoms suggestive of excessive catecholamine production such as fluctuating hypertension (measure vanillyl mandelic acid) flushing and palpitations, but this is actually very rare.

Treatment: Not all tumours should be removed because most of these are benign. However, young healthy patients benefit from tumour excision (Figure 12.30). Patients who are having symptoms but are at high risk for surgery may respond to localized radiotherapy.

Glomus jugulare/glomus tympanum These paragangliomas arises around the jugular ganglion and tend to manifest with deafness and cranial nerve palsies. They rarely manifest as neck lumps.

FURTHER READING

Soames JV, Southam JC. *Oral pathology*, 4th ed. Oxford: Oxford University Press, 2005.
This eminently readable oral pathology text has the background information on almost all the conditions described.
Watkinson JC, Gilbert R, eds. *Stell and Maran's textbook of head and neck surgery and oncology.* 5th ed. 2012. CRC Press. New York.
This is a very good general head and neck text. Chapter 11 on benign neck disease is informative and easy to read.
Specific literature includes the following:
Brewis C, Pracy JP, Albert DM. Treatment of lymphangiomas of the head and neck in children by intralesional injection of OK-432 (Picibanil). *Clin Otolaryngol Allied Sci* 2000;25:130–4.
Chapelle KAOM, Stoelinga PJW, De Wild PCM, Brouns JJA, Voorsmit RACA. Rational approach to diagnosis and treatment of ameloblastomas and odontogenic keratocysts. *Br J Oral Maxillofac Surg* 2004;42:381–90.
Kanatas A, Mücke T, Houghton D, Mitchell DA. Schwannomas of the head and neck. *Oncol Rev* 2012;3:107–11.
Patlola R, Ingraldi A, Walker C, Allie D, Khan IA. Carotid body tumour. *Int J Cardiol* 2010,143:e7–10.
Stoelinga PJ. Excision of the overlying, attached mucosa, in conjunction with cyst enucleation and treatment of the bony defect with Carnoy solution. *Oral Maxillofac Surg Clin North Am* 2003;15:407–14.
Stoelinga PJ. The management of aggressive cysts of the jaws. *J Maxillofac Oral Surg* 2012;11: 2–12.

13

Paranasal sinuses

Contents

Aims

- To achieve an understanding of the anatomy, physiology and pathology of the maxillary sinus.
- To understand basic surgical principles of maxillary antral surgery.

Learning outcomes

For undergraduates:

- To be able to list the possible complications of maxillary tooth removal in relation to the maxillary sinus.
- To be able to describe and differentiate the signs and symptoms of maxillary sinusitis and dental pain.
- To describe the first-line treatment of a newly created oroantral communication.

For postgraduates:

- To be able to describe the signs and symptoms of pansinusitis.
- To be able to describe nonsurgical management of pansinusitis and orbital cellulitis and be in a position to discuss effective management with colleagues.
- To describe the steps in the surgical management of oroantral fistula.
- To be able to describe the signs and symptoms of malignant disease of the paranasal sinuses.

Introduction

There are four paired paranasal sinuses, which are essentially extensions of the nose. These are the frontal sinus, the sphenoid sinus, the ethmoid air cells and the maxillary sinus.

The frontal sinus is not present at birth, but it pneumatizes throughout the frontal bone in life and drains through the frontonasal duct.

The sphenoid sinus rapidly enlarges around puberty. This is the deepest of the paranasal sinuses and is of great significance because of its close relationships with dura, the pituitary fossa and the cavernous sinus.

The ethmoid sinuses are a delicate labyrinth of cavities lying between the medial walls of the orbits. These are of particular importance in maxillofacial surgery with regard to medial wall blowout injuries of the orbit.

The maxillary sinus is the paranasal sinus of greatest significance to oral and maxillofacial surgery because it lies in direct contact with the teeth in the upper jaw. This is of most direct relevance with regard to finding symptoms of pathology that may arise in the mouth and appear to manifest in the maxillary sinus (also known as the antrum) and *vice versa*.

Virtually all paranasal sinus disease will manifest through the nose because this is the final drainage site and the site of ventilation of the sinuses. Symptoms arise as a result of obstruction of this site.

Sinusitis

Sinusitis can be acute or chronic, and it is defined as the inflammation of the lining of the paranasal sinuses. This may be restricted to one sinus (e.g. maxillary sinusitis) or may occur in all sinuses, as seen in pansinusitis.

Acute sinusitis

This is usually caused by relative obstruction to the ostea of the sinuses or in the presence of a foreign body. The mechanism of the pathology is usually fairly evident in that patients either have a recent history of viral upper respiratory tract infection that has led to defunctioning of the cilia and mucosal inflammation, which results in stagnation within the sinuses and bacterial superinfection, or they have had recent dental pathology or surgery of some description that has resulted in placement of a foreign body in the maxillary sinus.

In instances of pansinusitis, aggressive emergency treatment is indicated if the frontal sinus is involved because this gives rise to very severe frontal headache, and the proximity of the brain in the anterior cranial fossa can result in frontal abscess, cerebral abscess, encephalitis and meningitis. Treatment of acute sinusitis centres on reestablishing ventilation of the sinuses by using decongestants such as xylometazoline and oxymetazoline. The classical ephedrine is less effective and more difficult to deliver. Systemic antibiotics effective against *Haemophilus influenzae* and *Staphylococcus aureus*, usually co-fluampicil or Co-amoxyclav (amoxycillin and clavulanic acid) in high doses, and symptomatic relief using analgesia and possibly steam inhalations are essential. The advantages of inhalations are dubious. Most cases of acute sinusitis resolve with this medical therapy. It is comparatively rare to have to drain the sinuses surgically. Patients who fail to respond to outpatient management or who have orbital cellulitis or acute frontal sinusitis should be managed by hospital admission, coronal computed tomography (CT) scanning, intravenous antibiotics and drainage if required, usually endoscopically. Children can develop a rapid form of orbital cellulitis secondary to pansinusitis and also need admission and a paediatric version of the foregoing.

Chronic sinusitis

Repeated bouts of acute sinusitis or failure to treat it adequately can result in chronic sinusitis, particularly in patients with established sinonasal disease. This can manifest as facial pain. The classical pain of sinusitis is worse when the head is moved forward and gives rise to a panmaxillary toothache. The management of chronic sinusitis has been revolutionized by the advent of functional endoscopic sinus surgery, which is a specialized subdiscipline of ear, nose and throat surgery, and patients with established chronic sinusitis should be referred for assessment for this kind of treatment. The one exception to this is patients who have repeated bouts of acute sinusitis secondary to a foreign body or a persisting oroantral fistula (Figures 13.1 and 13.2) or a retained root.

The most common cause of an oroantral communication is the extraction of single standing

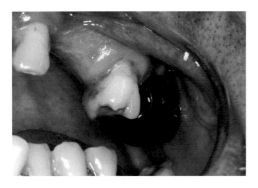

Figure 13.1 Clinical view of antral lining prolapsing through an oroantral communication.

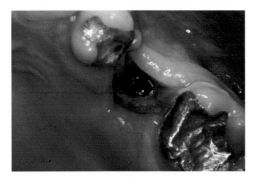

Figure 13.2 Typical oroantral fistula. The communication has now become lined with epithelium.

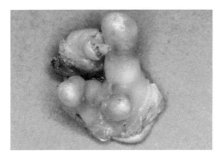

Figure 13.3 Multirooted, single standing upper molars are the typical cause of oroantral communication.

multirooted upper molars (Figure 13.3). Endoscopic sinus surgery with antrostomy is the technique of choice in the treatment of chronic sinusitis. The canine fossa puncture technique has been advocated, but this has an element of reinventing the wheel because this was the site of the traditional Caldwell-Luc approach.

Retained roots in the maxillary antrum

This complication is often created when a root fractures during removal of a maxillary molar tooth, and rather than carry out transalveolar removal of the root, injudicious probing in the socket forces the root up into the antrum. Many roots are found actually lying underneath the antral mucosa and not lying loose in the antrum. In this case they tend to cause local infection rather than significant sinusitis. Most of these retained roots should be removed. Other pathology found in the maxillary antrum includes the entirely innocuous antral mucocele, antroliths and tumours. Antral malignancy is dealt with in Chapter 22.

There are basically two techniques for removing foreign bodies from the antrum. One is to use the point of entry, which is usually a tooth socket.

Procedure for removing retained roots

Give additional local anaesthesia if you are continuing from immediately fracturing the tooth. Use a vasoconstrictor for haemorrhage control. Mark out a broadly based two- or three-sided flap (a three-sided flap should be used if you wish to mobilize the mucosa for a buccal advancement flap). Elevate the flap subperiosteally. Retract the flap and remove the bone with a round burr (see Chapter 6). Remove any obstructing interdental septa that will obscure your view. It is essential that an adequate view is obtained; if the root is lying underneath the antral mucosa it will be comparatively easy to see and can be picked out. If the antral mucosa has been disrupted a fairly large amount of bone will have to be removed to create an adequate visual inspection hole through the socket. If this is the case use the buccal fat pad flap and an advancement flap to close the defect because it will be significant.

The second way to remove foreign bodies is to approach the maxillary antrum via the Caldwell-Luc operation. This has the advantage of providing a wide portal of entry into the maxillary antrum. It is illustrated in Figures 13.4 to 13.8.

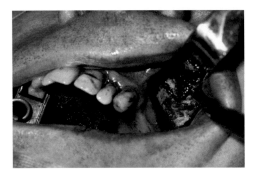

Figure 13.4 Caldwell-Luc approach. A subperiosteal flap is raised along the gingival crevice of the upper premolars.

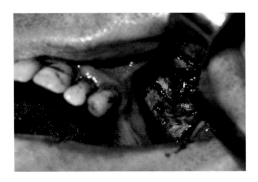

Figure 13.5 A window in the thin bone is made.

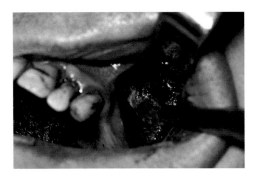

Figure 13.6 Antral lining or pathology is removed with forceps.

Caldwell-Luc procedure

The classical description is to create a linear incision above the maxillary premolar teeth where the bone lining the antrum is relatively thin. This is probably a mistake because it means that the

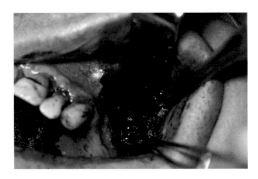

Figure 13.7 The antrum is cleaned out if indicated.

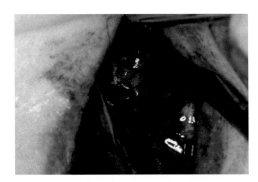

Figure 13.8 The residual defect. This can bleed considerably.

scar is placed over an area with no bony support. One way of avoiding this is to ensure that you create an approach to avoid placing the incision line over a bony defect. Raise a classical three-sided flap by using the gingival sulcus and two relieving incisions (Figure 13.4). This allows wide exposure and also creates the option of raising an osteoplastic flap (where the bone is elevated intact with the periosteum and retaining vascularity). Another classical description is to gain access to the antrum for the Caldwell-Luc procedure by using a series of hand-held trocars thrust through the thin antral wall; this is a fairly brutal technique. Another way of doing this is to use a dental fissure burr and cut a bony window as an osteoplastic flap or simply a bony window that can be lifted out (Figure 13.5). The maxillary antrum is then opened (Figure 13.6), and the entire sinus can be inspected for foreign bodies, retained roots or any other pathology that happens to be present. Generally speaking, the antral lining should be left unless it is grossly diseased, in which case it should be completely stripped out (Figure 13.7).

If it is necessary to strip out the antral lining completely, significant bleeding may occur into the sinus (Figure 13.8), resulting in epistaxis. It is possible to minimize this bleeding by placing a pack in the antrum either via the Caldwell-Luc procedure or by bringing it out through the nose via an intranasal antrostomy. A simple way to do that is to use balloon catheters in the antrum. The catheters are then simply deflated the day after and are taken out.

Oroantral communication

The most common cause of an oroantral communication is the removal of a single standing maxillary molar tooth with hypercementosis. It is worthwhile in the assessment of such teeth for exodontia to obtain a radiograph to see whether the roots of the tooth are in close proximity to the antrum. This does not mean that the tooth should not be removed or even that the patient has to be referred to a local oral surgeon; you simply should be aware when removing the tooth of the high chance of creating an oroantral communication.

Treatment of a primary oroantral communication

Treatment of a primary oroantral communication consists simply of removing the tooth and any fragments of bone. Mobilize local gingivae and primarily suture the socket. This should allow a healthy clot to form within the area of communication. There is a high likelihood that this will heal. The patient should be advised of the communication and instructed to avoid nose blowing. The patient should also be provided with a nasal decongestant such as xylometazoline or oxymetazoline for the reasons given before and a broad-spectrum antibiotic (e.g. amoxycillin 250 to 500 mg three times daily). Review the patient to ensure that this site has healed and that an oroantral fistula (a fistula has occurred where there is an epithelial lining to the communication rather than a simple communication between the antrum and the mouth) has not formed (Figure 13.9).

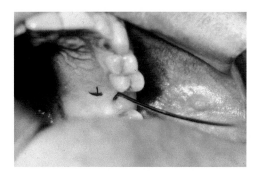

Figure 13.9 An oroantral fistula. A fistulous lining is an established oroantral communication that is lined with epithelium.

Established oroantral fistulae

Once the fistula is established treatment will require formal excision of the fistulous tract to gain healing both of the antral lining and of the oral lining. There are various ways of achieving this.

Patients with established oroantral fistulae will suffer from bouts of recurrent maxillary sinusitis, complain of a foul taste in their mouth and may have fluids passing from the mouth through the fistula and out the nose. The fistula can be demonstrated by asking the patient to occlude the nose and blow out through the nose; air will be seen to bubble out of the fistula. In some instances hyperplastic antral lining may prolapse out through the established fistula (see Figure 13.1).

Investigations

The only investigation required is a plain radiograph to ensure that there are no retained roots in the sinus. Small fragments of multirooted teeth are the likely cause of persisting postextraction sinusitis.

Treatment of established oroantral fistula

The principles of treatment are as follows:

1. Complete excision of the epithelial lined tract (Figure 13.10).
2. Removal of any foreign bodies.
3. Mobilization of tissue on the oral side and closure using an incision line that is capable of healing by primary intention. This means that it must rest on healthy bone or another layer of vascularized tissue. This can be achieved in the following three basic ways:

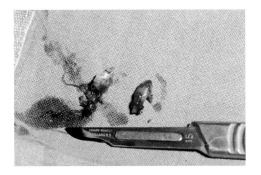

Figure 13.10 It is essential to excise the fistulous tract before closure of an established oroantral fistula.

Buccal advancement flap (as described by Rehrmann)

This procedure uses a three-sided advancement flap of buccal mucosa that is mobilized by making an incision through the periosteum to allow the flap to be stretched without tension over the defect (Figure 13.11). It is essential that the suture line rests on sound bone; otherwise, this flap will inevitably dehisce. The disadvantages of the buccal advancement flap are a relatively shallow sulcus postoperatively and the risk of flap dehiscence because it is a single-layer closure and must be closed over bone (Figure 13.12).

Buccal fat pad flap

This procedure is approached using a similar incision to the buccal advancement flap, but when the periosteum is incised, an artery clip is passed into the submucosa to identify the buccal fat pad (Figure 13.13). This is an axial fat flap that lends itself beautifully to the closure of oroantral fistulae. It can be used as an isolated flap where the vascularized fat fills the defect and is held in place with vertical mattress sutures, thus allowing the raised buccal flap to be repositioned in the buccal sulcus to maintain sulcus depth (Figures 13.14 through 13.18).

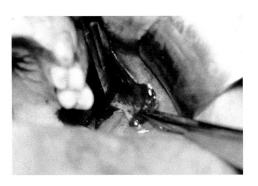

Figure 13.11 A buccal advancement flap is raised and mobilized by incising the periosteum. This also allows access to the buccal pad of fat.

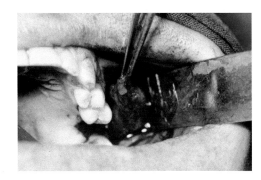

Figure 13.13 The buccal pad of fat, a vascularized, mobilizable entity which can be repositioned as a flap.

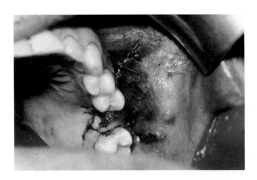

Figure 13.12 Simple buccal advancement flap closure.

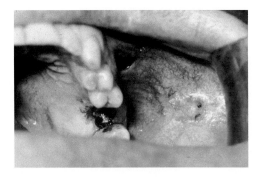

Figure 13.14 Technique for buccal fat pad flaps – relieving incisions.

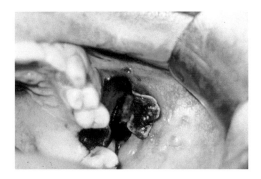

Figure 13.15 Subperiosteal flap elevated.

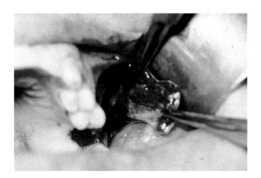

Figure 13.16 Buccal fat pad exposed by periosteal incision.

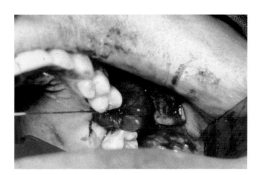

Figure 13.17 Fat pad delivered and used as sole reconstruction to maintain sulcus depth.

A combination of buccal fat pad and buccal advancement flap is probably the most effective way to close an oroantral fistula. The advantage of this technique is that the vascularized buccal fat pad fills the defect below the buccal advancement flap, which provides mucosal closure and thereby creates a double layered vascularized closure that has virtually no chance of dehiscence and breakdown (Figures 13.19 through 13.22).

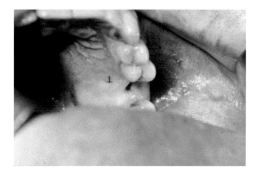

Figure 13.18 Postoperative healing showing preserved cheeks and sulcus.

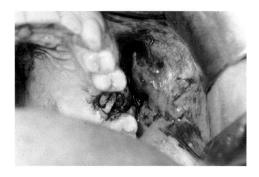

Figure 13.19 Combination approach using the buccal fat pad and the buccal advancement flap technique.

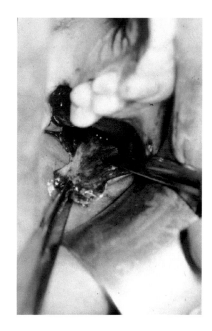

Figure 13.20 Flap elevated.

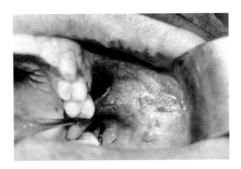

Figure 13.21 Flap mobilized.

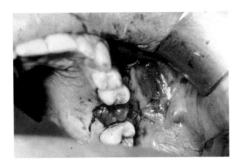

Figure 13.22 Fat pad inset, mucosa partially advanced.

Palatal finger flap

This is the third technique for closing chronic or persisting oroantral fistula where buccal advancement flaps or fat pad flaps are not appropriate. The palatal finger flap is based on the greater palatine artery. The palatal flap is a very stiff and immobile flap, although it provides extremely robust, well-vascularized tissue. The disadvantages of the palatal flap are that it leaves a raw defect on the palate that requires some form of palate coverage because it is extremely painful for weeks afterward and it is difficult to rotate the flap into position. This flap is one of those procedures that look very straightforward when it is drawn on a diagram but in reality, because of the stiffness of the palate, is actually extremely awkward to achieve.

As with closure on initial oroantral communications, the patient should avoid nose blowing and should be provided with a nasal decongestant and an antibiotic.

Other antral pathology

The maxillary antrum is a site of oral cancer. Persisting oroantral fistula (Figure 13.23) may

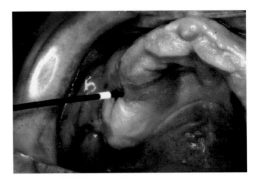

Figure 13.23 Chronic oroantral fistula. Beware; these can (rarely) be a sign of underlying malignancy.

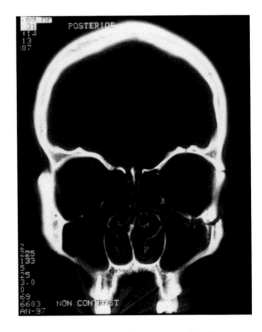

Figure 13.24 Computed tomography demonstrating a right antral polyp and a left antral haematoma from a zygomatic orbital fracture.

indicate underlying malignancy (see Chapter 22). Facial trauma (Figures 13.24, 13.25 and 13.26) (see Chapter 16), particularly zygomatic and midface fractures, inevitably involve the maxillary antrum.

Common antral pathology such as sinusitis has already been described, and common antral radiographic findings include the antral mucocele, which is a well-circumscribed, slightly radiopaque lesion usually arising from the floor of the antrum. Antral malignancy is slightly more difficult to detect, and it is worth bearing in mind the cardinal

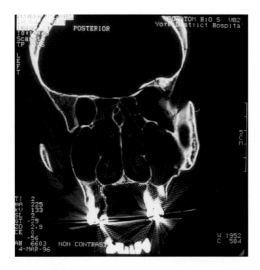

Figure 13.25 Traumatic blindness resulted from this fracture. Computed tomography demonstrates the anatomy of the orbits and sinuses.

signs of malignant disease of the maxillary sinus because early detection has a significant influence on the outcome.

Alarm bells

The signs of malignant disease include the following: painful unilateral sinusitis with discharge, particularly if it is associated with maxillary tooth movement; swelling in the buccal sulcus or palate; oral ulceration; unilateral epistaxis or persistent offensive nasal discharge or swelling over the cheek, particularly if it is associated with erythema; or altered sensation of the infraorbital nerves. Trismus and diplopia are very late signs of antral malignancy.

Elective operations affecting the maxillary sinus

Functional endoscopic sinus surgery is mainly the province of the experienced rhinologist. The sinus lift procedure (Figure 13.27) is a common technique for augmenting maxillary alveolar height before implant insertion (see Chapter 15). Clinicians must keep in mind the potential adverse effects of endosseous dental implant placement such as penetration of the sinus.

Epistaxis

Epistaxis (nosebleed) is common in children and in elderly patients but rarely serious. Occasionally it may be associated with an underlying condition (bleeding disorders, telangiectasia and tumours), and so recurrent episodes need to be investigated. Bleeding usually occurs from the anterior nasal septum (Little's area) and can be controlled simply by cauterization or pinching the nose. In most cases the bleeding stops quickly with first aid measures.

Major bleeding requires more aggressive treatment, particularly in elderly patients, in whom

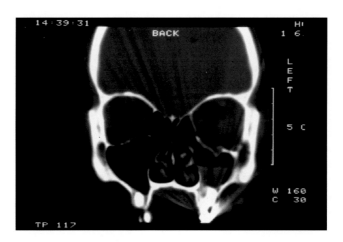

Figure 13.26 Orbital blow out fracture demonstrating the 'hanging drop' sign.

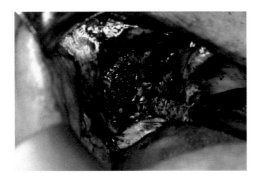

Figure 13.27 Sinus lift procedure. Bone graft is fixed beneath antral lining to increase bone depth for implant placement.

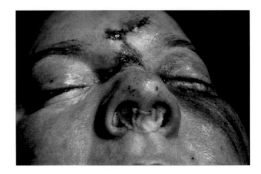

Figure 13.28 Nasal packing with petrolatum (Vaseline) gauze.

the site of bleeding may be the sphenoethmoidal recess, which is farther back in the nasal cavity. Bleeding from that site cannot be stopped by compression and may require endoscopic ligation.

Epistaxis associated with midfacial trauma can be extremely difficult to manage. However, it is rarely a cause of hypovolaemic shock in itself, and any patient in shock should have another cause searched for (e.g. abdomen, chest, pelvis) Following trauma it must be remembered that midface fractures may involve the anterior cranial fossa. Overzealous packing may perforate the fragile skull base at the ethmoids, and all packing introduces a risk of infection.

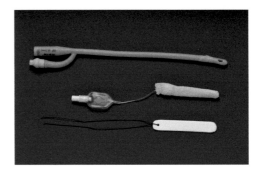

Figure 13.29 Range of equipment that can be used to tamponade nasal haemorrhage.

Management

Minor bleeding requires only simple measures (sitting forward and pinching the nose), or the bleeding points may be cauterized using silver nitrate sticks. When the source of bleeding cannot be seen, the nose can be packed using ribbon gauze impregnated with petrolatum (Vaseline) (Figure 13.28) or bismuth iodoform paraffin paste (BIPP). If this does not work, a soft, specially designed catheter (Brighton Balloon, Rapid Rhino) can be inserted through the nose until it is visible at the back of the throat.

The balloon is then inflated and gentle traction applied, 'wedging' the balloon between the soft palate and the nasopharynx. The second balloon can be inflated anteriorly. Alternatives include commercially available nasal 'tampons' or urinary catheters (Figure 13.29).

Patients may need fluid replacement and occasionally a blood transfusion. Elderly patients can be difficult to manage because of their poor physiological reserve and coexisting medications such as beta blockers.

In rare instances when haemorrhage cannot be controlled by packing, vessel ligation may be necessary either via the neck and orbital approach (external carotid artery, anterior ethmoidal artery) or endoscopically through the nose (sphenopalatine artery). Alternatively, embolization may be carried out if facilities for acute interventional radiology are available in your hospital.

FURTHER READING

Albu S, Baciut M, Opincariu I, Rotaru H, Dinu C. The canine fossa puncture technique in chronic odontogenic maxillary sinusitis. *Am J Rhinol Allergy* 2011;25:358–62.

Bomelli SR, Branstetter BF 4th, Ferguson BJ. Frequency of a dental source for acute maxillary sinusitis. *Laryngoscope* 2009;119:580–4.

Felisati G, Chiapasco M, Lozza P, Saibene AM, Pipolo C, Zaniboni M, Biglioli F, Borloni R. Sinonasal complications resulting from dental treatment: outcome-orientated proposal of classification and surgical protocol. *Am J Rhinol Allergy* 2013;27:e101–6.

Najm SA, Malis D, Hage ME, Rahban S, Carrel JP, Bernard JP. Potential adverse events of endosseous dental implants penetrating the maxillary sinus: long-term clinical evaluation. *Laryngoscope* 2013;123:2958–61.

Pokorny A, Tataryn R. Clinical and radiographic findings in a case series of maxillary sinusitis of dental origin. *Int Forum Allergy Rhinol* 2013;12:973–9.

14

Temporomandibular joint and facial pain

Contents

Aims and learning outcomes

For undergraduates:

- To be able to describe the distinguishing features of individual disorders of the temporomandibular joint (TMJ).
- To be able to discuss the common conditions that do not require surgical intervention.
- To be able to list the common, effective, non-invasive treatments for TMJ dysfunction.
- To be able to list serious conditions that may be confused with TMJ dysfunction.

For postgraduates:

- To be able to describe a treatment strategy for the patient with a TMJ disorder.
- To be able safely to exclude or instigate treatment for serious conditions that may be confused with TMJ dysfunction.
- To be able to identify cases in which surgery may be helpful.

- To be able to describe the steps of basic useful operations.

By far the most common condition is TMJ pain dysfunction syndrome (TMJPDS)/facial arthromyalgia (3% to 5% of the population will seek treatment).

Introduction

The TMJ is a synovial joint in which the mandibular condyle articulates with the base of the skull at the glenoid fossa and articular eminence. Interposed between the two is the articular disc or meniscus, the function of which is to contribute to the smooth action of the joint. The disc is also believed to be involved in many of the disorders commonly seen. The disc is divided into three zones – a thick posterior band, a thin intermediate zone and a slightly thicker but narrow anterior band.

TMJ pain is to the maxillofacial surgeon what low back pain is to the orthopaedic surgeon and irritable bowel syndrome is to the general surgeon – common, often difficult to treat and not fully understood. It is important to understand that many 'TMJ' patients have dysfunction of the muscles of mastication as a secondary manifestation of psychosocial conditions, and the effect on the joint itself is tertiary. **Only a small proportion of patients will benefit from surgery.** All three components (muscle pain, disc dysfunction and psychological aspects) are commonly seen in the same patient. It has been estimated that approximately 5% of the population will seek treatment, and of these approximately 1 in 20 will undergo some form of surgery. It is worthwhile noting that although a female predominance exists (female-to-male ratio of 3:1 to 8:1) in patients requesting treatment, the incidence from population studies is equal between the sexes.

The TMJ nerve supply arises from the mandibular division of the trigeminal nerve. The auriculotemporal nerve innervates most of the TMJ mainly anterolaterally, and small branches of the masseteric and deep temporal nerves supply the posterior aspect. Its vascular supply arises from the external carotid artery via the internal maxillary artery and the superficial temporal artery.

Frequency of temporomandibular joint disorders

Common disorders

Disorder	Frequency
TMJ pain dysfunction syndrome/facial arthromyalgia.	Up to 75% of population has signs.
Internal derangement.	Up to 25% has symptoms.
Fractures and dislocation.	See Chapter 16.

Uncommon disorders

- Degenerative joint disease.
- Inflammatory joint disease.
- Ankylosis.
- Condylar hyperplasia or hypoplasia.
- Idiopathic condylar resorption.

Rare disorders

- Infective arthritis.
- Tumours of the TMJ.

Normal joint function

Normal movement in the TMJ should be smooth and pain free. Both joints are almost (bone does have some plasticity) rigidly linked together by the horseshoe-shaped mandible and therefore move together – it is not possible for one joint to move without affecting the other. Consequently, any disorder of movement involving one joint will by necessity have an effect on the opposite one.

Initial mouth opening (up to 1 cm) involves a hinge-type movement, analogous to that seen in the knee or phalanges. However, the remainder (and the majority) of mouth opening involves a bodily shift, or translation, of the condyle as it moves down the articular eminence. Closure is essentially the reverse of this. Side to side movements of the mandible involve a mixture of rotation of each condyle through a vertical axis and a minor degree of lateral shift.

In the normal TMJ the meniscus is placed on top of the condyle and the two move in harmony as the mandible moves. Movement of the disc is possible because of its elastic attachments and the attachment of the lateral pterygoid – an important muscle in mouth opening. It is this relationship that is disrupted in the condition known as internal derangement (discussed later).

Symptoms and signs of abnormal joint function

Symptoms

Symptoms arising from the TMJ and its associated muscles are common and include:

- **Pain** – this is probably the most common symptom resulting in patients seeking help. Pain may arise from the joint capsule, "retrodiscal" tissues or associated muscles such as the lateral pterygoid or masseter. Often it can be well localized to the joint making diagnosis relatively straightforward; however, referred pain or pain arising within the muscles can be experienced elsewhere. Pain aggravated by chewing or stressing the joint points heavily to a musculoskeletal cause.

Signs

These are elicited on clinical examination.

- **Joint noises** – these are usually experienced as clicking and grating. They can occur in otherwise asymptomatic joints. Grating noises may be experienced by patients as a result of some destructive processes resulting in loss of the smooth articular surfaces and irregular joint movement. In mild cases no cause can be found, although arthroscopically there may be evidence of mild degenerative changes with debris in the synovial fluid. Otherwise, asymptomatic joint noises do not require any treatment. The noises can be heard by the clinician without the use of stethoscope amplification.
- **Limitation of mouth opening** – it is important to draw a distinction between limitation of movement resulting from some kind of obstruction within the joint and that caused by muscle spasm (Figure 14.1).
- **Deviation on mouth opening** – normal mouth opening should be symmetrical and pain free; interincisal opening should approach 40 mm, although this varies with height, occlusion and dentition (Figure 14.2). Deviation may result from mechanical interference or pain. When deviation is prolonged, this new movement becomes subconscious and automatic and may continue after the initial cause has resolved (Figure 14.3).
- **Clicking** – see the later section on internal derangement.
- **Locking** – see the later section on internal derangement.

Trismus

Unfortunately the indistinct mishmash labelled 'TMJ disorders' can manifest with much less

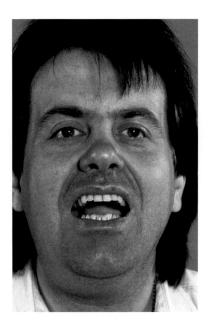

Figure 14.1 Example of trismus, opening less than 40 mm.

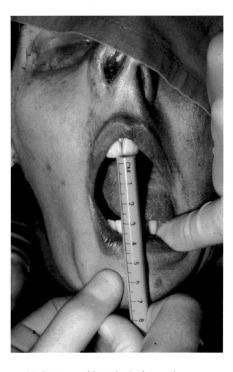

Figure 14.2 Normal interincisal opening.

specific symptoms including headaches, neck pain and earache. In these cases other causes need to be considered. Stress, anxiety, depression or significant life events are also often related. Although it

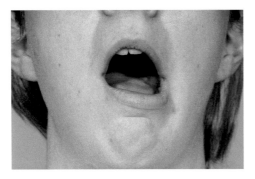

Figure 14.3 Deviation on opening.

is not immediately curative to draw the patient's attention to this, some patients are helped by awareness of this cause. In patients with sleep disturbance and parafunctional habits, dosulepin 75 mg or amitriptyline 10 to 25 mg at night can help. Selective serotonin reuptake inhibitors ([SSRIs] e.g. sertraline 50 mg, paroxetine 20 mg in the morning) are better if there is no evidence of sleep disturbance or if 'lassitude' is an additional complaint.

Occlusion and occlusal wear patterns amplify this limitation of mouth opening as a result of muscle spasm (usually, but not always painful). Trismus therefore implies an *inflammatory* process involving one or more of the muscles of mastication. As a symptom, take it seriously – not all cases are caused by 'TMJ' problems. Causes of trismus include:

- Infection and/or inflammation in or near the TMJ (e.g. acute pericoronitis, suppurative arthritis, osteomyelitis, cellulitis, and parotitis) (see Chapter 10).
- Abscesses or infection in the pterygoid, lateral pharyngeal, submasseteric or submandibular fascial spaces (see Chapter 10).
- Trauma (condyle neck fracture, muscle spasm following direct blow or an inferior alveolar nerve block) (see Chapter 16).
- Tetanus (risus sardonicus) – history of dirty wound, no prophylaxis.
- TMJ pain dysfunction syndrome.
- Drugs (e.g. phenothiazines, metoclopramide especially in young women).
- An infiltrating tumour (rare; either directly into muscle, usually pterygoids, or skull base affecting V_C) (Figure 14.4).

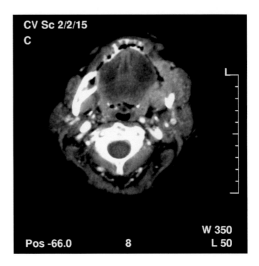

Figure 14.4 Scan of a maxillary tumour invading the pterygoid muscles. The patient presented with trismus and was referred as a temporomandibular joint problem.

Imaging studies

Although plain radiographs are relatively easy to obtain in the clinic they really play a minor role in detecting TMJ pathology (Figures 14.5 and 14.6). The TMJ is a complex three-dimensional structure, and conventional radiographs show only a two-dimensional view through one particular part of the joint. Only gross pathology can be picked up in this way (Figure 14.7). TMJ arthrography, which involves the direct injection of contrast medium into one or both of the joint spaces, provides

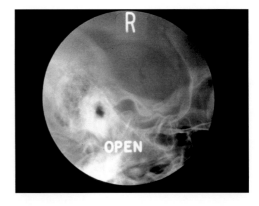

Figure 14.5 Transcranial plain radiograph of a normal temporomandibular joint with the mouth open.

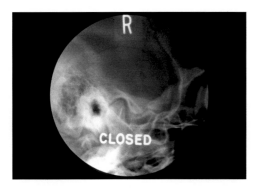

Figure 14.6 Transcranial plain radiograph of a normal temporomandibular joint with the mouth closed. Neither view (open or closed mouth) is consistently easy to interpret.

information on joint function, particularly that of the meniscus (Figure 14.8), but it is technically demanding. Magnetic resonance imaging (MRI) has increasingly been used in the study of the TMJ because it is particularly useful for visualizing the associated soft tissues (e.g. disc, lateral pterygoid). It is also useful in studying the vascularity of the condyle. MRI is currently considered to be the imaging modality of choice, although reports are now suggesting an increasing role for ultrasound in imaging of the joint.

Facial pain syndromes

Classification

Idiopathic facial pain makes up a significant workload in oral and maxillofacial practice. In 1994 the International Association for the Study of Pain revised its classification of chronic pain. This now includes:

- Dental-type pain.
- Odontalgia (toothache!).
- Pulpitis (inflammation of the dental pulp).
- Periapical periodontitis and dental abscess.
- Atypical odontalgia (toothache, in the absence of detectable dental disease).
- Cracked tooth syndrome.
- Glossodynia and sore mouth (also known as 'burning mouth' or oral dysaesthesia).
- Trigeminal herpes zoster and postherpetic neuralgia.
- Trigeminal neuralgia (tic douloureux).
- Glossopharyngeal neuralgia.
- Secondary neuralgia (from central nervous system lesions).
- TMJ pain dysfunction syndrome.
- Rheumatoid arthritis of the TMJ.

Idiopathic facial pain

Idiopathic facial pain makes up a significant portion of outpatient attendances. This less extensive classification describes four major symptom complexes and may be more practical in day to day dealings with these problems. Four symptom complexes are as follows:

- Facial arthromyalgia (or TMJ dysfunction syndrome [TMJPDS]).
- Atypical facial pain (nonjoint or nonmuscle pain).
- Atypical odontalgia.
- Oral dysaesthesia (oral sensory disturbances).

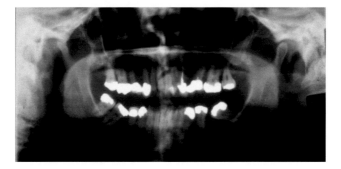

Figure 14.7 Dental panoramic radiograph showing severely resorbed right condyle.

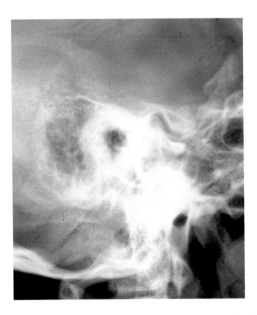

Figure 14.8 Lower joint space arthrogram of the temporomandibular joint, a difficult but interpretable investigation.

Idiopathic (i.e. cause unknown) facial pain is a very real entity and not just a manifestation of psychological problems, although they are sometimes associated. All forms should remain a diagnosis of exclusion (i.e. all other causes of facial pain, notably arising from the teeth, sinuses, neuralgias and headaches should be considered and if necessary investigated). Patients need to have a thorough history and examination taken including examination of the cranial nerves. In selected cases computed tomography (CT) or MRI may be necessary to exclude serious pathology. This is important because vague pain can on occasion be the presenting symptom of life-threatening disease. A high index of suspicion is therefore necessary, particularly in those patients who fail to respond to conventional treatments. Periodic reassessment is also advisable for this reason. Occasionally some forms of idiopathic facial pain (e.g. oral dysaesthesia) are associated with deficiencies in iron, vitamin B_{12} or folic acid.

Aetiology

It has been suggested that these symptoms may be interrelated and form part of a whole body pain syndrome involving the neck, back, abdomen and skin. Adverse life events, 'stress' and impaired coping ability are the strongest known associated factors.

The aetiology of idiopathic facial pain is (by definition) unknown – the physiology of pain is very complicated. In TMJPDS evidence suggests that stress-induced inflammation within and around the joint causes local production of various chemicals, including free radicals, that result in pain and in susceptible patients possibly destructive changes. Some of these chemicals may also develop in muscles and teeth and may account for the different anatomical locations for pain. Neuropeptides have been demonstrated within the TMJ capsule. Free radicals, in addition to causing pain, may also have an effect on the synovial fluid, thus impairing its lubricating ability and resulting in adhesions across the joint. Other pain mediating agents, including 15-hydroxyeicosatraeinoic acid (15-HETE) and substance P, have been identified. It has been suggested that these chemicals may be present in other nerve endings, and that may help to account for dental-type pain in the absence of obvious dental disease (odontalgia).

Management

Often the ill-defined nature of the patient's pain results in unnecessary dental work. In light of the association of atypical facial pain with neuroses, particularly depression, and the belief that this pain essentially has a psychogenic basis, emphasis has been placed on the use of antidepressant therapeutic agents as the main treatment option. For instance dosulepin, a tricyclic antidepressant, has been shown to be effective in reducing the painful symptoms. Amitriptyline is an alternative. It is thought that these drugs alter the sensory discrimination component of pain independently of its antidepressive effect. The possibility of the use of SSRIs to interfere with serotonin metabolism in the brainstem (a known effective treatment of monopolar depression) has yet to be clarified by any trials. Pregabalin, which is a neuropathic analgesic with secondary anxiolytic effects, may have a role in some of these patients.

Atypical facial pain

This is pain which does not fit into any other diagnostic categories (e.g. diseases of the teeth, sinuses, ear, TMJ). It is essentially a diagnosis of exclusion.

Atypical facial pain is often characterized by its bizarre and inconsistent nature. Symptoms may be related to those of atypical odontalgia, which, it has been suggested, is a localized variant of atypical facial pain. It may be described as an intense, deep, constant burning or aching pain. Patients usually have difficulty in localizing it and may point to various sites. As a rule of thumb, organic pain (e.g. from infection, trauma, tumours, nerve irritation) does not cross the midline. Despite the reported severity of the symptoms patients are not kept awake at night by them. Other symptoms (e.g. dysaesthesia, paraesthesia, tingling and numbness) may be described, and these patients must be carefully assessed to make sure there is no underlying disease such as multiple sclerosis or tumours. As with TMJPDS, stress, anxiety and depression are often associated.

Trigeminal neuralgia

Trigeminal neuralgia (tic douloureux) is described as 'a painful unilateral affliction of the face, characterised by brief electric shock-like (lancinating) pains limited to the distribution of one or more divisions of the trigeminal nerve'. Typically it occurs in middle-aged and elderly patients. The second and third divisions of the trigeminal nerve are usually affected. Episodes may occur occasionally or frequently over several weeks to months, often followed by pain-free intervals. Patients describe the pain as like a sudden electric shock, frequently triggered by trivial stimuli of the face such as with washing, shaving, chewing and talking. It may also occur spontaneously.

Usually, trigeminal neuralgia responds well to carbamazepine. Other drugs known to have an effect include gabapentin, pregabalin, amitriptyline and a muscle relaxant such as baclofen. Carbamazepine is usually the drug of choice, with approximately 70% of patients reporting significant relief. Side effects include drowsiness, confusion, vertigo, nausea, vomiting, aplastic anaemia and liver failure. Patients should be carefully titrated to the lowest dose required to control the pain and should have regular monitoring of liver function and plasma carbamazepine concentration. It is also advisable to withdraw therapy slowly to prevent acute psychosis associated with abrupt withdrawal. If medical therapy fails to bring about relief of pain, invasive techniques such as cryotherapy, peripheral nerve blocks and percutaneous destruction of the trigeminal ganglion may be indicated. Open neurosurgical procedures such as microvascular decompression of the trigeminal root (Jannetta) are an excellent option in those patients demonstrated to have a microvascular loop compressing the trigeminal nerve root; these cases are comparatively rare.

Other facial pain syndromes

Odontalgia

- Short-lasting diffuse pain resulting from dentinoenamel defects and evoked by local stimuli.
- Sharp or dull, mild to moderate pain lasting less than a second to minutes.
- Treatment – protect the defective area with a dressing or restoration, and administer simple analgesics.

Pulpitis

- Pain resulting from pulpal inflammation that is evoked by local stimuli.
- Sharp, dull ache, or throbbing pain, moderate to severe, lasting minutes or hours, with episodes that may continue for several days.
- Treatment – this includes extirpation of the pulp, extraction and combination analgesics (e.g. non-steroidal anti-inflammatory drugs [NSAIDs], paracetamol and codeine, Co-Dydramol).

Periapical periodontitis and abscess

- Severe throbbing pain arising from the periodontal tissues.
- Continuous, mild to intense aching, especially after hot or cold stimuli, that may last a few minutes to several hours.
- Treatment – this includes extirpation or extraction, antibiotics, NSAIDs, paracetamol and codeine.

Atypical odontalgia

- Severe throbbing pain in the tooth without major pathology.
- Often described as severe continual throbbing in teeth and gingivae. It may vary from mild pain to intense pain, especially with hot or cold stimuli. It may be widespread or well localized, frequently precipitated by a dental procedure and may move from tooth to tooth. It may last a few minutes to several hours.
- Possible symptom of hypochondriacal psychosis or depression, and there is often excessive concern with oral hygiene.
- Treatment – this includes counselling, cognitive behavioural therapy, avoidance of unnecessary pulp extirpations and extractions, antidepressants and phenothiazines.

Glossodynia and sore mouth (also known as 'burning mouth' or oral dysaesthesia)

- Burning pain in the tongue or mucous membranes.
- Burning, tender, nagging pain, usually constant, but may be variable, and increasing in intensity from morning to evening; occasionally associated with iron, vitamin B_{12} or folate deficiency.
- Treatment
  - Treat deficiency states. This condition sometimes responds to antidepressants.
  - Try B vitamin supplements or alpha-lipoleic acid–containing preparations if nothing else helps.
- Clonazepam used topically may be beneficial and minimizes the drug's systemic effects.

Cracked tooth syndrome

- Brief sharp pain in a tooth resulting from cusp flexion and 'microleakage'.
- Moderate pain on biting that lasts a few seconds.
- Treatment – repair the cracked portion of the tooth, and administer simple analgesics.

Trigeminal herpes zoster

- Acute herpetic infection in cranial nerve V.
- Burning, tingling pain with occasional lancinating components felt in the skin. Pain may precede or follow herpetic eruptions and last from 1 week to several weeks.

- Spontaneous permanent remission is common, although the condition may progress to chronic (postherpetic) neuralgia.
- Treatment – in the acute phase, stellate ganglion blocks using local anaesthetic (e.g. bupivacaine) are indicated for severe pain. Pregabalin, transcutaneous electrical nerve stimulation (TENS), capsaicin cream and tricyclic antidepressants are useful.

Postherpetic neuralgia

- Chronic pain with skin changes in the distribution of cranial nerve V following acute herpes zoster.
- Burning, tearing, itching dysaesthesia and crawling dysaesthesias in skin of affected areas of moderate intensity; exacerbated by mechanical contact. This may last for several years, and spontaneous subsidence is not uncommon.
- Treatment – combination therapy includes pregabalin, capsaicin cream, TENS, tricyclic antidepressants and cognitive behavioural therapy.

Secondary neuralgia from central nervous system lesions

- Pains in the distribution of one or more branches of cranial nerve V resulting from a recognized lesion (e.g. tumour, multiple sclerosis, aneurysm).
- May be indistinguishable from trigeminal neuralgia or be a constant, severe dull pain.
- Treatment – this involves treatment of the underlying cause. A combination of centrally acting drugs (e.g. carbamazepine, phenothiazines and tricyclic antidepressants) can help symptomatically, but the real point is to identify and treat the underlying condition.

Glossopharyngeal neuralgia

- Sudden, severe, brief stabbing recurrent pains in the distribution of the glossopharyngeal nerve.
- Sharp, stabbing bouts of severe pain felt deep in throat or ear, often triggered by touch or swallowing and by ingestion of cold fluids. Episodes may interfere with eating and can last for weeks to several months and subside spontaneously. Recurrence is common.

- Treatment – application of local anaesthetic to the trigger point relieves the pain. Carbamazepine and other drugs used for trigeminal neuralgia are not as effective but offer the best chance for symptom relief.
- Distinguish from Eagle's syndrome (elongation of the styloid process treated by excision of the calcified stylohyoid ligament).

Dry socket

- This disorder is discussed in Chapter 6.

Disorders of the temporomandibular joint

Temporomandibular joint pain dysfunction syndrome

'Temporomandibular joint pain dysfunction syndrome' is a descriptive term (which often means very little is known about it) relating to pain arising from the joint itself and the muscles of mastication. It is also known as facial arthromyalgia and myofacial pain.

It has been suggested that up to 70% of the population has, at some time, experienced at least one episode of painful symptoms that can be attributed to TMJ dysfunction.

The aetiology of TMJPDS is unknown, although stress, often associated with 'parafunctional habits' such as bruxism (teeth clenching) are common features. Headaches, neck ache and back pains are also commonly seen with this condition. Abnormalities in occlusion have long been held responsible for TMJPDS, but this is controversial and the evidence for this is conflicting. There does appear to be a subgroup of patients who do benefit from correction of a malocclusion; however, this is certainly not the case in all patients. Furthermore, it is important to identify TMJPDS in patients who are about to undergo orthognathic surgery because in some of these patients, surgery or even orthodontics will make things worse.

Three cardinal features exist:

- Pain.
- Joint noise.
- Restricted movement.

Pain is the most common presenting complaint and is by far the most difficult component to assess. It is characterized clinically by pain in and around the jaw joint, involving the muscles of mastication and often radiating to the temple, jaw and into the neck. Patients often describe a dull, deep ache around the joint, which they may call 'earache', along with a superimposed sharper component, which may radiate over the side of the face. Patients can also report clicking of the joints with limitation of the range of mouth opening. Joint noises, however, are quite common in asymptomatic people in the general population, and they are of little clinical importance in the absence of pain. When mechanical symptoms predominate, the term 'internal derangement' is sometimes used, implying that there is a problem with the meniscus. However, clicking is a common finding in the normal population, and in the absence of other symptoms it does not need treatment.

Clinical examination

Assess for tenderness in the muscles of mastication (Figure 14.9). Areas of tenderness, trigger points and patterns of pain referral should be noted. Place your fingertips in the preauricular region just in front of the tragus of the ear and ask the patient to open and close the mouth – the fingertip should fall into a depression left by the translating condyle. Listen for joint sounds.

Assess mandibular function by noting whether the mouth opens in a straight line or deviates with jerky movements. Normal painless maximal opening should be around 40 to 55 mm.

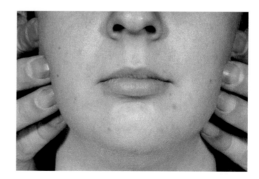

Figure 14.9 Clinical examination of muscles of mastication. The external muscles are straightforward. Remember gloves and watch out for teeth when palpating the medial and lateral pterygoid!

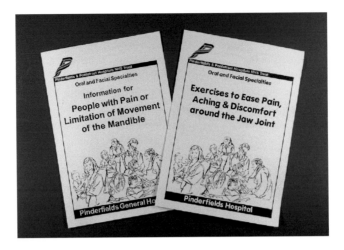

Figure 14.10 Self-help leaflets. Every department should have some.

Diagnosis is essentially based on clinical grounds. A history of limited mouth opening, which may be intermittent or progressive, is a key feature of TMJ disorders.

Differential diagnosis

- Dental pain.
- Disorders of the ears, nose and sinuses.
- Neuralgias.
- Headaches.
- Diseases of the major salivary glands.

Treatment

Many treatments are available, none of which have been consistently shown to be superior to the others. Because the clinical course does not reflect a progressive disease, the main goals of treatment are to reduce or eliminate pain and joint noises and to restore normal function. This is best achieved when contributing factors such as stress, depression and oral parafunctional habits (e.g. bruxism) are also addressed. Psychogenic factors are mostly found in patients with myofascial pain and dysfunction. These patients may need psychotropic medication and psychotherapy.

Nonsurgical treatment

Explanation and reassurance – these are probably among of the most important components of treatment. Explain to the patient the cause and nature of the disorder, and reassure him or her of its benign nature (Figure 14.10). Do this early to prevent the development of institutionalization and 'doctor dependency'.

Lifestyle changes – advise a soft diet and avoidance of heavy chewing, wide yawning, chewing gum and any other activities that would cause excessive jaw movement. Patients should also be advised to identify any remediable source of stress, and try and change their lifestyle accordingly.

Massage – massaging the affected muscles and applying moist heat will promote muscle relaxation and help soothe aching or tired muscles.

Biofeedback techniques – bioelectric feedback, which allows a patient to identify muscle overactivity, can be linked to learned technique of muscle relaxation. This is not usually available in the hospital environment.

Jaw exercises – retrusive jaw exercises are indicated in cases of parafunction and may prove useful for clicking joints, restricted mouth opening and recurrent anterior dislocation of the meniscus. Use an advice sheet that the patient can take home and study.

Analgesia – simple NSAIDs will relieve the pain and certainly reduce inflammation around the TMJ. These drugs also have an identifiable effect in improving the capacity of the synovial fluid to act as a lubricant.

Restorative and prosthetic rehabilitation – this provides occlusal balance, posterior support and correct vertical discrepancies.

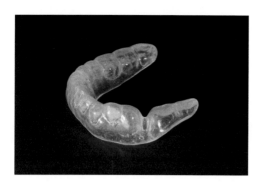

Figure 14.11 A lower soft bite raising appliance.

Splints – various occlusal splints have been suggested in the treatment of TMJ dysfunction (see later) (Figure 14.11).

Psychiatric support – psychiatric referral for assessment and consideration of suitable therapy should be considered in those patients in whom a psychogenic element may be seen. Dosulepin, amitriptyline and nortriptyline have all been shown to be useful, but close monitoring and appropriate patient selection are essential.

'Alternative therapies' – few, if any, controlled studies exist to support the benefit of such treatment modalities, but in refractory cases other possible treatment options include the following:

Ultrasound – this is popular, with a small evidence base supporting its role in symptomatic relief.

Laser (low-intensity laser treatment) – no follow-up evidence is available.

TENS – this was referred to previously.

Acupuncture – although not widely used for this condition, acupuncture has a definite and effective role in the management of some people's chronic pain.

Relaxation therapy – this is really an extension of self-help.

Hypnosis – although no real evidence is available to support this treatment in TMJ disorders, it has an established role in chronic pain.

Surgical treatment

Injectables The presence of muscle spasm in easily accessible muscles of mastication, particularly the masseter and temporalis, in patients with myofascial pain as the primary symptom has created interest in overcoming this spasm. Originally it was believed that this outcome was the main benefit of the soft coverage splint. Many clinicians believe that the presence of this 'irritant' between the teeth may actually encourage bruxism. The widely available botulinum-alpha toxin has become increasingly used (without any sound randomized controlled clinical trials) as a logical extension of an approach based on overcoming painful muscle spasm. This toxin is injected directly into the masseter and/or temporalis muscles, and a period of 3 to 6 months of enforced decreased muscle activity provides apparently effective analgesia in a group of patients.

Surgical procedures Around 5% of patients require surgery. Surgical procedures currently used range from arthrocentesis and arthroscopy to more complex open joint procedures. These are more useful in patients who have internal derangement with severe chronic pain or significant mechanical symptoms.

Internal derangement

As far back as 1992 the Consensus Conference for Temporomandibular Surgery defined internal derangement as 'a localised mechanical fault in the joint which interferes with its smooth action'. To complicate matters, however, internal derangement may also occur together with TMJPDS. It is essential therefore that the contribution of each condition to the patient's symptoms is assessed because one disorder may benefit from surgery, whereas the other will not.

Normally when the mouth opens and closes, the meniscus moves in harmony with the condyle as it translates along the articular eminence. In certain circumstances, however, this gliding movement is disrupted, and the disc may become adherent to the fossa either by fibrous adhesions or by the so-called suction cup effect. The disc may also change shape. As a result the mandibular condyle is unable to move smoothly and may have to 'jump' over the periphery of the disc to continue moving. This movement is felt by the patient as a click.

Why the disc becomes sticky in the first place is not known. There is, however, a mounting body of evidence suggesting that changes in the consistency of the synovial fluid as a result of inflammatory processes may be responsible. This may be caused by chronic pressure applied to the joint, as in those patients with constant bruxism.

Untreated, clicking may, but does not always, progress to locking, in which the disc becomes so abnormally shaped and displaced that it effectively acts like a door stop, preventing the mandibular condyle from undertaking a full range of movements. This results in 'locking' of the jaw, which may occur on either opening or closing of the mouth (open lock, closed lock) (Figure 14.12).

Pain may result from reflex muscle spasm or may arise from the joint itself. It has been suggested that in susceptible patients, alterations in the synovial fluid can also result in destructive arthropathy. These biochemical changes are similar to those seen in depression, and this helps to explain why improvement in symptoms can occur in patients who are *not* depressed and who take tricyclic antidepressant drugs. It is important to explain this rationale to patients at the outset of treatment because many will quickly realize that antidepressants have been prescribed and will assume they have been labelled as depressed or psychiatrically unwell.

Initial treatment is essentially along the lines of TMJPDS. For patients who do not respond and who have a clear internal derangement of the meniscus, 'lysis and lavage', achieved either by arthroscopy or by simple joint irrigation, are often helpful. If the condition relapses or locking is a major problem, meniscal placation or eminectomy can be effective.

A classification system of internal derangement (based on arthrographic findings) was produced by Wilkes and includes:

- **Class I** – painless clicking; no restricted motion, slight forward displacement of disc.

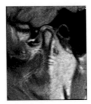

Figure 14.12 A parasagittal T1-weighted magnetic resonance image demonstrating an anteriorly displaced temporomandibular joint meniscus with the teeth in occlusion (closed view).

- **Class II** – occasional painful clicking, intermittent locking, headaches; slight forward displacement of disc.
- **Class III** – frequent pain, joint tenderness, headaches, locking, restricted motion, painful chewing; anterior disc displacement.
- **Class IV** – chronic pain, headaches, restricted motion; early to moderate degenerative changes, flattening of eminence, deformed condylar head, sclerosis.
- **Class V** – variable pain, joint crepitus, painful function; disc perforation, gross anatomic deformity of disc and hard tissues with degenerative arthritic changes.

Osteoarthrosis

Osteoarthrosis has been described as a degenerative (wear and tear) disease that commonly affects weight-bearing joints such as the hips and knees. However, more recently the underlying pathology has been questioned, and a degenerative cause is not so clear-cut. It is now believed to be a systemic disease with trauma contributing only at the onset of symptoms. Nevertheless, changes of osteoarthrosis can be detected in the TMJ at postmortem examination in more than 40% of middle-aged and elderly patients, and radiographically osteoarthritis is a common incidental finding. Despite this frequency, osteoarthritis seldom causes TMJ symptoms. Clicking and limitation of movement are the most common symptoms; however, pain is unusual unless the condition is advanced. Radiographs of the mandibular condyle show the typical changes of osteoarthrosis, namely osteophytic lipping and small subarticular radiolucent areas. As the condition progresses the articular surfaces become flattened, the articular cartilage becomes less elastic and cracks appear in the underlying bone. In localized areas there may be loss of cartilage with eburnation of bone.

Symptoms include:

- Crepitus.
- Difficulty in chewing.
- Reduced mouth opening.
- Chronic pain.

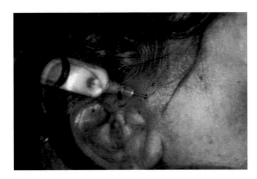

Figure 14.13 An intra-articular injection of triamcinolone acetate 40 mg into the lower joint space.

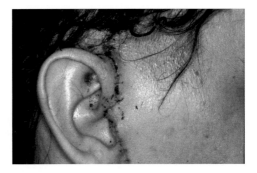

Figure 14.14 The preauricular approach to the temporomandibular joint just after suture removal at 6 days; the site allows an excellent aesthetic result.

Treatment in the first instance is essentially along the lines of TMJPDS. However, these patients may become candidates for joint replacements. Steroid injections are useful for pain relief, but they can damage the articulating surfaces further and may result in accelerated joint destruction (Figure 14.13).

Rheumatoid arthritis

This is a multisystem disease that predominately affects the joints, most commonly the hands, wrists and elbows. Progressive damage and significant symptoms tend to be uncommon in the TMJ (<5%). Of these the most common symptoms are crepitus and restriction of mouth opening. Rheumatoid arthritis undergoes acute phases of exacerbation followed by quiescent periods. Histologically there is overgrowth of the synovial lining associated with dense inflammation (pannus). This inflamed vascular mass spreads over and progressively destroys the articular cartilage, with resulting adhesions and limitation of movement. In severe cases this may progress to fibrous ankylosis. In the acute phase there may be pain and tenderness over the joints, which may be hot and look swollen and therefore appear infected. Patients frequently complain of a deep-seated, aching pain, particularly on moving the jaws. In advanced cases patients develop limitation of movement. In the acute phase, an acute infection must be excluded because this is severe and potentially life-threatening; however, it is rare.

Arthritis in children (juvenile arthritis), if severe, can damage the condyle's growth potential and can result in facial asymmetry, micrognathia and malocclusion.

Treatment in the first instance is essentially along the lines of TMJPDS. Steroid injections are useful for pain relief, but they can damage the articulating surfaces further and may result in accelerated joint destruction. Excision of pannus via a standard preauricular approach can relieve symptoms (Figure 14.14). Total condylar destruction may necessitate prosthetic joint replacement.

Infective arthritis

Infective arthritis has become rare since the advent of antibiotics. Most cases arose from the spread of infection from the ear (otitis externa, otitis media), which is now much better diagnosed and treated. However, infective arthritis is a potentially very severe condition because it may spread into the middle cranial fossa and result in intracranial sepsis. Symptoms include:-

- Pyrexia and systemic upset.
- Throbbing pain.
- Swelling.
- Erythema.
- Suppuration.
- Very restricted mouth opening.

Treatment includes antibiotics and drainage of any pus. Joint lavage may be required. In the young patient this can result in ankylosis, so aggressive physiotherapy and prolonged follow-up are usually necessary.

Ankylosis

Ankylosis is an abnormal union across a joint space. This may be either fibrous or bony in origin. Commonly, ankylosis is seen in the larger joints (e.g. the hips and knees following severe injuries or the spine in ankylosing spondylitis).

Normal mouth opening is said to be greater than 40 mm in adults. In addition it should be possible to protrude the mandible at least 7 mm and to move it side to side a similar amount. Untreated ankylosis results in permanent limitation of the mouth opening and may restrict development of the midface if it occurs in very young patients. Bony ankylosis results in the most severe limitation of opening. Ankylosis may be considered either extracapsular ('false' ankylosis) or intracapsular ('true' ankylosis).

Causes of extracapsular ankylosis

- Trauma resulting in periarticular fibrosis (e.g. lacerations, burns, dislocation).
- Chronic or untreated infection next to the joint.
- Tumours (e.g. fibrosarcoma, chondrosarcoma).
- Periarticular fibrosis (irradiation, prolonged immobilization of the jaws).

Causes of intracapsular ankylosis

- Trauma (intracapsular condylar fracture, penetrating wounds, forceps delivery at birth).
- Infection (otitis media, mastoiditis, osteomyelitis, pyogenic arthritis).
- Systemic disease (juvenile arthritis, psoriasis, rheumatoid arthritis, osteoarthritis).
- Tumours (chondroma, osteochondroma, osteoma, sarcoma, fibrosarcoma, synovial sarcoma).
- Miscellaneous (synovial chondromatosis).

Pseudoankylosis

This condition is a mechanical interference with mouth opening that does not directly involve the joint itself. Causes include:

- Trauma (e.g. depression of the zygomatic arch impinging on the coronoid or insertion of the temporalis muscle).
- Myositis ossificans within any of the muscles of mastication.

Treatment

The key to treatment is identification of at risk cases and prevention. When mouth opening is mildly limited, aggressive physiotherapy is required. Mechanical obstruction is addressed by surgery to the relevant part.

In adults the joint can be simply excised (gap arthroplasty) and an interpositional material placed to prevent recurrence of ankylosis. Many materials exist, including temporalis muscle, Silastic and ear cartilage. Alternatively, the joint can be completely replaced. In the growing face, the ankylosed segment may need to be excised, but it can be left, or replaced with a costochondral (rib) graft. The graft will actually grow, completely unpredictably (overgrowth, undergrowth or no growth equally likely). Total joint replacements using either stock or custom prostheses are increasingly recognized as predictable and long-lasting solutions.

In all cases aggressive mouth opening exercises are important. In long-standing cases bilateral coronoidectomies may also be necessary – as in any joint, if the muscles are not put through their full range of motion, they will contract and fibrose.

Splint therapies

A considerable amount of hot air is generated over the value of various forms of splints. Most district hospital practices restrict themselves to simple lower soft full occlusal coverage splints. Dental practitioners with a 'TMJ interest' often have a range of hard acrylic splints. (sometimes the same splint with a different name) that they believe in. No patient should undergo any permanent occlusal rehabilitation until it has been verified that their symptoms resolve with temporary ideal occlusion using a removable splint.

Lower soft 'bite raising appliance'

The lower soft bite raising appliance (BRA) is a thermoplastic polyvinyl full occlusal coverage splint. A lower alginate impression is taken, and the splint is fitted as early as possible. The patient wears it in the evenings and at night. Benefits are usually apparent after 1 to 2 months of wear. Quite how it works is a matter of conjecture; several theories have been proposed, including a placebo effect. The splint may absorb excessive occlusal forces; allow repositioning of the meniscus and restore muscle balance or even vertical dimension. Whatever the reason, it eases symptoms in 80% of patients. The practitioner should gradually wean the patient off the splint after 6 to 8 months.

Hard acrylic splints

Hard acrylic splints require considerably more refined dental techniques for manufacture and are multiple, depending on the 'occlusal theory' they are attempting to correct. They include the following: a localized interference splint, which is really just a habit breaker; the stabilization splint (also known as Turner, Michigan, Fox or CR splint), which aims to recreate an ideal occlusion; the anterior repositioning splint, which postures the mandible forward; and the anterior bite plane, which disengages posterior molar contact. The further reading section has details of these very dental approaches to TMJ pain and dysfunction. All these splints can give rise to occlusal changes, and patients need to provide informed consent and be monitored carefully.

Edentulous patients with TMJ disorders should receive essentially the same approach as dentate patients, with the obvious proviso that an adequate prosthesis may be helpful.

Currently used temporomandibular joint operations

Arthroscopy and arthrocentesis

This combined procedure involves a minimum of inserting an 'input and outlet' needle into the upper or lower joint space and irrigating the space with Hartman's solution or saline. The idea is that adhesions are broken down and inflammatory intermediaries are washed out. If a specially designed fibreoptic endoscope is placed instead of the input needles, the joint surfaces can be inspected; this is known as TMJ arthroscopy (Figure 14.15). Postprocedure injection with hyaluronic acid may be beneficial, but the evidence base is incomplete in a similar way to corticosteroids.

A number of microinstruments or fibreoptic lasers can be delivered this way. A simple and reliable landmark is a line between the midpoint of the tragus and the lateral canthus; 2 cm forward and 2 mm down will take a white needle into the upper joint space.

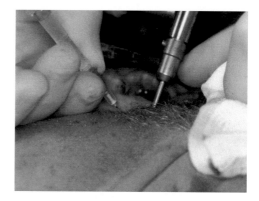

Figure 14.15 An arthroscope placed in the lower joint space. The outlet port allows irrigation outflow. This is the basis of 'lysis and lavage'.

High condylar shave

This term means approaching the condyle by open operation and resecting and reshaping the damaged joint surface (Figure 14.16).

There has been a vogue for preserving the meniscus to allow a new lower articulatory surface

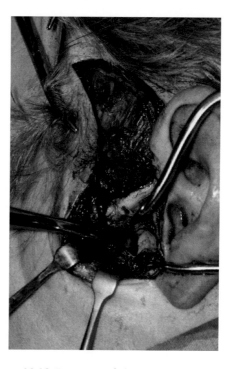

Figure 14.16 Exposure of the condyle via a preauricular approach for excision of a condylar osteoma.

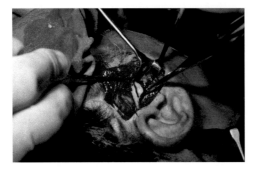

Figure 14.17 The bone cuts for an eminectomy. This is a particularly useful operation for recurrent dislocations.

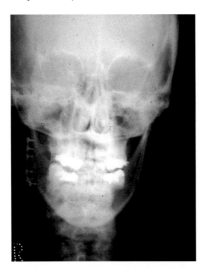

Figure 14.18 Postoperative radiograph of a costo-chondral rib graft total condyle replacement.

to form. Current thinking is moving in favour of excision of damaged meniscus, but a new articular fossa is usually implanted in these cases. Fat grafting following discectomy rather than fossa replacement has a number of advocates, particularly in North America.

Eminectomy

Eminectomy, removal of the articular eminence, is a favourite surgical approach to recurrent dislocation of the TMJ (Figure 14.17).

This procedure becomes popular for treatment of internal derangement approximately every 5 years. This is then followed by a period of condemning its use for exactly the same problem.

Joint replacement

Joint replacement is a significant operation for symptomatic, irreparably damaged joints. Costochondral rib grafts (Figure 14.18) or customized prosthetic joints are used. The unpredictability of costochondral rib (one third are stable, one third resorb and one third overgrow) and refinements to customized prostheses have moved almost all joint replacement for terminal joint damage to these devices (Figure 14.19).

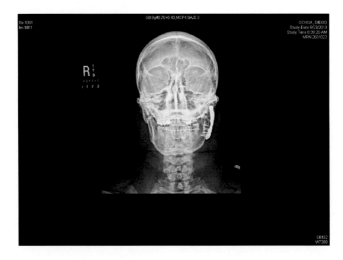

Figure 14.19 Customized total temporomandibular joint replacement.

FURTHER READING

Dolwick FM, Sanders B. *TMJ internal derangement and arthrosis.* St. Louis: Mosby, 1985.
Definitive guide to surgical procedures for internal derangement.

Gray R, Danes S, Quayle A. *Temporomandibular disorders: a clinical approach.* London: BDJ Books, 1995.
A practical well illustrated guide to TMJ disorders from a dental viewpoint.

Harris M, Feinmann C, Wise M, Treasure F. Temporomandibular joint and orofacial pain: clinical and medicolegal management problems. *Br Dent J* 1993;174:129–36.
A thoughtful and pragmatic review of TMJ dysfunction from a surgical and psychological perspective.

Idle MR, Lowe D, Rogers SN, Sidebottom AJ, Speculand B, Worrall SF. UK temporomandibular joint replacement database: report on baseline data. *Br J Oral Maxillofac Surg* 2014;52;203–7.

Pedlar J, Frame J. *Oral and maxillofacial surgery: an objective based textbook.* Edinburgh: Churchill-Livingstone, 2001, Chapters 17 and 18.
A clear and generally accepted guide to a frustrating subject.

Reston JT, Turkelson CM. Meta-analysis of surgical treatments for temporomandibular articular disorders. *J Oral Maxillofac Surg* 2003; 61 3–10.
Shows some limited evidence base for joint procedures, particularly arthroscopy.

Wilkes CH. Internal derangements of the temporomandibular joint: pathologic variations. *Arch Otolaryngol Head Neck Surg* 1989;115:469–77.

15

Implantology and preprosthetic surgery

Contents

Aims and learning outcomes

For undergraduates:

- To be able to list the range of preprosthetic procedures available.
- To be able to describe the principles, indications and steps of common implant procedures.
- To demonstrate an awareness of the less common procedures.

For postgraduates:

- To be able to describe the principles of all preprosthetic procedures.
- To be able to describe the steps of individual implant procedures.
- To demonstrate the ability to link individual preprosthetic problems to surgical and non-surgical solutions.

Introduction

The core problem in prosthetics is tooth loss. This may seem self-evident, but in relation to preprosthetic surgery it is the progressive loss of the residual alveolar bone at the rate of 0.5 to 1.0 mm/year following tooth loss that generates a patient's difficulties. This results in a progressive loss of bone stock and secondary soft tissue support for any prosthesis. To compensate for this loss of soft tissue support and to maintain the occlusal vertical dimension there is an increase in bulk of the dentures that leads to further instability. The initial healing of the extraction socket by secondary intention with the formation of myofibroblasts within the organizing blood clot also hastens this loss of bone stock. Finally, the pathological processes that have led to the initial loss of teeth may continue, thus leading to the progressive loss of remaining teeth.

Atraumatic exodontia

Taking the foregoing observations into account, surgery for prosthodontics begins with the extraction of teeth and the removal of retained roots and unerupted teeth (see Chapter 6). The need to preserve alveolar bone is paramount and is best achieved by atraumatic exodontia including socket compression. Socket compression reduces any expansion of the buccal plate and also reduces the residual blood clot within the socket. This blood clot may be further diminished by intraradicular radiculectomy and crush.

Intraradicular radiculectomy and crush

This technique reduces the socket dead space following multiple extractions, usually in the upper and lower labial segments. Following extraction, the bony septum between the sockets is removed by means of rongeurs (Figure 15.1). The buccal plate is then compressed manually and is in-fractured to reduce the socket space. The approximation of buccal and lingual/palatal plates of the socket allows the gingival margins to be sutured to maintain the compression. This technique is of particular benefit for the immediate insertion of dentures (Figure 15.2 (a) and (b)).

Surgery for conventional prosthodontics

Fixed and removable prosthesis

Fixed prostheses

Nonimplant fixed prostheses are predominately confined to crowns and bridgework. Surgery for these prostheses is invariably confined to periapical surgery (see Chapter 7) or to periodontal procedures.

Removable prostheses

Surgery for removable prostheses can be considered under soft tissue and hard tissue surgery. In either case, surgery is aimed at improving retention and stability of the prosthesis, improving the patient's comfort or removing pathological tissue. It should be considered best practice for the surgeon to work in close collaboration with the prosthetist in the joint management of these patients.

Soft tissue surgery

Common soft tissue procedures include:

- Fraenectomy.
- Ridge reduction.
- Removal of irritation ('denture') hyperplasia.
- Vestibuloplasty.

Fraenectomy

Large fraena or resorption of the residual ridge can interfere with the peripheral seal of the denture and lead to poor retention. The relief for such fraena may also result in repeat fractures of the prosthesis and discomfort. In these cases, fraenectomy may be carried out using a technique as for upper labial fraenectomy for orthodontic indications (see Chapter 9) (Figure 15.3).

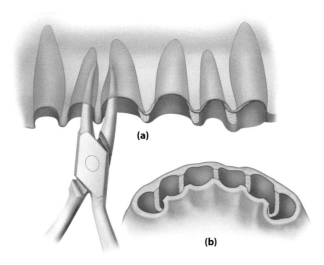

(a)

(b)

Figure 15.1 (a) and (b) Diagrams representing the removal of intrabony septa with rongeurs.

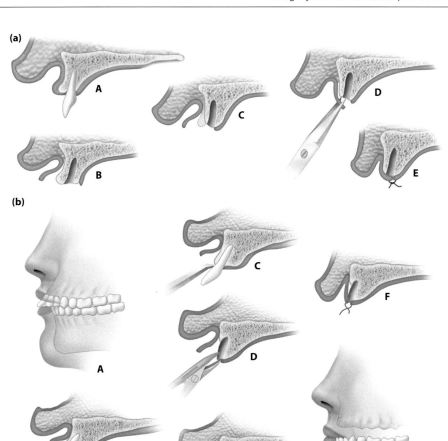

Figure 15.2 The first procedure (a) is socket reduction where a bony undercut needs to be reduced. (A) Vertically positioned tooth with prominent bony undercut. (B) Atraumatic removal of tooth. (C) Full-thickness mucoperiosteal flap and removal of bone. (D) Trimming of excess mucosa. (E) Suturing mucosa to seal socket. The second procedure (b) is socket reduction where excessive angulation of tooth and socket requires infracture of labial plate of socket. (A) Class II div I angulation of incisor teeth. (B) Full-thickness mucoperiosteal flap raised. (C) Atraumatic removal of tooth. (D) Infracture of labial plate of socket. (E) Repositioning of labial plate and trimming of mucosa. (F) Closure of wound. (G) Final alveolar bone shape and profile change.

'Flabby' ridge reduction – 'Schlotterkamm'

In patients who have tooth loss associated with advanced periodontal disease, the excess of soft tissue may result in a flabby ridge, which in turn causes poor denture stability. This commonly affects the maxillary tuberosity region and labial segments. The localized bone loss can be further accelerated if natural standing teeth oppose a denture. In these cases soft tissue reduction is carried out by excision of the underlying fibrous tissue while preserving, where possible, the attached mucosa (Figure 15.4). In these cases it is important to have a replacement baseplate in which a tissue conditioner can be placed to enable close adaptation of the mucosa to the underlying bony ridge.

Irritation (denture) hyperplasia

Resorption of the residual ridge continues after initial socket healing. The loss of bone height causes a previously adequately extended denture

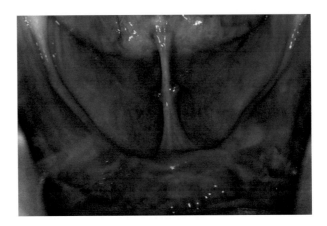

Figure 15.3 High fraenal attachments like the lingual attachment shown here can be simply divided. The tight 'bowstring' opens into a loose diamond shape which can be closed primarily. This automatically deepens the sulcus.

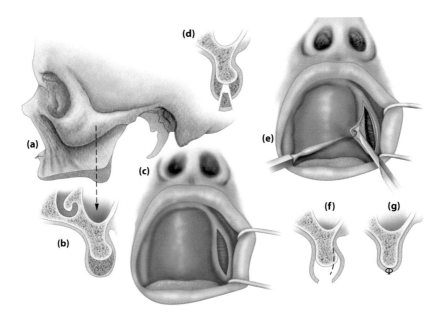

Figure 15.4 These steps illustrate the common region of the maxilla to have a 'flabby' ridge. (a) Tuberosity region. (b) Cross section showing antrum, alveolar bone, excessive fibrous tissue and attached gingivae. (c) Elliptical excision of attached gingiva exposes underlying excess fibrous tissue. (d) Wedge of excess tissue excised. (e) Residual excess fibrous tissue excised down to bone but preserving attached gingivae. (f) Excessive undercuts removed if necessary. (g) Attached gingivae sutured adherent to underlying bone.

to have a peripheral margin that is overextended, usually into the buccal or labial sulcus. This leads to a traumatic ulcer in the sulcus, which, with repeated trauma, produces an overgrowth of fibrous tissue. Initial management is by the drastic local relief of the flange of the denture and strict instructions to the patient to leave the denture out as much as possible ('social use only'). After a period of a few weeks, inflammation is reduced and the hyperplastic tissue decreases in size. In

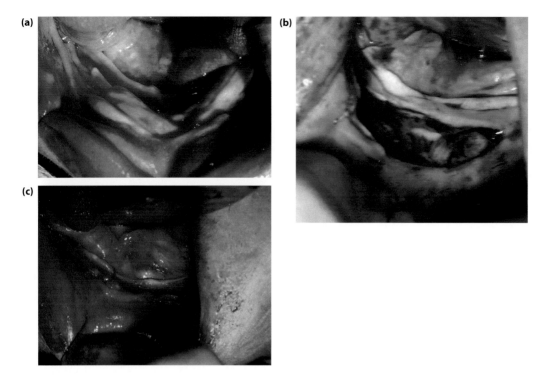

Figure 15.5 (a) Irritation hyperplasia; if leaving the lower full denture out does not allow the area to settle, excision is indicated. (b) Excision of irritation hyperplasia. (c) Mucosa should be preserved wherever possible.

many cases the reduction in size is such that the hyperplastic tissue will not interfere with new denture construction.

When the residual hyperplastic tissue will interfere with denture construction, excision is indicated (Figure 15.5 (a)). This may take the form of *simple excision* with elliptical excision of the excess tissue at its base. In large areas of hyperplasia, simple excision may create a shallow V-shaped sulcus. In these cases a *mucosal-preserving approach* should be attempted, by dissecting and preserving the buccal/labial mucosa while excising the remainder of the hyperplastic lesion, with the preserved mucosa inlaid as a graft to preserve sulcus depth (Figure 15.5 (b) and (c)). In this case a healing baseplate suitably lined with tissue conditioner is essential to try to maintain sulcus depth.

Vestibuloplasty

In areas where residual ridge height or sulcus depth has been lost, commonly because of loss of attached mucosa, vestibuloplasty may be beneficial. In these cases a supraperiosteal mucosal flap is reflected and sutured 'apically' in the sulcus.

Muscle attachments may need to be released to achieve the desired increase in sulcus depth. The exposed periosteum may be left to granulate; however, this may result in scarring and a narrow V-shaped sulcus, which the prosthetist may have difficulty using. Scar reduction may be achieved by grafting with palatal mucosal free graft or split-thickness skin graft. In either case a healing baseplate lined with gutta percha or a proprietary denture liner should be fixed in place for the initial healing period by means of heavy nonresorbable suture (or stainless steel wire) passed around the mandible or less often through the maxillary antrum or screws directly into the hard palate.

In the case of lingual vestibuloplasty, following release of the lingual muscle attachments, the new sulcus depth is created by a temporary baseplate secured by circummandibular wires or heavy nonresorbable sutures.

After initial healing, a temporary denture extended to the full depth of the new sulcus should be provided. Unfortunately, the benefits of vestibuloplasty are lost if subsequent prostheses do not make full use of the new sulcus depth.

Hard tissue surgery

Hard tissue surgery may be required in the form of *alveoplasty, ridge reduction, removal of tori* and *reduction in muscle attachments*. These procedures aim to reduce or remove hard tissue prominences that create excess undercuts that the prosthetist is unable to use, thus creating dead spaces. You should always remember that complete elimination of undercuts could render the patient in a worse condition postoperatively with a completely unretentive denture. It is even more important in hard tissue preprosthetic surgery that liaison is maintained with the prosthetist to agree on how much bone should be removed to achieve the maximum prosthetic gain.

Where there has been significant bone loss consideration may be given to *ridge augmentation*. This augmentation may be in the form of *onlay grafting, interpositional grafting* or *distraction osteogenesis*. All these techniques may be augmented by the use of growth factors derived from platelet-rich plasma (PRP).

Alveoplasty

Despite the most careful of extraction techniques, circumstances will occur in which the residual ridge heals to become irregular or feather edged. Pressure on these bony irregularities under the mucosa by a denture results in pain. Alveoplasty is the smoothing of these bony irregularities. Mucoperiosteal flaps are reflected using a subcrestal incision to expose the whole residual ridge. The irregular areas can be visualized or felt with the gloved finger and smoothed using hand instruments or well-irrigated burrs. Alveolar bone is precious, and the minimum amount of bone should be removed to achieve the desired result. When extensive smoothing is required, an intraoperative clear acrylic template may help demonstrate residual areas of irregularity by blanching of the underlying mucosa.

Ridge reduction

Where the residual ridge heals with excessive undercuts, reduction may be of benefit. In consultation with the prosthetist, the undercut is reduced or removed via a mucoperiosteal flap raised from a subcrestal incision. Presurgical planning demonstrating acceptable paths of insertion will dictate how much undercut should be removed to give maximal denture retention (Figure 15.6 (a) and (b)).

Removal of tori and muscle attachments

Palatal and lingual (mandibular) tori are normal anatomical variants. The lingual tori and prominent genial tubercles are often bony overgrowths at the site of muscle attachments. Because the lower full denture is inherently unstable, there may be benefits in retaining the lingual torus unilaterally to facilitate the use of the undercut to improve retention and stability. Prominent genial tubercles commonly occur in the atrophic mandible. They are removed on symptomatic grounds but may result in further loss of stability of the lower prosthesis. Lingual tori are removed via a lingual mucoperiosteal flap. Care should be taken in reflection of these flaps because the mucosa is friable. Particular care needs to be taken around the bony prominence as a result of undercuts. The bony prominence may be

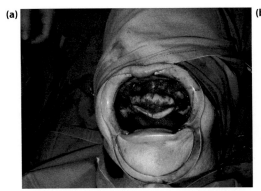 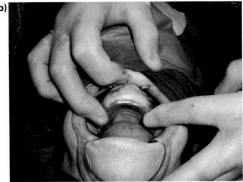

Figure 15.6 (a) Intraoperative view of ridge reduction technique. (b) Example of a surgical baseplate.

removed with burrs combined with hand instruments such as an osteotome. A wide flap is raised to protect the lingual nerve adequately because, idiosyncratically, a wide subperiosteal lingual flap is associated with a lower level of lingual nerve neurapraxia than a small (Howarth's periosteal elevator size) flap (see Chapter 8).

Palatal tori should be removed if they cause denture instability or repeated fracture or where there is soft tissue trauma. In this case the torus is removed via a split palatal mucoperiosteal flap, preserving the incisive neurovascular bundle, to expose the bony torus fully (Figures 15.7a and b). Reflection of the flap over the torus is often difficult because of undercuts. The torus is sectioned with a fissure burr, and each segment is removed with an osteotome or chisel. Final smoothing is with a large bone-cutting burr (acrylic burrs are often used for this final smoothing but these clog and overheat, so an ear, nose and throat 'mastoid' burr is perfect). Following closure a healing baseplate or pack may be placed to reduce the risk that a haematoma will form from the raw bone margins.

Ridge augmentation

The residual ridge may be built up using a variety of materials. These include *bone autografts* or *allografts* (or bone substitutes). The risks of viral and prion infections make the use of xenografts or cadaveric materials no longer acceptable. These grafts may be placed as either *onlay* or *interpositional grafts*.

The main complication of ridge augmentation is accelerated resorption of the graft. This is thought to be caused by the lack of an adequate soft tissue

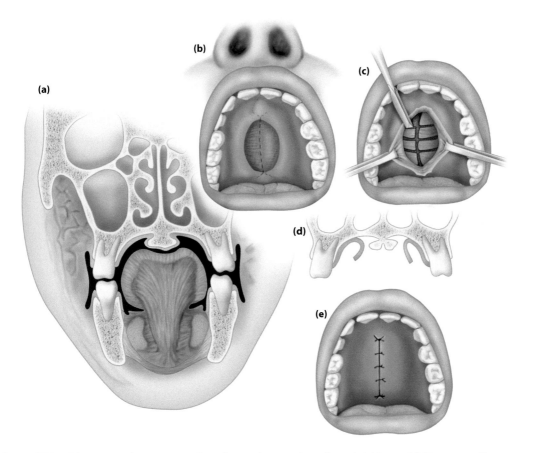

Figure 15.7a Diagrammatic representation of steps in resection of a palatal torus. (a) Diagrammatic cross section of the face showing a torus palatinus. (b) Schematic of incision to expose bony outgrowth. (c) The bone of the prominent palatinus is cut into smaller pieces in situ. (d) Diagrammatic cross-sectional view of sectioning the torus palatinus. (e) Schematic of wound closure.

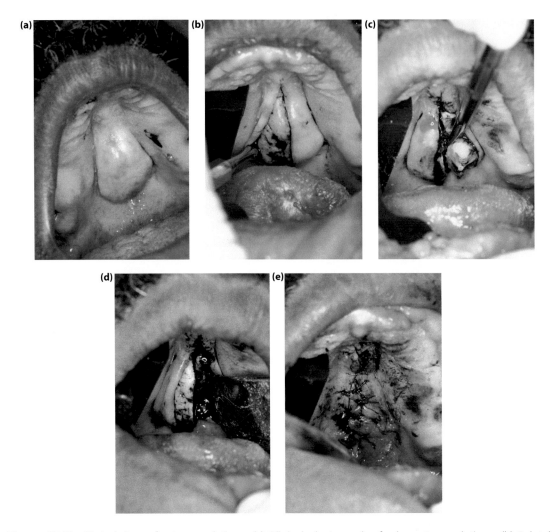

Figure 15.7b Clinical view of a torus palatinus. (a) Clinical photograph of a large torus platinus. (b) Palatal subperiosteal flap being raised. (c) Sectioning and removing the bone. (d) Bleeding from the base of the bone, half the torus has been removed. (e) Wound closure with resorbable sutures.

envelope resulting in little space for graft placement. The consequent tight tissue envelope is thought to produce loss of the graft. Techniques to improve the soft tissue space (e.g. periosteal release) can lead to loss of sulcus depth and attached mucosa. This means a later vestibuloplasty and graft to allow full use of the ridge height gained. A brief experiment with intraoral tissue expansion was never followed through, although it provided a theoretical technique to overcome this problem.

Complications of ridge augmentation

In addition to the general postoperative complications of bleeding, bruising, swelling and infection,

ridge augmentation may be associated with special complications. These may include:

- Accelerated bone loss as discussed earlier.
- Nerve injuries – surgical approaches close to the infraorbital and mental nerves may cause transient or long-standing altered sensation. Harvest of bone graft from the chin may damage the branches of the incisive nerve to cause paraesthesia of the gingivae of the lower labial segment. Harvest of bone from the retromolar region may involve the inferior alveolar neurovascular bundle with resultant mental paraesthesia.

- Fracture – in the severely atrophic mandible, osteotomies for distraction osteogenesis may predispose to a pathological fracture.
- Loss of soft tissue support – extensive stripping of the tissues around the chin can lead to loss of the muscle attachments. The result can be that the chin is no longer supported and is displaced inferiorly, giving an unacceptable profile ('witch's chin').

Autografts

When choosing the donor site for autografts consideration should be given to the volume of bone required, the need for particulate or corticocancellous block and the ease of harvest. There is evidence to suggest that donor bone of the same embryological type gives better results with less resorption. The bone of the residual alveolar ridge is membranous in origin. This supports the use of the retromolar regions or the chin as intraoral sites, which are readily available using outpatient local anaesthesia and are membranous in origin. Where large shaped corticocancellous blocks are required, anterior or posterior iliac crest proves the most suitable site, even though this is of endochondral origin.

Allographic materials are inorganic bone substitutes. These may be calcium phosphates or hydroxyapatites. There is significant experience using bovine bone, which has been treated to remove all organic material. These materials can be used alone or as a bulking agent for bone autografts (Figure 15.8).

These graft materials may be augmented by the use of PRP. The principle behind the use of

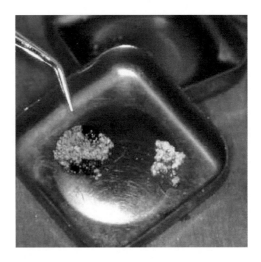

Figure 15.8 Hydroxyapatite synthetic bone substitute.

PRP is the concentration of growth factors (endothelial-derived growth factor [EDGF]; vascular endothelial growth factor [VDGF]; transforming growth factor-β2 group, including bone morphogenic protein [BMP]) in platelets. A sample of the patient's blood is manipulated in a centrifuge to give 5 to 9 mL of plasma, which contains 2 million platelets. The effect of this PRP is to give earlier vascularization of the bone graft, which allows earlier and better bone consolidation. There are also soft tissue effects with improved healing (Figure 15.9).

An alternative is to use commercially prepared BMP, although this is expensive and excites a significant inflammatory response.

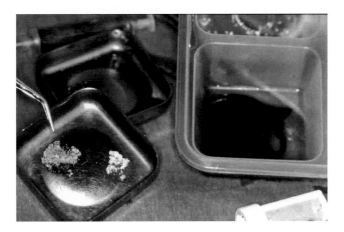

Figure 15.9 Platelet-rich plasma and hydroxyapatite.

In Germany the most commonly used bone substitute material is Bio-Oss, produced by Geistlich Company. Bio-Oss is derived from bovine material, which makes it a xenograft. There is a strong lobby by the pharmaceutical companies for allografts and xenografts in Germany. Patients are receptive of the idea of using bone substitute material because it prevents donor site morbidity.

Distraction osteogenesis

The advent of distraction osteogenesis applied to the facial bones using the principles originally developed by Ilizarov is an alternative method of ridge augmentation that may overcome some of the problems associated with onlay or interpositional ridge augmentation. The surgical technique involves an osteotomy of the residual ridge to create a mobile segment. A distraction appliance is fitted and the wound closed. After a latency period the device is activated to increase the alveolar bone height along a predetermined vector. Once the planned amount of bone height increase has been reached, the device is left for a period of up to 2 months before it is removed. The advantages of this approach are the removal of the need for a second donor site and risks associated with the use of allografts. In addition to distraction osteogenesis, there is also distraction histogenesis increasing the soft tissue envelope and thus reducing the risk of resorption. This technique does require two surgical procedures and the use of specialist devices with associated costs. Careful patient selection is necessary because sufficient bone must be present to allow the initial osteotomy. The rate of distraction is critical in these cases. If the distraction rate is too fast, wasting of the bone will occur – too slow and the transport disc will fuse prematurely. This can be overcome by placing a PRP/bone graft interposed at the osteotomy site.

Orthognathic surgery in preprosthetic surgery

In patients with an existing skeletal anomaly, this can be further exaggerated by bone resorption. In particular, resorption of the maxilla is both vertical and horizontal. Ridge augmentation alone may not be sufficient to allow for the satisfactory construction of conventional dentures. In these situations consideration may be given to a combined augmentation and maxillary repositioning procedure. This will involve a Le Fort I advancement osteotomy with the insertion of an interpositional horseshoe corticocancellous bone graft to down-graft the residual ridge and give ridge augmentation. The planning of this procedure is similar to that for orthognathic surgery in the dentate patient (see Chapter 19), but it is modified to take account of the proposed positioning of the incisal tips of the prosthesis.

Mandibular prognathism may be corrected by conventional setback osteotomies. There is a change in blood supply to the mandibular bone following the loss of teeth and the potential effects this may have on healing. The advent of distraction osteogenesis has probably cast procedures such as the visor osteotomy to the history books.

Implants

The principle behind implantable materials for prosthodontics is to use the underlying bone for support of the prosthesis. Implants can be classified as *submucosal, subperiosteal, endosseous* and *transosseus.*

The earliest forms of implant were either submucosal or subperiosteal. In both cases soft tissue flaps were reflected, and impressions were taken of the underlying bone surface. As intimated by their classification, submucosal implants were placed below the mucosa but were supraperiosteal, the theory being that this would protect the blood supply to the underlying basal bone, which at this stage would be predominantly centripetal from the periosteum. Subperiosteal implants were placed under a mucoperiosteal flap. In both cases this was a two-stage procedure with a cast stainless steel or chrome/cobalt framework spreading the loads of the prosthesis onto the underlying bone. These implants tended to fail because of soft tissue encroachment around the metal framework that led to mobility and low-grade infection. They are of historical interest only.

Endosseous implants are placed within the residual bone of the alveolar ridge. These are either *osseointegrated* or *nonosseointegrated.* The nonosseointegrated implants derived from the submucosal/subperiosteal implants. In this technique metal implants (stainless steel, gold and, later, titanium) are placed into the alveolar process. These implants are retained by the mechanical design of the fixture (e.g. holes placed within the implant to allow bone ingress during healing). An example is the blade implant, which still has the occasional advocate for its use.

Osseointegrated implants use the unique biocompatibility properties of titanium. Branemark, while studying the blood flow in rabbit bones, noted that he had difficulty in removing the titanium viewing chambers on sacrifice of the animal. Further study showed that, contrary to understanding at that time, the bone had grown onto the pure titanium surface. From this discovery Branemark developed his dental implant system, and the first patient had implants in the early 1960s. Although there are now numerous implant systems available, they all are based on the same principle of osseointegration into the residual alveolar bone, thereby transmitting the forces of mastication directly to the underlying bone.

Principles for implant placement

Planning with a prosthodontist (or maxillofacial technician for extraoral implants) is essential. Perhaps obviously this has led to an expansion of many restorative dentists into surgical implantology, and in some countries dental implantology has become a subspecialty of its own.

Surgical templates that relate the position of the implants to the prosthesis are prepared in the laboratory. The choice of implant is made based on individual preference and on the site and depth of available bone. Implants come in a variety of shapes and sizes. The most common are cylindrical or tapered. Specific instructions, including indications, contraindications, conditions and techniques specific to that implant system, are individualized to each company's product.

Planning for the rehabilitation of the dentition with osseointegrated implants requires close collaboration between prosthodontist and implantologist, if they are not the same person. In some instances they are, but generally the surgical skills, particularly for more complex cases, of a trained surgeon are needed. Equally, the construction of superstructure and prosthesis is a specialist skill in its own right, almost never included in oral and maxillofacial surgical training. To achieve success the implants have to be placed in an ideal position to satisfy the mechanics and aesthetics of the prosthesis but also in bone of adequate quantity and quality to support the implant. Various methods can be used to evaluate the quality and quantity of bone before implant placement, but the most effective is helical computed tomography (CT) scanning linked to three-dimensional implant planning computer software (Figure 15.10). This software allows for the virtual placement of implants in varying positions to give alignment and implant size before surgical placement. Once this process is completed, it is possible to download the final plan to have custom made surgical templates constructed. Some controversy exists about the advantages and disadvantages of cone beam CT scanning over conventional CT scanning and three-dimensional reconstruction in this field.

The imaging and assessment of the potential implant sites indicate to the implantologist/prosthetist the sites where preliminary preimplant

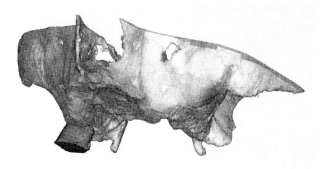

Figure 15.10 Three-dimensional computed tomography reformat.

surgery will be necessary. The preimplant surgery may include removal of teeth or roots, removal of intrabony pathology and bone grafting.

The removal of teeth and roots is covered elsewhere (see Chapter 6). In the case of preimplant surgery these teeth or roots should be removed, preserving as much alveolar bone as possible. In this case the use of specialist instrumentation such as the periotome can be helpful. Similarly, the removal of residual intrabony pathology (e.g. residual cysts) should preserve bone where possible.

Surgery for osseointegrated implants

Bone grafting is often required to provide sufficient height and or width of the alveolus to allow implant placement. The most common grafting procedures are *sinus lifting* and *onlay grafting*.

Sinus lifting is necessary when the floor of the maxillary antrum invaginates the residual alveolar ridge in the premolar region and reduces the amount of bone height required for placement of implants in this area. The surgical technique is similar to a Caldwell-Luc approach to the maxillary antrum. In the case of sinus lifting, the bone window is retained attached to the antral lining (Figure 15.11 (a) to (c)), which is carefully elevated from the antral floor to create a mucoperiosteal pocket. Bone is placed into this pocket and thus raises the antral floor. Indirect closed sinus lifting can also be carried out at the time of implant placement if the amount of additional bone required is small. In this case the bone is prepared for the implant in the normal manner, taking care not to perforate the antral lining. The antral lining is lifted through the hole and bone graft is packed into the prepared hole immediately before fixture placement. In the process of placing the

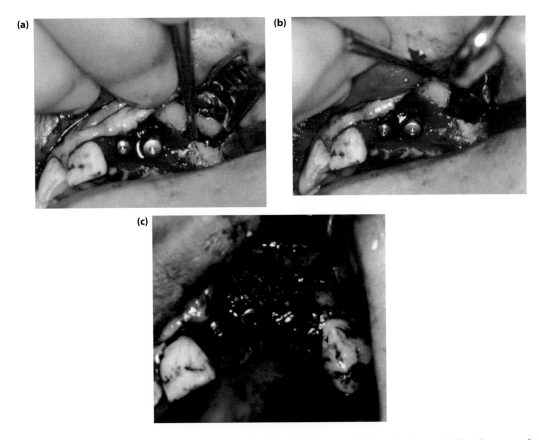

Figure 15.11 (a) Incision and exposure for the sinus lift. (b) The antral lining is elevated. (c) A bone graft is placed and secured between bone of the antral floor and the elevated lining.

fixture, the bone graft is forced under the antral lining to give the necessary support for the newly placed fixture.

Onlay grafting is required to increase residual alveolar ridge width and height. The anterior alveolus in particular resorbs both vertically and distally and thereby provides a narrow palatal or lingually placed residual ridge. Onlay grafting allows for the restoration of normal ridge width and eliminates concavities, which may result in exposed implant threads.

Other techniques to increase residual bone height and width include corticocancellous block grafts and segmental distraction osteogenesis. Segmental distraction osteogenesis can be performed either before implant placement or, with special distraction implants, following fixture placement.

Individual implant placement

This procedure is usually performed using local anaesthesia with or without sedation. The residual alveolar ridge is exposed by a crestal incision, and mucoperiosteal flaps are raised medially and laterally. The bone is prepared by drilling at slow speed with meticulous irrigation to avoid osteocyte death caused by bone overheating. The implant site is prepared by sequentially increasing twist drill size to reach one just under the maximum diameter of the implant. Depending on bone density and implant design, the bone is tapped (prepared for a thread) before placing the implant. This is also under coolant irrigation (Figure 15.12). It is essential to avoid contamination of the pure titanium surface of the implant with stainless steel instruments or soft tissue. The implant is screwed into the bone at slow speed until the maximum torque is reached. Do not overtighten because this can strip the implant from the bone. Sometimes exposed threads are seen on the buccal/labial aspect of the implant on final placement. If there is primary stability, the majority of implants will integrate despite exposed threads (Figure 15.13). These threads can also be covered by bone harvested by a surgical filter or bone substitute. Semipermeable membrane covering this can promote healing by guided tissue regeneration (Figure 15.14). A cover screw is fitted over the internal threads of the implant (Figure 15.15), and the wound is closed. The patient is advised not to

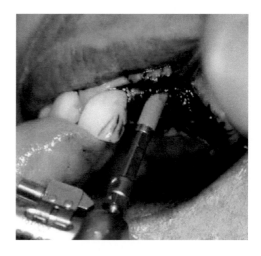

Figure 15.12 Implant socket preparation.

wear the prosthesis for 7 to 10 days, followed by occasional wear only.

The time taken for integration depends on the quality of bone available at the implant site. It is generally accepted that an implant will integrate in 3 months in the mandible and in 3 to 6 months in the maxilla. Titanium oxide coatings on the threads of implants have reduced the integration time in the maxilla.

At second stage surgery, a small mucosal window is cut over the cover screw, and the cover screw is removed. Any covering bone is removed.

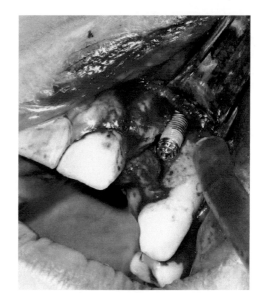

Figure 15.13 Exposed implant threads.

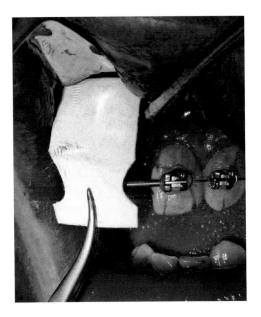

Figure 15.14 Material used for guided tissue regeneration.

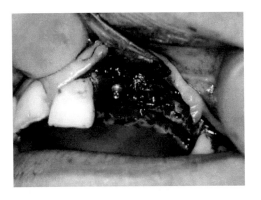

Figure 15.15 Dental implants in place with cover screws visible.

A temporary 'healing' abutment is placed to the size that will allow suitable protrusion through the mucoperiosteum. This is left in place for a minimum of 2 weeks to allow the mucosal cuff to heal around the healing abutment. Once healing has occurred, the prosthodontist places a final abutment and takes impressions of the fixture head for construction of the definitive prosthesis.

Special cases

The technique for implant placement is essentially the same for single and multiple implant restorations. Special considerations and modifications take place for *Same Day Teeth,* the *custom bar prosthesis* and *transmandibular implants.*

Same Day Teeth and custom bar prostheses

Same Day Teeth (Branemark Novum; Figure 15.16 (a) and (b)) and *custom bar prostheses* are modifications of an immediate loading technique relying on the cross bracing of the implants by a preformed titanium bar. In the case of the Novum Same Day Teeth prosthesis, a bone platform is created and three implants are placed according to a standardized jig. Because the framework for the prosthesis is prefabricated, the prosthodontics can be taken to try-in stage, with the final bite registration taken following placement of three fixtures and the preformed lower bar. The lower prosthesis is constructed on a preformed upper bar, which is screwed onto the framework by means of four screws. This technique is principally directed toward those cases with significant loss of bone height that must be replaced by

(a)

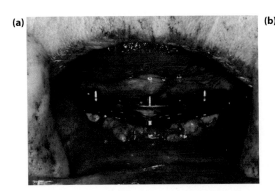

(b)

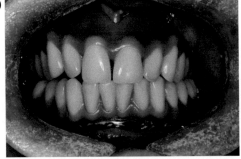

Figure 15.16 (a) The Branemark Novum system implants with a custom bar. (b) Prosthesis *in situ.*

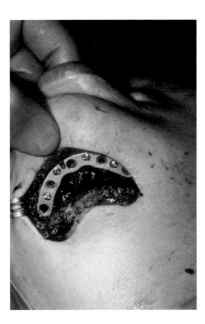

Figure 15.17 The submental approach for insertion of the transmandibular implant.

the prosthesis, which forms a bridge removable by the dentist. When the arch form of the anterior mandible does not allow placement of the implants in the positions determined by a jig or when there is sufficient bone, four fixtures may be placed and immediate impressions taken for implant head position so that a custom made titanium lower bar may be constructed and fitted at a later stage for early loading. This technique does not appear to have been as successful as initially hoped.

Transmandibular implant

The transmandibular implant (TMI Bosker) uses transmandibular gold fixtures screwed into a baseplate (Figure 15.17), which is secured to the lower border of the anterior mandible. The principle behind this is that a load is transmitted down the transmandibular fixtures and is disseminated along the lower border basal bone. This is particularly of benefit in patients with severe resorption of the mandible (Figure 15.18). Where there is the potential for pathological fracture, extension bars can be fitted distally. Serial postoperative radiographs have shown that in these cases regeneration of bone density and height has occurred. It must be stressed, however, that in these cases, the transmandibular implants are not strictly osseointegrated, and the popularity of these implants has waned since 2000.

More recent developments have used the bone volume of the root of the zygoma for placement of implants (Branemark Os Zygomaticus was the first such). This implant allows fixtures in the upper tuberosity region. This is of particular benefit for patients who have lost significant amounts of bone because of disease or trauma.

Extraoral craniofacial implants and bone anchored hearing aids

The principles of osseointegration can also be applied to the remaining bone of the facial skeleton and skull where there has been significant loss of hard and soft tissue as a result of congenital deformities, disease or trauma. Fixtures may be placed in the skull or periorbital region to support the prosthesis to replace the eye, nose and ears (Figure 15.19). The advantage of an implant-retained prosthesis over conventional techniques is the superb stability achieved that allows for fine moulding at the edges of the prosthesis against natural skin by the maxillofacial technician, thereby giving excellent and durable aesthetics.

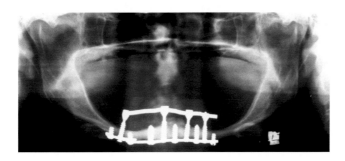

Figure 15.18 Radiographic example of the transmandibular implant *in situ*.

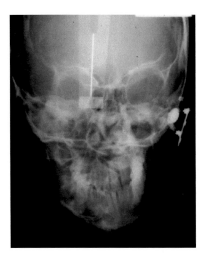

Figure 15.19 Posteroanterior radiograph of an osseointegrated implant-borne prosthetic ear from a patient with hemifacial microsomia.

The integration of the fixtures into the bone of the skull can also be used to support a bone-anchored hearing aid (BAHA). In this situation the implant is used to facilitate bone conduction of sound to allow hearing in patients with severe conductive deafness.

Surgery for prosthodontics in patients with cancer

Surgery for prosthodontics in patients with head and neck cancer should be considered at the time of planning for the ablative surgery. The eventual rehabilitation of the patient has to be considered at the time of initial resection and reconstruction, but it must not compromise the principles of oncological surgery (see Chapters 22 and 23). Planning of flaps to restore tissue volume should take into account the eventual prosthetic rehabilitation with regard to appropriate bulk and preservation, where possible, of appropriate bone and soft tissue undercuts. It is with this planning for reconstruction in mind that there has been debate on the appropriateness of placement of osseointegrated implants at the time of initial ablative surgery. Because many of these patients will receive adjuvant radiotherapy, there is a much higher risk of implant failure with the real risk of osteoradionecrosis. The effects of radiotherapy on bone are lifelong, with the potential for development of osteoradionecrosis following minor trauma or surgery. There is a fine balance between the potential need for implants for rehabilitation and the inconvenience and costs of hyperbaric oxygen therapy for the prevention of osteoradionecrosis (if, indeed, the long-term evidence validates this strategy). Not all patients having radical ablative surgery will require or be suitable for osseointegrated implants. However, when appropriate, the use of osseointegrated implants in the rehabilitation of patients with head and neck cancer does have a significant part to play in improving quality of life. The use of osseo-integrated implants should form part of the initial treatment planning for these patients and should not be an afterthought or a treatment modality of last resort.

Complications of osseointegrated implants

Apart from the traditional perioperative complications associated with any minor oral surgical procedure (i.e. bruising, swelling, risk of infection and bleeding), there are a few special complications. In the placement of implants in the anterior mandible, in particular when using the Same Day Teeth technique, the preparation of the bone for the implant often involves perforation of the cortical bone of lower border of the mandible. In this situation patients need to be warned about the possibility of localized cutaneous bruising. Similarly, in placement of the implants in the anterior maxilla, the cortical bone of nasal floor is often used. Patients need to be warned of the possibility of bruising around the nose and nasal stuffiness.

In all cases, there is the possibility that the implant will fail to integrate. This is usually detected at the time of second stage surgery and when attempts to remove the cover screw lead to unscrewing of the implant. In this situation the bone is allowed to heal, and the implant can usually be replaced after allowing 3 months for bone to regenerate.

A small amount of bone loss around implants in the order of less than 0.1 mm per year is normally expected. In patients with excessive loading of the implant-retained prosthesis or exceptionally poor oral hygiene, inflammation of the mucosal cuff around the implant abutment may be seen with localized bone loss at the pocket formation. This peri-implantitis is usually reversible with judicious oral hygiene measures and scaling, although it may lead to eventual implant loss.

United States perspective

In the United States (and likely elsewhere where the costs can be transferred to the patient rather than subtracted from a centralized total, as in a state- or taxation-funded system like the UK National Health Service), if implant placement following extraction is planned, thought is often given to socket preservation grafting. In these cases care is taken to remove the tooth as atraumatically as possible, often using periotomes. The socket is then grafted with an allogeneic material such as demin-eralized bone matrix. The socket may be covered with a collagen membrane when primary closure is not possible. This combination of relatively minor procedures enables maximal alveolar bone preser-vation and attached gingiva for implant insertion and long-term preservation.

Posterior implants in very atrophic mandibles may require lateralization of the inferior alveo-lar nerve. This is a technique updated from a similar approach used when progressive alveolar resorption caused the mental nerve to be pain-fully compressed by the often ill-fitting lower full denture. The use of piezosurgical instru-ments makes this both safer and easier in the twenty-first century.

FURTHER READING

Hopkins R. *A colour atlas of preprosthetic oral surgery.* London: Wolfe Medical Publications, 1987.

An old book but absolutely full of techniques other than implants and well worth a glance for those who are interested.

Anyone with an interest in implant surgery should go on an introductory course on this subject. At that point you will get a feel for which type of system you wish to use and can follow the specific recommendations for that system.

Specific references of interest include:

Altintas NY, Senel FC, Kayipmaz S, Taskesen F, Pampu AA. Comparative radiologic analyses of newly formed bone after maxillary sinus augmentation with and without bone graft-ing. *J Oral Maxillofac Surg* 2013;71:1520–30.

Basegmez C, Karabuda ZC, Demirel K, Yalcin S. The comparison of acellular dermal matrix allografts with free gingival grafts in the augmentation of per-implant attached mucosa: a randomised controlled trial. *Eur J Oral Implantol* 2013;6:145–52.

Dandekeri SS, Sowmya MK, Bhandary S. Stereolithographic surgical template: a review. *J Clin Diagn Res* 2013;9:2093–5.

Lorean A, Kablan F, Mazor Z, Mijiritsky E, Russe P, Barbu H, Levin L. Inferior alveolar nerve transposition and reposition for dental implant placement in edentulous or par-tially edentulous mandibles: a multicentre retrospective study. *Int J Oral Maxillofacial Surg* 2013;42;656–9.

16

Maxillofacial trauma – hard tissue

Contents

Aims and learning outcomes

For undergraduates:

- To be able to describe the principles and techniques of Advanced Trauma Life Support.
- To be able to describe the aetiology of hard tissue maxillofacial trauma.
- To be able to describe the typical clinical presentation and principles of management of hard tissue injury.
- To list the markers of successful outcome of treatment.

For postgraduates (in addition to the foregoing):

- To be able to describe the main steps in treatment of maxillofacial hard tissue injuries.
- To describe the common maxillofacial emergencies.
- To be able to discuss appropriate management of the common maxillofacial emergencies.
- To be able to discuss a range of facial hard tissue injuries and their treatment.

Principles of trauma care (Advanced Trauma Life Support)

Modern trauma resuscitation is based on the Advanced Trauma Life Support (ATLS) course for doctors that was devised and is updated by the American College of Surgeons Committee on Trauma. This system has established an accepted international reputation as the gold standard for trauma resuscitation.

It follows a logical sequence of care that is designed to maximize the efficiency of assessment of the trauma victim, as well as provide priority ranking of potential, life-threatening problems and simultaneous resuscitative interventions. The sequence of ATLS is as follows:

Preparation

This is divided into a *prehospital phase* essentially limited to first aid in the field of injury and an in-hospital phase. A matching system exists for paramedics and field physicians (PreHospital Trauma Life Support [PHTLS]). **Triage,** which is a sorting of patients based on the urgency of need of treatment and the available resources to provide that treatment, may be carried out in both prehospital and in-hospital phases. This is based on the principle that the most severely injured patient requires the more urgent treatment, and the less injured patient can receive treatment after a slight delay by using the ABCs described here. Battlefield triage modifies this by introducing an element of 'usefulness' to the injured individual (Battlefield Advanced Trauma Life Support [BATLS]), and appropriate modifications are made to this protocol for those operating behind enemy lines (Covert Advanced Trauma Life Support [CATLS]).

The second phase of preparation is the *in-hospital phase* in which the patient has been brought to the hospital where he or she can be managed according to the extent of injury.

Primary survey

The primary survey is the rapid but thorough assessment of patients' treatment priorities based on their injuries, their vital signs and the injury mechanism. It follows the ABCs of trauma care and identifies life-threatening conditions by adhering to the following sequence:

A – Airway maintenance with cervical spine protection.
B – Breathing and ventilation with maximum flow oxygen.
C – Circulation with haemorrhage control.
D – Disability; neurological status assessment.
E – Exposure/environment control – Completely undress the patient but prevent hypothermia.

A – Airway maintenance with cervical spine protection

After ensuring personal safety, assess the patient's airway. Look, listen and feel for air movement. Grunting, snoring or absence of breath indicates an obstructed airway. Talking, swearing or screaming, conversely, indicates a patent airway. This rapid assessment should include inspection for foreign bodies and facial, mandibular or tracheal/laryngeal fractures that may result in airway obstruction.

Measures to establish a patent airway, if needed, should be instituted while protecting the cervical spine. (Loss of airway kills fastest, but creating a quadriplegic in the process does not help the patient.) Initially, manually clearing the airway and using the chin lift or jaw thrust manoeuvre are recommended, and these measures may be reinforced in the unconscious patient with an oral airway or, in the rousable patient, a nasopharyngeal airway. These airway adjuncts do not secure the airway (that requires a secured, cuffed tube in the trachea), but they may be adequate until a secure airway can be safely achieved by nasal, oral or surgical intubation. A reduced level of consciousness or blunt injury above the clavicle *in a polytrauma patient* carries a 10% risk of cervical spine injury. Immobilization in the neutral position minimizes the risk of further morbidity.

B – Breathing and ventilation

Airway patency alone does not *ensure* adequate ventilation – adequate gas exchange is required to maximize blood oxygenation and carbon dioxide elimination. Ventilation requires adequate function of the lungs, chest wall and diaphragm. Each component must be examined and evaluated rapidly. If the patient is not breathing adequately, immediately remediable problems (e.g. tension pneumothorax, displaced tube or cardiac tamponade) are addressed. If there is no effort or adequate effort at self-ventilation, then manual or mechanical ventilation must be started. Give high-flow oxygen in any case (with a reservoir bag if by facemask).

C – Circulation with haemorrhage control

Stop obvious external bleeding by direct pressure. Establish two wide-bore intravenous cannulae, take blood and give a fluid challenge (2 litres of warmed Hartmann's solution; lactated Ringer's solution and normal saline are more commonly quoted than Hartmann's in the United States).

Monitor pulse, respiratory rate and blood pressure. All trauma shock is initially managed as haemorrhagic shock until proven otherwise. Look for bleeding in the chest, abdomen and pelvis, and get help. In the case of maxillofacial trauma, fractures of the midface (Le Fort I, II and III) can lead to torrential haemorrhage and, rarely, immediate specialist maxillofacial resuscitation is needed (see the later section on that topic).

D – Disability and neurological evaluation

A rapid neurological evaluation is performed to assess the patient's level of consciousness, pupillary size and reaction. The Glasgow Coma Scale is the international gold standard (see Chapter 5).

E – Exposure/environment control

Special effort must be made to keep the patient from developing hypothermia during the early stages of trauma care. Exposure (removing clothing to ensure that no other injury is missed) is carried out in a warmed environment.

Secondary survey

The *secondary survey* does not begin until the primary survey (ABCDE) is completed, resuscitation has been successful and the patient is demonstrating normalization of vital functions. This survey is essentially a head to toe evaluation that looks at head injury, cervical spine and neck injury, chest injury, abdominal injury, perineum and rectal/vaginal injury, musculoskeletal injury, peripheral neurological injury and maxillofacial injury. Assessment of maxillofacial trauma is part of the secondary survey when it is not compromising the airway or leading to significant haemorrhage. As discussed earlier, if maxillofacial trauma is compromising the patient's airway or is causing significant

Despite the evidence, particularly from recent warfare experiences and common use in UK emergency departments, giving tranexamic acid as an infusion has not yet translated into ATLS protocols.

haemorrhage, then this is noted in the primary survey and acted on at that time. Many lives have been saved by healthcare workers who have stuck rigidly to this tried and tested methodology.

Specialist maxillofacial resuscitative techniques

Resuscitation is initially based on airway preservation and adequate ventilation to maintain oxygenation and prevent hypoxia (decreased partial pressure of oxygen) and hypercarbia (increased partial pressure of carbon dioxide). These factors are critical in managing the trauma patient, especially if a head injury has been sustained. Maxillofacial trauma demands aggressive airway management. High-impact trauma to the midface produces fractures with displacement and oedema that will obstruct the nasopharynx, oropharynx and hypopharynx. Facial fractures may be associated with haemorrhage, increased secretions and dislodged teeth causing additional problems in maintaining a patent airway. Fractures of the mandible, especially bilateral mandibular body fractures, may cause loss of normal tongue support and may lead the tongue to fall backward and block the airway. Airway obstruction can also result because post-traumatic oedema develops rapidly. The problem can be exacerbated if the patient is in a supine position (the position favoured in ATLS resuscitation) because secretions, blood and the abnormally heavy tongue can fall to the back of the mouth.

Patients who refuse to lie down may be demonstrating difficulty in maintaining their airway or handling secretions and should not be presumed to be uncooperative in the first instance. This situation creates a dichotomy between allowing the patient to maintain his or her own airway in an upright position and securing the airway in the supine position. Common sense, clinical judgement and proceeding using the skills and abilities you are personally most comfortable with are the solution.

Airway maintenance techniques

Even in the nontrauma patient with decreased consciousness, the tongue may fall backward and obstruct the hypopharynx. This form of obstruction can be corrected by a *chin lift* or *jaw thrust* manoeuvre. The airway can then be maintained with an oropharyngeal or nasopharyngeal airway. These manoeuvres must always be done with in-line immobilization of the cervical spine if the cervical spine has not yet been cleared of any injury by clinical and radiological methods and an appropriately trained individual.

Chin lift

The fingers of one hand are placed under the patient's mandible, which is gently lifted upward to bring the chin forward while the thumb of the same hand lightly depresses the lower lip to open the mouth. The thumb may be placed behind the lower incisors to help pull the chin forward. The chin lift manoeuvre should not hyperextend the neck. This manoeuvre is useful for the trauma victim because it does not risk compromising a possible cervical spine fracture or converting a fracture without spinal cord injury into one with spinal cord injury.

Jaw thrust manoeuvre

This manoeuvre is performed by grasping the angle of the mandible with one hand on each side and displacing the mandible forward. When this method is used with the facemask or an anaesthetic bag valve device, a good seal and adequate ventilation can be achieved.

Oropharyngeal airway

An oral airway is inserted into the patient's mouth behind the tongue. The preferred technique is to insert the tube upside down and then rotate it over the back of the tongue. The device lifts the tongue forward off the hypopharynx and allows air to pass through the lumen of the oropharyngeal airway.

Nasopharyngeal airway

This airway is inserted into one nostril and passed into the posterior nasopharynx. Beware obstruction of this (or any) tube (Figure 16.1). This airway is better tolerated in the conscious patient.

Needle cricothyroidotomy

There are common misconceptions about this technique. It does **not** secure the airway. It does maintain some form of airway that can allow insufflation of the lungs and preserve life for about 30 minutes until a secure airway is achieved (see the next

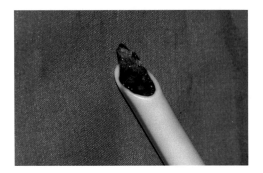

Figure 16.1 Beware the unexpected. Nasopharyngeal airways and endotracheal tubes can become occluded, in this case by an inferior turbinate.

paragraph). It is performed by inserting a wide-bore intravenous cannula (12 or 14 gauge) through the cricothyroid membrane (above the cricoid cartilage and below the thyroid cartilage – feel it on yourself). Aspirate to confirm that the cannula is in the trachea. Connect to oxygen at 12 to 15 L/minute via a Y connector or cut a hole in the tubing. Occlude the hole for 1 second to 'inflate' the lung, and then turn off the oxygen for 4 seconds to allow the lung to deflate. Remember the 'off for 4' rule or you will blow the lungs up like a balloon.

The foregoing mechanisms are merely temporary *airway maintenance techniques* and do not represent a definitive airway. A secure airway has not been obtained until an endotracheal tube has been placed with the cuff inflated and the tube secured. The tube is connected to some form of high-flow oxygen (12 to 15 l/minute). If the patient has difficulty in breathing, either remove the mechanical obstruction (pneumothorax, tamponade) or provide assisted ventilation (Ambu bag, ventilator).

Definitive airways

These are of three varieties – orotracheal tube, nasotracheal tube and surgical airway (cricothyroidotomy or tracheostomy; Figure 16.2). A definitive airway is required if the patient is going to undergo surgical correction of facial fractures and treatment of other associated injuries. It is also indicated if the patient is destined to spend a long time recovering from head injury or requires a prolonged period of artificial ventilation in an intensive care unit. Orotracheal intubation and

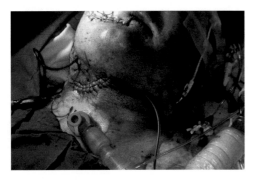

Figure 16.2 A secured, definitive surgical airway – a cuffed tube in the trachea.

nasotracheal intubation are specialized techniques, best performed by those trained and experienced in them. Hypoxia can result while inexperienced personnel attempt to place these tubes. The rule to remember is to maintain oxygenation by the most effective method your skill level allows while getting help.

Cricothyroidotomy

Cricothyroidotomy is an emergency procedure and can be done in the field, accident and emergency setting or in a ward setting as long as the surgeon has the ability to perform the procedure. This involves making a cut through the skin and the cricothyroid membrane and introducing a cuffed tracheostomy tube (size 6) into the trachea to allow oxygen delivery.

Tracheostomy

A tracheostomy is not an emergency surgical airway and should not be done in the acute trauma airway emergency setting. It requires controlled operating theatre equipment and lighting to ensure a successful procedure. It takes longer and involves displacement or incision of more structures. Tracheostomy involves incising the skin, dissecting fat to expose the strap muscles and separating these muscles. The thyroid gland is identified and either is displaced or the isthmus is ligated and divided. A hole in the trachea in the region of the second to fourth cartilaginous rings is created either as a slit (in children) or by cutting out a circle of trachea or creating an inferiorly based flap (Bjork's flap) and passing a tube into the tracheal lumen.

End tracheostomy is the stoma created when laryngectomy is performed and is quite different from these temporary airway operations.

Specific maxillofacial emergencies

Laryngeal injuries

The larynx is a semirigid structure made up of the hyoid and several cartilages interconnected by fibrous tissue. This framework is lined by mucosa, which can become grossly swollen following injury. In young patients, the larynx is elastic and tends to flex and spring back to its normal position rather than fracture following traumas. The epiglottis may become avulsed. In older patients, the cartilages become calcified and fractures are more likely. Rarely the trachea can be avulsed. This is usually fatal at the time of injury.

Flow varies according to Poiseuille's law (flow is proportional to radius of tube to the power of 4), which effectively means that only small changes in the radius are necessary to affect the flow of air through it significantly. This is seen particularly after thermal inhalation in which oedema of the whole upper respiratory tract results in rapid reductions in airflow. Early intubation is often necessary.

Cause of obstruction

- Blunt injuries
  - Road traffic accidents.
  - Sports (e.g. contact sports, martial arts).
  - Assaults.
- Penetrating injuries
  - Knife wounds.
  - Firearms.
  - Shrapnel (including human body parts common with improvised explosive devices or suicide bombs).
- Thermal injuries
  - Inhalation of smoke, hot air or steam.
- Blast injury.

Clinical features

- Dyspnoea.
- Stridor.
- Pain.
- Localized tenderness.
- Hoarse voice.
- Dysphagia.
- Surgical emphysema.
- Displacement of the larynx.

Management

Rapid identification is essential because patients can quickly deteriorate if the airway is not secured. This is particularly the case in burn victims. With minor injuries, humidified air and steroids may be all that are required. However, these patients must be kept under close observation and frequently reassessed. Patients who have had major laryngeal disruption need the airway secured. This can be done by intubation, cricothyroidotomy or tracheostomy. Surgical repair may be required in patients with:

- Tracheal injuries.
- Laryngeal displacement or disruption.
- Excessive swelling of the laryngeal soft tissues.
- Most cases of surgical emphysema.

Vision-threatening injuries

Eye injuries are commonly associated with damage to the upper midface; in some studies, up to 90% of patients had some form of ocular injury. However, in most cases these are relatively minor and require no treatment. The term *vision-threatening injuries* refers to those injuries that, if untreated, rapidly result in loss of sight. These are relatively rare but are reported in up to 10% of patients who have significant facial injuries (e.g. panfacial injuries, high-velocity injuries, gunshot wounds).

The three common vision-threatening injuries are:

- Retrobulbar haemorrhage (now considered part of orbital compartment syndrome).
- Penetrating ocular injuries.
- Optic nerve compression.

Diagnosis is usually straightforward, but these injuries can be missed in the unconscious or uncooperative patient. The eye must be inspected, but care must be taken not to press on the globe in case there is a penetrating injury. Visual-evoked potential is an experimental method of evaluating the visual pathways that has shown much promise. However, it does not identify any specific causes.

Retrobulbar haemorrhage (orbital compartment syndrome caused by bleeding)

Bleeding and gross swelling behind the eye may occur following trauma (or surgery) to the orbit, which is effectively a rigid, closed 'box', with the globe forming one of its 'walls'. Any swelling therefore causes raised pressure behind the eye, with resulting compression and spasm of the ciliary vessels. In addition, the eye itself becomes pushed forward (proptosed). This combination has compressive effects on the vasa nervorum of the optic nerve and creates direct neurological damage that can quickly become irreversible. Retrobulbar haemorrhage is rare, with a reported incidence of around 0.3%. It commonly occurs within a few hours of the injury, although patients presenting up to 5 days following injury have been reported.

Signs may include:

- Proptosis.
- Ophthalmoplegia.
- Chemosis and pain.
- Relative afferent papillary defect (RAPD) (this can indicate either optic nerve or severe retinal disease).
- Papilloedema.
- Raised intraocular pressure.
- Lack of central retinal artery pulsation.
- Pale optic disc (late sign).
- Cherry red macula.

Blindness is believed to result from spasm of the optic and retinal blood supply secondary to a high tamponade pressure. The difference between this condition and the 'benign' retrobulbar bleeding seen in 2% of cataract extractions is thought to be related to location and tamponade pressure.

Retrobulbar haemorrhage requires immediate surgical decompression if vision is to be restored. This simply involves removal of all sutures in the area in operated patients. In trauma patients who have not yet been operated on, an incision around the eyelid is made to allow access to the lateral canthal ligament (really an area of denser fascia). This is incised and released to allow blunt dissection, passing behind the periorbita to enable decompression of the haematoma.

When delays in surgery are unavoidable, short-term measures include:

- Dexamethasone – 8 mg intravenously.
- Acetazolamide (carbonic anhydrase inhibitor, reduces production of aqueous humour) – 500

mg intravenously and then 1000 mg orally over 24 hours.

- Mannitol – 100 mL 20% infusion (doses for a standard 70-kg adult without medical contraindications).
- Lateral canthotomy and cantholysis – this involves division of one of the supporting ligaments attaching the eyelids to the orbital rim. It can be carried out using local anaesthesia. This procedure provides a little 'breathing space' by allowing the eye to pop forward and reduce the pressure in the orbit.

Optic nerve compression

Displaced fractures that involve the orbital apex (panfacial, skull fractures) can sometimes press on the optic nerve. Often those structures passing through the superior orbital fissure are also traumatized, resulting in the orbital apex syndrome. The management of this disorder is controversial and involves either surgical decompression or high-dose steroids. When there is direct impingement of the optic nerve by bone or other penetrating fragments, removal of these rarely results in an improvement in visual acuity. When there is no identifiable hard tissue, surgery can be positively harmful, and medical reduction of swelling is more appropriate.

Penetrating neck injuries

These injuries are often very dramatic in appearance, but in many cases they may miss vital structures. Penetrating injuries *deep to the platysma* muscle should not be explored using local anaesthesia in an emergency department setting.

When assessing patients with neck wounds, think about the following, depending on the point of entry and direction:

- Major vessels (carotid artery, internal jugular vein).
- Lung apex.
- Upper airway.
- Oesophagus.
- Vagus nerve.
- Phrenic nerve.
- Thyroid gland.

All penetrating foreign bodies should be left *in situ* until the patient is anaesthetized and has secure intravenous access. Surgical removal can be then undertaken in an operating theatre. Generally this is by directly reversing the path of insertion but with wide visualization and access to surrounding vital structures.

Specialist maxillofacial techniques for arresting haemorrhage

In a few cases, exsanguinating haemorrhage from facial fractures requires direct intervention in the primary survey. This is usually because of bleeding from the nose or maxillary fractures.

Nasal bleeding can be dealt with by bilateral anterior and posterior nasal packing using specially designed inflatable catheters (Brighton balloons, Epitek catheters, Rapid Rhino) or urinary catheters in the postnasal space with conventional anterior nasal packing.

Bleeding from the maxilla can be arrested by manual reduction and immobilization with a conventional dental rubber mouth prop.

Temporary splinting of open fractures can be achieved with the 'bridle wire', which is a direct wire ligature passed around teeth on either side of a fracture and tightened by twisting clockwise.

Diagnosis of facial fractures

As with all trauma diagnosis, think about:

- Mechanism of injury.
- Symptoms.
- Signs.
- Special investigations.

In general an underlying facial fracture is recognizable clinically based on symptoms of pain, malocclusion and diplopia. Signs are malocclusion, visible deformity, sublingual haematoma, subconjunctival haemorrhage, epistaxis and abnormal mobility (Figure 16.3). Site and specific fracture pattern details are confirmed by plain films at right angles and computed tomography (CT) scan, usually coronal or three-dimensional (3-D) reformatted.

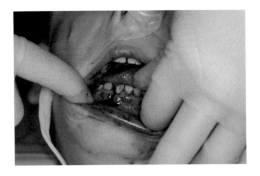

Figure 16.3 Abnormal mobility, bleeding and inter-dental space characteristic of a mandibular fracture.

Mandibular fractures

The mandible is a rigid horseshoe of bone with a modified hinge joint at either end. It is much more sensitive to lateral than frontal impact (it takes around 190 kg frontal impact to consistently fracture condyles in cadavers).

Common fracture patterns are shown diagrammatically in Figure 16.4. These percentages change with age, as do the specific types of fractures seen between paediatric and adult mandibles and dentate and edentulous mandibles.

Intracapsular fractures of the condyle are more common in childhood because of a short ramal neck, whereas condylar neck fractures are more common in adults. Body fractures of the edentulous mandible are more common than in the dentate mandible because the loss of bone height and density after tooth loss is greatest at that point.

Incidence

Fractures of the mandible account for 20% of all facial bone fractures; 80% of these are in male patients.

Aetiology

In Britain, 75% of mandibular fractures are caused by interpersonal violence, usually involving alcohol. Sports injuries (10%), road traffic collisions (8%) and falls (4%) are the next most common factors. These percentages vary internationally, particularly in relation to the availability of intoxicants and the presence or absence of civil unrest. A study in Aachen, Germany of mandibular fractures in 370 patients between 1995 and 2007 found the following: interpersonal violence, 40%; falls, 20%; road traffic collisions, 14%; bicycle accidents, 10%; and sports injuries, 5%. These findings suggest variation even within Northern Europe.

Symptoms

The patient may complain of pain in the bottom jaw, abnormal bite, bleeding from the mouth, loose teeth, numb lip, pain in the temporomandibular joint region, limited mouth opening, swelling

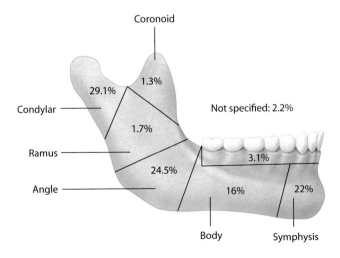

Figure 16.4 Relative frequency of sites of mandibular fractures.

of the floor of mouth and swelling of soft tissues around the mandible. Immobility of the mandible is usually in an effort to prevent pain, but it can be caused by spasm of the muscles of mastication.

Signs

Clinical examination of the mandibular fracture may well show, depending on the level of fracture displacement and fracture pattern, no evidence of disruption of the mandibular body and essentially a normal occlusal contact pattern. These fractures represent undisplaced hairline fractures of the mandible and are confirmed by radiological investigation. Examination of a displaced mandibular fracture shows disruption of the occlusion and subtle or obviously mobile fragments. Beware sharp bony fragments or fractured teeth during intraoral examination.

Lingual haematoma is seen as a swelling and bruising on the floor of the mouth adjacent to the fracture site. Fractures of the ascending ramus and condyle may manifest with no gross clinical signs. Always examine the external auditory canal for bleeding, which may be from a base of skull fracture or, more commonly, a condylar neck fracture connecting with the external ear canal.

Mandibular fracture patterns

The condyle is the most common site of fracture of the mandible, but the type varies with the patient's age. These fractures can be intracapsular or extracapsular, displaced, undisplaced or dislocated.

Bilateral condylar fractures are classically seen in falls and road traffic collisions, in which a large frontal impact can occur. The classical 'Guardsman's fracture' involves fracture of bilateral mandibular condyles, with or without symphyseal fracture, caused by a fall or blow to the point of the chin (the term comes from UK royal palace guards who faint in the 'attention' stance and land on their chins).

The angle and the parasymphyseal regions are commonly weakened by the presence of third molars in various stages of eruption and the canine teeth, respectively. These are the most common sites of fracture resulting from a lateral impact, more usually caused by a blow.

Combinations of fractures are possible and should be always looked for.

Investigations

The combination of both dental panoramic tomogram (DPT; Panorex in the United States) (Figure 16.5) and posteroanterior plain radiographs (Figure 16.6) gives adequate diagnostic information for most mandibular fractures. If the patient is unable to stand in the DPT machine, left and right lateral oblique mandibular views will give good imaging of the body of the mandible. If the patient has multiple complex maxillofacial fractures, a CT scan (coronal and axial images with or

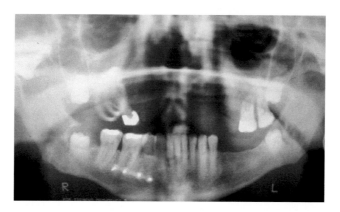

Figure 16.5 Dental panoramic tomogram showing bilateral mandibular angle fractures. Note the previous parasymphyseal fracture repair, which used a single body plate with a tension band to avoid the risk of mental nerve damage associated with the traditionally recommended two plates.

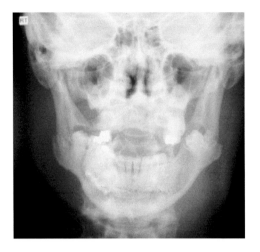

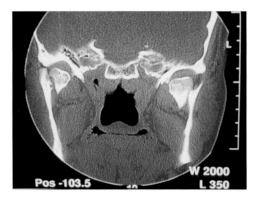

Figure 16.8 Computed tomography scan of bilateral condylar fractures. Note the overlap of fragments.

Figure 16.6 Posteroanterior radiograph of bilateral angle fractures (see the comment in the Figure 16.5 legend).

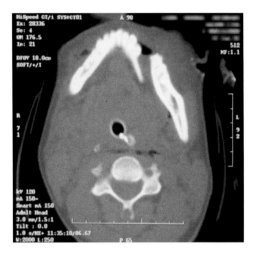

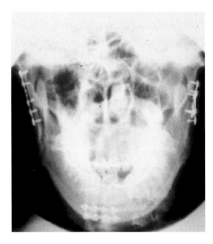

Figure 16.9 Posteroanterior radiograph demonstrating reduction and fixation of both condyles and symphyseal fracture repair.

Treatment

Figure 16.7 Computed tomography scan showing a displaced mandibular fracture.

without 3-D reformat) is helpful (Figure 16.7). The CT scan will help assess condylar fracture position, angulation and any fractured dislocation of the condylar head (Figure 16.8). It can also image multipart mandibular body fractures. The imaging will help the surgeon plan the operation, find and realign the fragments and avoid missing a fracture segment when operating (Figure 16.9). The 3-D formatting is increasingly available and may be helpful in demonstrating injuries to patients and support staff.

Immediate treatment in the primary survey is rare and is discussed previously. Early treatment involves analgesia, either in the form of nonsteroidal anti-inflammatory drugs or opioids. Start oral or intravenous antibiotics because, by definition, all mandibular fractures passing through the tooth-bearing segment and periodontal ligament are compound fractures into the mouth and are therefore contaminated. (Condylar fragments and fractures which do not communicate with the periodontal ligament are *closed* injuries and do not require antibiotics. However if there is a cutaneous wound caused by the fracture fragment, or by penetration of a foreign body, they are compound fractures and so require antibiotics.)

Displaced, mobile fractures are very painful. The placement of temporary stabilizing wires around the teeth adjacent to the mandibular fracture will immobilize the fracture and make the patient more comfortable while awaiting definitive surgery using general anaesthesia. This technique can help to reduce the need for analgesics in the preoperative period.

Treatment planning

Mandibular fractures with altered occlusion are best treated by surgery (excluding condylar fractures – see later). Fracture treatment involves reduction of bone ends and stabilization to allow healing. Some minimally or undisplaced hairline fractures can be treated without surgery as long as the occlusion is not altered. Sometimes the patient will elect not to have surgery and will accept the slightly altered occlusion. Informed choice must be respected and documented in this instance. Close follow-up is advised, although the reality of follow-up in trauma patients in most countries and in most published series is that these patients comprise a very reluctant cohort when it comes to hospital attendance.

Preoperative consent

Preoperative assessment of inferior alveolar nerve injury must be documented because it may become worse postoperatively. Patients must be informed of this possibility during the informed consent process.

Access to fracture sites and fixation must be described. Most mandibular fractures are approached transorally. External approaches are used particularly for edentulous body fractures and condylar fractures. The scar caused by these incisions and the small risk of damage to the facial nerve must be outlined. Placement of plates (whether they are intended to be permanent or removed), loss of teeth, intermaxillary fixation (IMF), if used, and where the patient will wake up (intensive treatment unit, recovery, ward) should be described.

Fracture repair

Definitive surgery usually involves open reduction and internal fixation (ORIF) with the patient under general anaesthesia, ideally with nasoendotracheal intubation. This allows the patient's mouth to be closed and the teeth to be manipulated into their normal occlusion. This manipulation helps reduce the mandible into the prefracture bone position. Temporary IMF is applied using a variety of techniques (trainee's hand, eyelets, transalveolar screws [Figures 16.10 and 16.11], 'rapid IMF', arch bars). This fixation helps to hold the fracture in its reduced position. Placing a bridle wire or tension band around the teeth can help reduce and temporarily fix the fracture.

Under direct vision via buccal sulcus incisions, the mandibular fracture is exposed and reduction is confirmed (Figure 16.12). Fixation is undertaken with titanium mandibular plates. According to *Champy's principles,* in the mandibular symphyseal and parasymphyseal region two mandibular plates are required, one just below the level of incisor/premolar apices and above the mental foramen and one as low down on the buccal surface as possible parallel to the lower

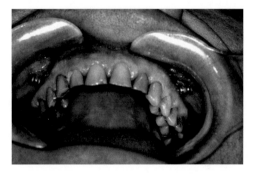

Figure 16.10 Transalveolar screws in place in the maxilla.

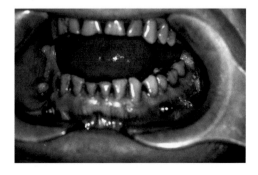

Figure 16.11 Transalveolar screws in place in the mandible.

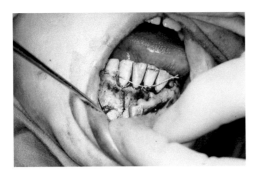

Figure 16.12 Open reduction and internal fixation of the mandible, with a buccal sulcus incision, subperiosteal dissection and tension band in place.

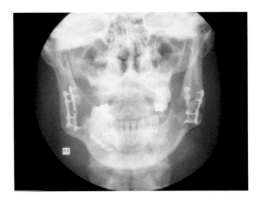

Figure 16.14 Posteroanterior radiograph showing reduction and fixation.

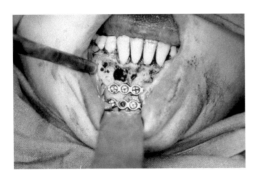

Figure 16.13 Fixation with two monocortical titanium plates.

border of the mandible (Figure 16.13). In the region of the angle of the mandible, a single plate is adequate to allow healing. In practice many surgeons now supplement this (or even replace it) with a transbuccally placed lateral plate that prevents lateral displacement of the lower border of the mandible often seen with the Champy external oblique ridge technique. All these techniques use monocortically placed matching titanium screws to retain the plates that immobilize the fracture sites. Long-acting local anaesthetic regional block provides good postoperative analgesia, and prophylactic broad-spectrum antibiotics are given preoperatively. Intraoral wounds are closed with resorbable sutures. If the occlusion is fully restored and stability of the fracture is ensured by the plates, IMF can be removed. The patient is placed on a soft diet for 2 to 4 weeks to ensure that the plates are not overstressed during the healing period. The fracture is sufficiently healed after this period to allow normal

mandibular function. The plates, now obsolete, remain *in situ* without causing problems. In the immediate postoperative period a strict oral hygiene regimen is implemented, in the form of 0.2% chlorhexidine gluconate mouth rinses and tooth brushing. Postoperative radiographs are taken (DPT and posteroanterior radiographs) to ensure correct placement of plates and screws and accurate realignment of mandibular fragments. It is also important to reassess the position of the condyles following ORIF because malpositioning can lead to temporomandibular problems later on (Figure 16.14).

Mandibular fractures in children

Fractures in children up to 6 years of age normally receive conservative treatment. An indication for osteosynthesis may be a simple or multiple fracture with displacement, especially when the possibilities of conservation fixation are limited.

In such cases two aspects that may be taken into account include, first, that a single 1.5-mm microplate is normally sufficient for the stabilization of the fracture, and second, because of the position of the teeth germs, the microplate should always be placed at the lower border of the buccal side. Fractures of the jaw in children 6 to 13 years old require attention to the tooth germs.

Mandibular fractures in elderly patients

Atrophic 'pencil thin' or 'pipe stem' mandibular fractures are common in elderly edentulous patients and can be devastating to the elderly patient (Figure 16.15). Malunion and even

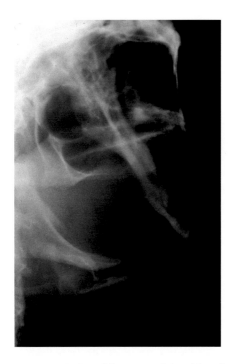

Figure 16.15 Displaced fracture of the thin edentulous mandible.

nonunion are common, and eating and nutrition deteriorate rapidly. Fracture repair is best done by keeping the maximum possible amount of periosteum intact and plating via an extraoral approach using a more rigid plate with bicortical screws that confer far greater rigidity and stability to the fracture site (Figures 16.16 and 16.17). This carries a greater risk of damage to the inferior alveolar neurovascular bundle but is balanced by the far higher success rate compared with conservative or monocortical plating techniques.

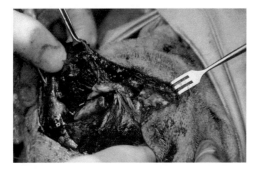

Figure 16.16 Compound mandibular fracture showing the genial muscle points of attachment.

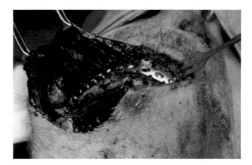

Figure 16.17 Continuity restored with a 2.4-mm reconstruction plate and direct suturing of genial muscles.

Treatment of fractures of the atrophic edentulous mandible

Fractures of the atrophic mandible have unfavourable conditions for healing, such as:

- Reduced cross-section and smaller contact area of the fractured ends.
- Usually dense and sclerotic bone that is poorly vascularized.

Classification of fractures of the edentulous atrophic mandible is as follows:

- Class I – 16 to 20 mm.
- Class II – 11 to 15 mm.
- Class III – <10 mm.

However, because in extremely atrophic mandibles the subperiosteal plexus is probably the major blood supply to the bone, a *supraperiosteal* dissection was suggested by Bradley, and a supraperiosteal placement of plates and screws was recommended by Luhr. (Personal experience with this technique showed it to be totally unhelpful because soft tissue ingrowth from the periosteum loosened the screws far too early.)

The advantage of rigid fixation is that it makes any postoperative maxillomandibular immobilization unnecessary. It allows free movement of the mandible, normal speech and immediate uptake of a soft, solid diet and thus provides greater comfort for the patient.

Condylar fractures

Condylar fractures are treated conservatively in children up to 12 years old with soft diet, analgesia and function. Young adults (12 to 18 years old) are also treated conservatively in the majority of cases. Adults (>18 years old) are treated with 7 to 10 days of heavy elastic IMF, and the occlusion is reassessed. If malocclusion persists, then ORIF of the condyle is undertaken. Overlap of fragments greater than 5 mm and angulation greater than 37° are postulated to warrant ORIF (Figures 16.18 and 16.19). Logically the function rather than the radiographic appearance should predicate the decision to undertake ORIF.

Subclassification of fractures of the condylar process of the mandible

Definitions are as follows (Loukota et al. 2005):

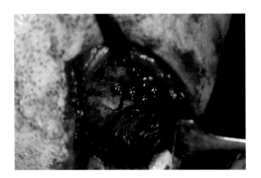

Figure 16.18 Open reduction and fixation of a fractured mandibular condyle.

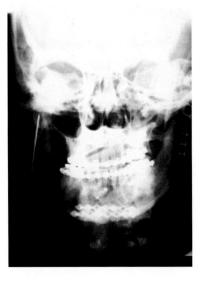

Figure 16.19 Radiograph of reduced and fixed condylar fracture showing two techniques.

1. Diacapitular fracture (through the head of the condyle) – the fracture line starts in the articular surface and may extend outside the capsule.
2. Fracture of the condylar neck – the fracture line starts somewhere above line A and in more than half runs above the line A in the lateral view (line A is the perpendicular line through the sigmoid notch to the tangent of the ramus).
3. Fracture of the condylar base – the fracture line runs behind the mandibular foramen and, in more than half, below line A.

The term *minimal displacement* is taken to be the definition that is used in the multicentre study – that is, displacement of less than 10° or overlap of the bone ends of less than 2 mm, or both.

Surgical treatment options

A trend is emerging in the surgical literature that confirms the superior functional results following ORIF of condylar fractures, where this is indicated. This trend is supported by existing level I evidence.

Endoscopic assistance, performed transorally, may also provide an alternative means for treating a subset of these injuries, thus reducing visible scar formation and possibly facial nerve damage.

The retroauricular approach initially popularized in Munich remains in vogue in some areas.

There are still areas of condylar trauma surgery that some surgeons consider controversial – condylar head fractures and displaced paediatric fractures. The use of resorbable osteosynthesis techniques may be of benefit in both these clinical settings.

Promising outcomes have been anecdotally reported following fixation of such fractures in children as young as 6 years of age. This finding is contrary to most accepted guidance, which recognizes extensive condylar remodelling in children less than 12 years old.

Indications for open reduction and internal fixation of mandibular condyle fractures

Absolute indications are applicable to children and adults (Zide et al. 1983):

1. Displacement into the middle cranial fossa.
2. Impossibility of obtaining adequate occlusion by closed reduction.

3. Lateral extracapsular displacement of the condyle.
4. Invasion by foreign body (e.g. gunshot wound).

Relative indications apply to adults with condyles displaced out of the fossa and associated malocclusion:

1. Bilateral condylar fractures in an edentulous patient when a splint is unavailable or when splinting is impossible because of alveolar ridge atrophy.
2. Unilateral or bilateral condylar fractures when splinting is not recommended for medical reasons (e.g. seizures, psychiatric problems).
3. Bilateral condylar fractures associated with comminuted midfacial fractures.
4. Bilateral condylar fractures and associated gnathologic problems (e.g. retrognathia or prognathism, open bite with periodontal problems or lack of posterior support).

Although condylar ORIF procedures are heavily endorsed by some surgeons, it is worth looking carefully at the published examples – all too often cases are shown that are relatively easy to access and fix, whereas others are quietly left as 'technically not feasible'. The old adage 'the ability to do an operation is not an indication' is worth keeping in mind in this area of facial traumatology.

Morbidity associated with open treatment of mandibular condyle fractures
Complications from open treatment (Ellis et al. 2000):

- Haemorrhage.
- Infection.
- Facial nerve weakness.
- Auriculotemporal nerve dysfunction.
- Frey's syndrome.
- Unsightly scar.

There are very few intraoperative or postoperative complications.

- At 6 weeks, 17.2% of patients had VII nerve weakness. This had resolved by 6 months
- The scars were judged either wide or hypertrophic in 7.5% of cases.

Open versus closed treatment of fractures of the condyle
Eckelt and colleagues (2006) conducted a prospective randomized multicentre study:

- Entry criteria: displaced fractures angulated more than 10° or ascending ramus was shortened by more than 2 mm.
- Results: correct anatomical position of the fragments was achieved significantly more often in the operative group in contrast to the closed treatment group. Therefore, differences were observed between both groups.

OPEN VERSUS CLOSED TREATMENT GROUPS

	Mouth opening	Lateral excursion	Protrusion
Open	47 mm	16 mm	7 mm
Closed	41 mm	13 mm	5 mm

- Regarding pain: Less pain in the operative treatment group.
- Conclusion: Both treatment options for condylar fractures of the mandible yielded acceptable results. However, operative treatment, irrespective of the method of internal fixation used, was superior in all objective and subjective functional parameters.

Indicators of successful outcome
Successful outcome is determined by:

- Restoration of the pretraumatic mandibular appearance.
- Restoration of pretraumatic occlusion.
- Normal function and mastication.
- Normal mandibular movement.
- Normal speech.
- Absence of chronic infection.
- Absence of pain and iatrogenic nerve injury.

Indicators of unfavourable mandibular fracture outcome

- Failure to restore pretraumatic appearance.
- Failure to restore pretraumatic occlusion.
- Difficulty with mastication or speech or limited mandibular movements.

- Mandibular malunion/nonunion.
- Chronic infection.
- Chronic pain.
- Failure of recovery of sensory dysaesthesias.
- Iatrogenic damage to trigeminal nerve (cranial nerve V, third division mental/inferior dental nerve). or creation of iatrogenic motor nerve injury (facial nerve) during extraoral incisions.
- Unacceptable facial scarring.
- Dental trauma and other pathology not identified preoperatively.
- Infected plates.
- Iatrogenic injury to tooth roots by screw placement.

Morbidity associated with open reduction and internal fixation of the fractured condyle by the transparotid approach. Downie and associates (2009) described morbidity with the transparotid approach:

- Temporary weakness – using the transparotid approach – of the facial nerve occurred in 14%. The buccal branch was affected in all cases. In some patients the zygomatic branch was also affected. No patient had permanent weakness.
- In a retromandibular approach where the parotid is avoided, temporary weakness of the facial nerve was 8%. In that study the marginal mandibular branch of the facial nerve was affected.

Comparing the traditional retromandibular approach with the transparotid approach, the latter provides good access and allows direct visualization of the fracture. It ensures that the plates can be well adapted and the screws placed at 90° to the bony surface, to give a maximal mechanical advantage that is not always possible with the more traditional retromandibular approach. It also gives an easier approach to the difficult area of the condylar neck with minimal surgical access.

Zygomatic complex fractures

A zygomatic complex fracture is a fracture of the zygomatic bone (zygoma). The zygomatic bone forms the cheek bone prominence, the lateral orbital wall, the lateral aspect of the orbital floor and the buttress of the maxilla. Because of this, fractures in this region are often referred to as the zygomatico-orbital (and sometimes zygomatico-maxillary) complex fractures. The zygoma also has a posterior extension (temporal process) that joins the zygomatic process of the temporal bone to form the zygomatic arch. Fractures in this region are referred to as zygomatic arch fractures.

Incidence

Fractures of the zygoma account for 25% of facial fractures and are the second most common; 80% occur in male patients.

Aetiology

Of these fractures, 35% result from interpersonal violence, 25% from road traffic accidents, 20% from sports injuries and around 10% from falls. Again, these percentages vary internationally.

Symptoms

Patients often complain of numbness of the cheek and side of nose on the affected side. The teeth in the corresponding upper quadrant may also feel numb. They may mention an altered bite (in extreme cases the maxilla is pushed down, causing posterior premature contacts) or inability to open their mouth (caused by the zygomatic arch impacting on the coronoid process), a flattened cheekbone and, in cases where the orbit is involved, double vision.

Zygomatic fractures with gross displacement can disrupt the orbital volume and eye suspensory ligaments leading to hypoglobus (lowered eye level) and enophthalmos (sinking of the eyeball into the socket). Globe displacement and trapping or later fibrosis of the periorbital fat and muscle can also cause diplopia (double vision), usually on upward gaze. Patients notice these signs themselves and may report them at presentation.

Signs

Inspection reveals facial asymmetry, loss of cheek prominence and indentation of the zygomatic arch

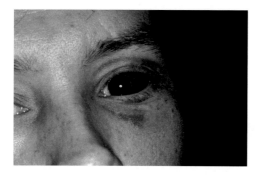

Figure 16.20 Black eye showing complete lateral subconjunctival haemorrhage.

(dimpling over fracture), although these signs can be masked by swelling. Subconjunctival haemorrhage (Figure 16.20) suggests direct trauma to the eye or fracture of the orbital walls or floor. A complete lateral subconjunctival haemorrhage usually indicates a zygomatic fracture. Medial subconjunctival haemorrhage implies naso-orbital fracture. Look for eye position from in front of, below and above the patient; subtle changes may not be seen if swelling is marked.

Palpation reveals facial asymmetry by comparing the normal and the injured side. Palpation of the infraorbital margin shows a palpable step and discontinuity of the bone. Palpation in the upper labial sulcus may reveal a fractured lateral maxillary wall, which feels boggy because of the presence of a haematoma. Sometimes a sharp laterally overlapping bone fragment is felt. Usually the fracture is impacted and therefore not mobile.

Testing sensation reveals loss of nerve function in the distribution of the infraorbital nerve. Document the extent of loss because it will be used to gauge nerve recovery in the months after trauma by repeat assessment.

Ocular involvement of zygomatico-orbital complex fractures

It is imperative that the visual acuity of the eye is fully assessed and recorded at initial presentation:

- Pupillary reaction, consensual reflex and accommodation.
- Visual acuity using a Snellen chart.
- Visual fields.
- Eye movements in an 'H' shape.

Any abnormality in acuity mandates discussion with an ophthalmologist (Figure 16.21). Abnormalities of movement as seen in orbital 'blow-out' fractures necessitate formal assessment of ocular movement (Hess chart) by an orthoptist.

Retrobulbar haemorrhage is a surgical emergency. The classic signs are pain, proptosis, dilated pupil, ophthalmoplegia and decreasing visual acuity. Immediate surgical intervention to prevent permanent loss of visual acuity is necessary.

The mechanism behind retrobulbar haemorrhage in orbital trauma is believed to be arterial bleeding rather than the venous bleeding seen in retrobulbar blocks. Surgical decompression by lateral canthotomy and drainage of intraconal haematoma

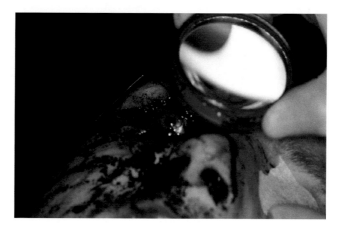

Figure 16.21 Perioperative ophthalmic examination of the eye.

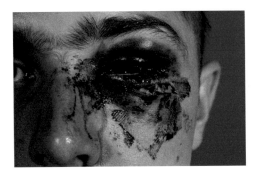

Figure 16.22 Decompression of a retrobulbar haemorrhage.

comprise the treatment of choice (Figure 16.22). Medical management is described earlier.

Orbital apex compression by oedema may respond to high-dose steroids. Damage by fragments of bone is not reversible, and the prognosis is poor.

Patterns of zygomatic fractures

Many patterns are possible. The classical 'tripod' fracture involves fractures in the frontozygomatic region, infraorbital margin and zygomatic arch. Displacement can be marked in one direction, rotated or in a combination of movements. Comminuted fracture patterns pose a difficult reconstructive challenge and usually occur in high-impact injuries such as road traffic collisions.

Classification of fractures is shown in Table 16.1 (as described by Killey et al. 1957). Many classifications exist (Henderson's was popular for a while), but few are used outwith prospective research trials.

Investigations

Plain film occipitomental (OM) views (OM 15° and OM 30°) generally give sufficient diagnostic information. In combination they give good imaging of the zygomatic complex and can be used to determine the level of displacement and fracture pattern. A teardrop appearance into the maxillary antrum suggests an isolated orbital floor fracture (blow-out orbital fracture; Figure 16.23). Identification of this fracture mandates a coronal CT and Hess chart test.

Table 16.1 Classification of zygomatic fractures

Fracture type	Degree of displacement
1	Undisplaced fractures
2	Fractures of the zygomatic arch
3	Rotation around the vertical axis
	(a) internal
	(b) external
4	Rotation around the longitudinal axis
	(a) medial
	(b) Lateral
5	Displacement of the complex *en bloc*
	(a) medially
	(b) Inferiorly
	(c) Laterally (rare)
6	Displacement of the orbitoantral partition
	(a) inferiorly
	(b) Superiorly (rare)
7	Displacement of orbital rim segments
8	Complex comminuted fractures

Isolated zygomatic arch fractures are best visualized on a submentovertex view; however, an adequate view of the fracture is usually visible on OM radiographs (Figure 16.24).

In the case of comminuted and badly displaced zygomatico-orbital complex fractures, the use of coronal and 3-D reformatted CT scans of the orbit

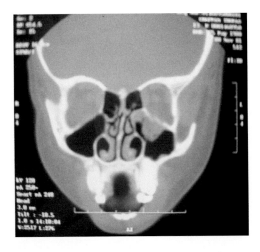

Figure 16.23 A coronal computed tomography scan showing a 'blow-out' fracture of the orbital floor.

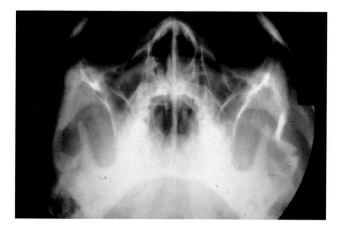

Figure 16.24 Depressed fracture of the zygomatic arch causing trismus.

will give the best imaging possible to aid planning of fracture repair.

Treatment

Aims of treatment

- Restoration of facial appearance.
- Restoration of orbital volume and globe position and prevention of enophthalmos.
- Repair of orbital floor fractures with reduction of herniated orbital contents and release of trapped inferior rectus muscle.
- Decompression of infraorbital nerve, thus promoting recovery of sensation.
- Restoration of full range of mandibular movements.
- Restoration of a normal occlusion by reduction of zygomatic and tuberosity displacement.

Treatment planning

Surgery is ideally carried out after most of the swelling has resolved, around 7 to 10 days after injury. Earlier surgery in the presence of oedema tends to create a higher risk of scarring, difficulty in access and ectropion. General anaesthesia with oral intubation is usual (a small risk exists of significant bleeding after some zygomatic fracture reductions, so a cuffed tube rather than a laryngeal mask is preferable). The aim of surgery is to **reduce** the fracture to restore the bone to its normal position. The bones are then **fixed** so that they heal in this position (ORIF). Occasionally the fracture

locks into a stable position after reduction, and no fixation is required. The time between injury and operation should be used to work up the patient fully by ensuring that Hess chart results, CT scans and so forth are obtained and acted on.

Preoperative consent

Advise patients about possible scarring, plate insertion, orbital floor repair and eyelid scarring. Chemosis (gross swelling of the conjunctiva) is common after transconjunctival incisions if that incision is used in accessing the infraorbital rim and floor. Discuss the risk of developing a retrobulbar haemorrhage after surgery.

Zygomatic fracture repair

Incisions to gain access to the fractures and place plates to stabilize the fracture after reduction include a temporal Gillies incision (Figure 16.25),

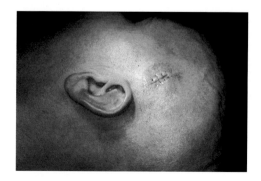

Figure 16.25 Temporal incision for the Gillies approach to elevation of a zygomatic fracture.

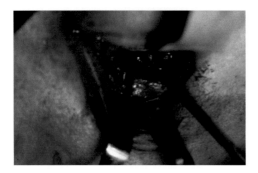

Figure 16.26 Lower eyelid incision to approach the infraorbital rim.

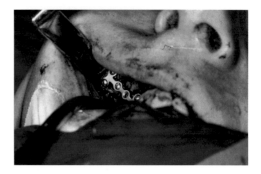

Figure 16.27 Miniplate sited at the zygomatic buttress.

upper lateral blepharoplasty incision, crow's foot incision, lateral brow incision, infraorbital incision (Figure 16.26), transconjunctival incision, subciliary incision and intraoral buttress incision.

In Germany there is neither a Gillies incision nor a Gillies approach.

Zygomatic fractures including zygomatic arch fractures are reduced by inserting a hook under the body of the zygoma caudally in a vertical line from the lateral canthus. The hook is named after Stromeyer. Interestingly, these surgical variants can be seen from unit to unit in the United Kingdom and internationally.

Reduction of a zygomatic fracture can be carried out in three ways:

1. Temporal approach – the incision is made in the hairline two fingerbreadths above the tip of the pinna. Dissect through skin, temporoparietal fascia and temporalis fascia. Try to avoid superficial temporal vessels but ligation of these, if needed, is not a disaster. An elevator is inserted just deep to the temporal fascia. It is passed along the lateral surface of the temporalis muscle and enters the natural space beneath the zygomatic arch deep to the zygoma.
2. Percutaneous approach – a small stab incision made in the cheek allows access for a bone hook to carry out the reduction.
3. Intraoral approach (Keen approach in the United States) – an incision is made in the upper buccal sulcus to expose the fracture at the buttress (Figure 16.27).

The direction of reduction (elevation) is to reverse the direction of the movement of the zygoma resulting from the impact. This is generally in an upward and outward direction opposite to that causing the fracture in the first instance. The aim of reduction is to restore the bone fragments to their symmetrical preinjury position. This is assessed by visually inspecting the patient after satisfactory elevation unless the fracture lines are being directly exposed and visualized. Elevation is generally easily achieved during the first 14 days after injury. After this time the fracture has started to heal in its incorrect position, and elevation can be more difficult. Simple fracture patterns may allow the fracture to be reduced into a stable position and require no formal fixation. If the fracture falls back into abnormal position after gentle palpation, it is considered unstable and requires fixation. This fixation takes the form of low-profile titanium or resorbable plates (usually 1.0, 1.3 or 1.5 mm thick, but this is changing as technology improves) placed across one or more of the fracture sites (frontozygomatic, infraorbital or buttress). Titanium has been the material of choice since 2000. Resorbable plates and screws have more recently become available but have not yet displaced titanium as the material of choice (Figure 16.28).

Small, asymptomatic orbital floor defects require no treatment. If the patient has persistent diplopia, enophthalmos or significant herniation of orbital contents into the antrum, repair is indicated. A bone graft from the outer table of skull (Figure 16.29) or the anterior wall of maxilla, artificial resorbable material, titanium mesh, preformed titanium plates, a Gore-Tex sheet, lyophilized dura and cartilage have all been used. The repair allows orbital volume to be maintained and encourages bony healing to restore the orbital defect. Care must

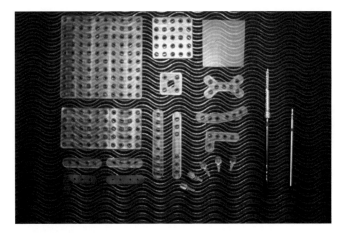

Figure 16.28 Bioresorbable plate.

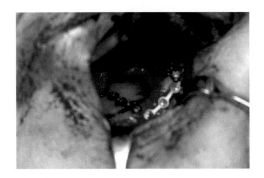

Figure 16.29 Split cranial bone graft fixed to reconstruct the orbital floor.

be taken to ensure that none of the extraocular muscles become trapped in the fracture or under the repair because this would cause even worse diplopia. The *forced duction test* is classically described as the test for ensuring that this has not happened. The surgeon rotates the patient's eye upward by pulling on the inferior rectus muscle to ensure that there is no limitation of passive eye movement.

The patient is advised not to blow his or her nose for a period of 2 to 2 weeks postoperatively; this is helped by using nasal decongestants for the first postoperative week. The reason to avoid nose blowing is to reduce the risk of surgical emphysema forming in the soft tissues of the periorbital and zygomatic region.

Postoperative care

Antibiotics are given intravenously during surgery and for two postoperative doses if plates are used. Radiographs are taken to confirm good reduction of the fractures and satisfactory plate and screw positioning, although published audit would suggest that these films rarely influence treatment. Topical chloramphenicol ointment is applied to skin and conjunctival wounds to promote healing and make suture removal easier. If necessary, eye exercises are prescribed to encourage mobility of the globe. Sutures are removed after 5 days.

Indicators of successful outcome

Restoration of facial appearance, restoration of eye position and function, recovery of infraorbital nerve function, minimal scarring and the absence of pain or infection associated with plates all indicate a successful outcome (Figure 16.30).

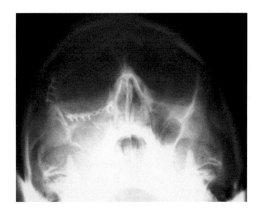

Figure 16.30 Postoperative radiograph of a reduced and fixed zygomatic fracture.

Indicators of unfavourable outcome

- Abnormal facial appearance.
- Lack of symmetry.
- Eye problems, persistent double vision.
- Heavy scarring, eyelid scarring.
- Temporal hollowing from temporalis muscle atrophy.
- Persistent numbness
- Infected plates or chronic pain in plates.
- Migration of orbital floor repair material.

Further advice

Advise the patient of a possible dull pain in the region of the fracture during winter months, slow recovery of the infraorbital nerve and the requirement to avoid fighting and contact sports for 6 to 8 weeks after fracture repair. Patients with persistent diplopia require a specialist ophthalmological opinion. They may require prescription of prism lens, eye rehabilitation and potential use of corrective eye muscle surgery.

Post-traumatic orbital reconstruction – anatomy

- 'Safe distances' (those distances within which it is considered safe to dissect within the orbit) have been derived from measurements made from intact orbital rims in dried adult skulls and are of limited value in cases of severe orbital disruption (Evans et al. 2006).
- In high-energy injuries, the subperiosteal plane can be difficult to identify or may be completely absent because of the extent of disruption of the orbit. The plane is often absent in old injuries, in which the surgeon may be attempting to correct post-traumatic enophthalmos.
- Despite the accuracy of modern imaging, the size of the defect on CT is often smaller than the size of the defect encountered at the time of operation.
- The anatomical landmarks of the deep orbit are both hard and soft tissue structures:

  1. Infraorbital nerve.
  2. Inferior orbital fissure.
  3. Greater wing of the sphenoid.
  4. Orbital plate of the palatine bone.

Orbital fractures in children

Blow-out fractures of the orbital floor are rare in children less than 5 years old. (Cobb et al. 2012) The very young are more likely to have a fracture of the roof. The investigation of choice is a CT scan (Drage et al. 2009). Approaches to the facial skeleton may include the subtarsal approach that gives good access for reconstruction of the medial canthal ligament and is less likely to damage the lacrimal system. Fractures of the roof and supraorbital rim are approached through a coronal flap. Access to the frontozygomatic suture in this series is via a horizontal upper lid blepharoplasty.

Management of orbital blow-out fractures in children

Fractures of the orbital floor are rare in children less than 8 years old. It is more likely that these fractures would involve the anterior orbital floor and be associated with diplopia. Classic presentation of an orbital blow-out fracture in a child is with no subconjunctival haemorrhage, a 'white eye blow-out fracture' with upgaze diplopia and general malaise caused by the oculovagal reflex. There is marked restriction of motility in upward and downward gazes and may be little evidence of disruption to the orbital floor on CT – only a small crack or trapdoor defect with little bony displacement. The greenstick trapdoor of bone in the orbital floor or medial wall in children tends to spring back after fracture and trap inferior orbital soft tissues, typically the inferior rectus muscle. If it is not released quickly, it may cause permanent ischaemic necrosis and potentially a Volkmann ischaemic contracture and permanent impairment.

The oculovagal reflex manifests with bradycardia associated with traction on the extraocular muscles or compression of globe. (Atropine may be necessary.) Refractory vomiting is also a feature of the reflex in children, and this may be uncontrollable until the child is anaesthetized. It's worth noting that a less severe set of symptoms can be seen in adults with posterior but otherwise similar white eye blow-out fractures.

Nasal fractures

Incidence

Fractures of the nasal bones account for 50% of all facial fractures. They are often regarded as trivial injuries, and poor outcomes of some of the more displaced fractures are seen as a result of this viewpoint.

Aetiology

Of nasal fractures, 40% are caused by interpersonal violence. Falls (25%), sports injuries (20%) and road traffic collisions (10%) account for the rest.

Symptoms

Difficulty in breathing, nosebleeds and appearance are the main problems.

Signs

Deviation of the septum and nasal bones occurs, as do flattening, dislocation and obstruction. Look for a septal haematoma because this should be evacuated early to prevent cartilage necrosis.

Pattern of nasal fractures

These were described by Stranc.

- **Plane 1 injury** – injury lies anterior to a line joining the nasal bones and the anterior nasal spine and is confined to the cartilaginous nasal skeleton.
- **Plane 2 injury** – injuries are limited to the external nose, not involving the orbital rims.
- **Plane 3 injury** – this plane represents nasoethmoid and nasoorbital fractures. These injuries involve the orbital walls and anterior cranium.

Investigations

Plain films are of limited diagnostic value. Complex fractures of nasoethmoidal bones warrant CT scanning to assess the extent of injury.

Treatment

Treatment aims

- To restore normal anatomy and function.
- To correct associated orbital, cranial or ethmoidal deformity.

Initial treatment

A septal haematoma must be evacuated by needle aspiration or incision as soon as possible after it is identified to prevent septal ischaemia and necrosis.

Plane 1 and 2 injuries

These are treated by closed manipulation using local or general anaesthesia to reduce the deformity (Figures 16.31 and 16.32). Nasal packs and an external splint are then placed to hold the nose in position.

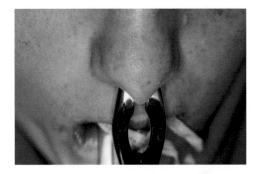

Figure 16.31 Reducing the nasal septum.

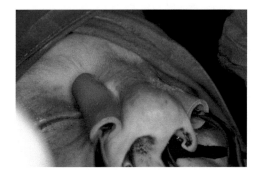

Figure 16.32 Reducing nasal bones with Walsham's forceps.

A long-standing deformity may require a submucosal resection or septoplasty. Complex residual deformity may require post-traumatic rhinoplasty.

Plane 3 injuries

Fractures involving the nasoethmoidal and naso-orbital complex are more demanding. Fractures here can lead to loss of nasal projection, widening of the intercanthal distance (distance between the eyes), unsightly appearance of the nasal bridge and considerable breathing difficulties. If the intercanthal distance is greater than 40 mm, an ORIF procedure of the nasoethmoidal complex is required to reattach the medial canthal ligament. This usually means fixing the bony attachment of the medial canthus rather than the canthus itself, although a specific piece of fixation apparatus is available to fix the ligament in rare instances.

Access for this operation is by coronal incision, to avoid scarring in the forehead region or local lacerations or scars. The bones are then elevated with intranasal forceps and are fixed in place with microplates. Reconstruction of the nasal bridge with an autogenous bone graft may be required. Profuse bleeding can occur perioperatively but is controlled by anterior nasal packs placed at the end of the procedure.

Indicators of favourable outcome

- Haemostasis.
- Normal nasal anatomy.
- Acceptable aesthetics.
- Good nasal air entry.

Indicators of unfavourable outcome

- Failure to control haemorrhage.
- Nasal deformity.
- Nasal obstruction.
- Patient dissatisfaction.

Midface fractures

Incidence

Midface fractures, which are less common than the other bony injuries, account for 5% of facial fractures in the United Kingdom. The introduction of seatbelt and crash helmet legislation and improved industrial health and safety have been held responsible for this. In countries where this legislation is not enforced (e.g. the Persian Gulf and Middle East), a higher incidence is seen.

Aetiology

Road traffic collisions are still the cause of around 50% of all midface injuries, with falls (20%), sports injuries (15%) and interpersonal violence (15%) accounting for the remainder. The force required to create these injuries accounts for the differences seen between midface fractures and the more common injuries.

Symptoms

These symptoms include pain, swelling, bruising, mobility of the upper teeth (feel soft to bite), altered occlusion (usually an anterior open bite) and bilateral numbness in the distribution of the infraorbital nerve.

Signs

The following are often present: swollen face, palpable fractures, mobile maxilla (Le Fort I); mobile maxilla and pyriform aperture (Le Fort II); mobile midface with zygoma and separation at fronto-zygomatic suture and base of skull (Le Fort III); bilateral black eyes (panda eyes); and bilateral numbness of the infraorbital nerves (Le Fort II). Premature contact of the posterior teeth causing anterior open bite can be seen. High-impact trauma can cause the palate to split down the midline and create multipart fractures of all facial bones. Bleeding from the nose can be torrential. Major displacement produces the classical 'dished-in face' appearance.

Patterns of midface fractures

Midface fractures are classified as follows (Figure 16.33):

Le Fort I fracture – involves disjunction of the left and right maxilla.

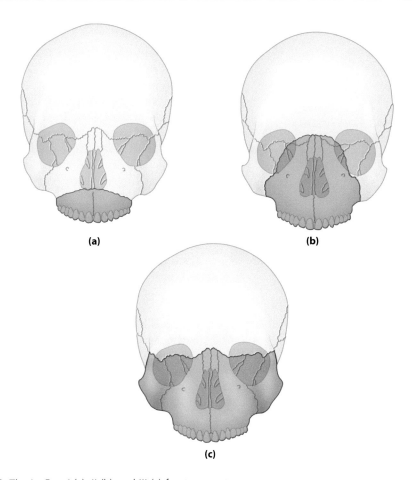

Figure 16.33 The Le Fort I (a), II (b) and III (c) fracture patterns.

Le Fort II fracture – involves fractures through the orbital floor and medial orbital wall and lateral maxillary wall.

Le Fort III fracture – involves disjunction of the mid facial skeleton from the base of skull. The fracture is through the pterygoid plates, zygomatic arch, frontozygomatic region and frontal nasal process bones and superior aspects of the medial and lateral orbital walls.

Investigations

OM views will give some information, but a much more accurate assessment of the extent of the fracture can be obtained from CT scans (Figure 16.34). CT scans also allow 3-D reformatted images of

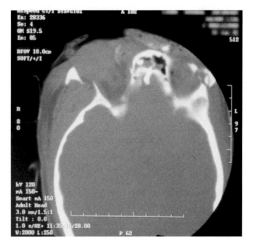

Figure 16.34 Computed tomography scan of a midface fracture.

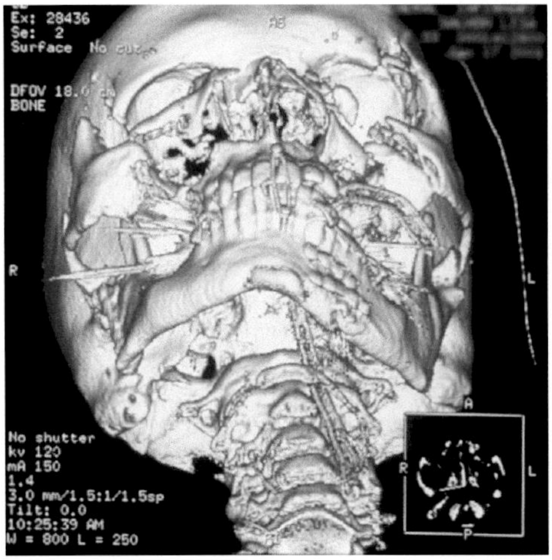

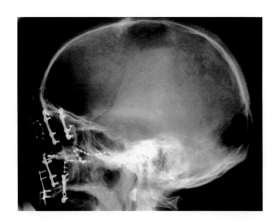

Figure 16.35 Three-dimensional reconstruction of a midface fracture.

the facial skeleton to be produced (Figure 16.35). Study models allow the patient's premorbid occlusion to be assessed and are helpful to have in the operating room because they allow the surgeon to visualize the correct occlusion before fixation. They can also be used to construct custom arch bars that will be used for IMF during surgery and postoperatively. Obtaining impressions on a seriously injured patient in the acute phase is, however, not always possible or even humane. It may simply be necessary to work with the scans and the surgeon's understanding of normal anatomy. If timing permits, models can be generated without the trauma of taking impressions by milling from 3-D CT reformatted information. Several commercial organizations offer this service.

Treatment

Treatment aims

- To restore facial appearance and occlusion.
- To stabilize fractures to allow healing.
- To reduce any fractures of the palate and prevent oronasal fistula formation.

Preoperative consent

Warn about facial scarring, possible IMF application, the possibilities of a temporary tracheostomy and nasal packs.

Fracture repair

Simple undisplaced fractures can be treated conservatively as long as there is no derangement of the occlusion or alteration of the facial profile. Complex displaced fractures with significant facial and occlusal change require ORIF of fracture fragments. All fracture repairs are carried out with the patient under general anaesthesia with nasal intubation ideally. In nasal intubation is not possible, temporary tracheostomy or a guarded flexible orotracheal tube is used.

The first manoeuvres during fracture repair are disimpaction and restoration of the fracture fragments to their premorbid position. Le Fort I fractures are treated by simply disimpacting the fracture and then closing the patient into their normal occlusion. Once the occlusion has been restored, temporary IMF is applied. An incision in the maxillary buccal mucosa allows access to the buttresses and pyriform aperture. The fracture is then exposed and miniplates placed. Two plates are normally placed on each side to stabilize the fracture (Figure 16.36).

The Le Fort II fracture requires buccal sulcus incisions and infraorbital incisions and fixation at the level of the infraorbital margin as well as the buttress region.

The Le Fort III fracture involves frontozygomatic repair, frontonasal fracture repair and zygomatic arch repair. Zygomatic arch fracture repair is best approached through a coronal incision, which gives good access to the zygomatic arch. It is imperative that the arch is returned to its pretrauma position

Figure 16.36 Postoperative reduced and fixed midface fracture.

because this determines the anteroposterior projection of the face and prevents any postoperative facial deformity. The zygomatic arch tends to 'telescope' under the force of the initial impact, thus shortening the anteroposterior facial dimension.

Special situations

1. Le Fort II and III fractures often involve disruption of the orbit and orbital floor; medial and lateral wall repair is an integral part of the operation.
2. If midface fractures occur in conjunction with complex mandibular fractures and condylar fractures, it is imperative that a logical sequence of repair is taken. Mandibular condylar height must be restored to ensure the overall *posterior facial height* does not change. Once the condyle is repaired, the frontozygomatic suture and zygomatic arch can be repaired, thus setting the outer facial frame. The next fracture to approach is the lateral orbital wall, then the maxillary buttress and finally the inner circle of the medial orbital wall and piriform fossa. Adhering to this sequence of repair allows achieved logical sequence, rational stepwise reduction of the fractures and optimizes the chances for a return to premorbid position (Figure 16.37).

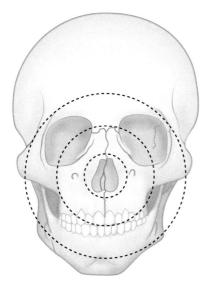

Figure 16.37 Diagram illustrating the rings of facial reconstruction.

Postoperative care

Postoperative analgesia, antibiotics and meticulous oral hygiene are required. Condylar height and midfacial position should be confirmed on postoperative radiographs. Skin sutures are removed at 5 days and coronal flap staples are removed at 7 days. Temporary IMF with elastic bands should be placed to reinforce the occlusal position for at least 7 days. Soft diet is recommended to ensure that the plates and the reduced fractures do not move. The patient is advised to avoid contact sports for approximately 3 months postoperatively.

Indicators of a favourable outcome

- Restoration of occlusion.
- Restoration of facial appearance.
- Restoration of eye function.
- Good healing without infection.
- Absence of palatal fistulae.

Indicators of unfavourable outcome

- Deranged occlusion.
- Flattened, 'dish face' appearance.
- Lack of nasal projection.
- Persistent diplopia.
- Shortened face.
- Infection of plates, exposed palatal bone and development of an oronasal fistula.
- Hypertelorism (i.e. wide eye separation).

Frontal bone fractures and frontal sinus fractures

Incidence

These are relatively rare fractures and are seen by both neurosurgeons and maxillofacial surgeons. Data regarding incidence are sparse and inaccurate.

Aetiology

These fractures involve considerable force, usually resulting from road traffic collisions, industrial accidents and assaults.

Symptoms

In the acute setting in association with head injury, these fractures are incidental findings. Patients may present following injury with concerns over appearance or recurring bouts of frontal headache (from frontal sinusitis), alterations in their sense of smell or nasal discharge.

Signs

The fracture involves the anterior wall of the frontal sinus and is often associated with orbital roof fracture, nasoethmoidal fracture, posterior wall fracture and complex cranial vault fracture. A dural tear can lead to cerebrospinal fluid (CSF) rhinorrhoea. A simple test to confirm CSF is to look for the presence of glucose on BM or multisticks. Reliable laboratory assay testing for CSF-specific proteins is also available.

Preoperative assessment is often difficult because the patient may well have a significant head injury. The patient is often on the operating table under the care of the neurosurgical team when maxillofacial surgical involvement is requested.

In the case of a nonacute setting, frontal sinus fracture leads to cosmetic deformity of the frontal bone. If the frontal sinus mucosa is damaged or the ventilation system of the frontal sinus is impaired, a history of recurring infection may be given.

Investigations

Plain films will give only a vague idea of the extent of the injury. CT scans are mandatory, allowing accurate assessment of the fractures; they do not provide any information on sinus function but show fluid collection within the sinus. It therefore becomes very difficult to plan treatment with any evidence base, and individualized 'best guess' treatment depending on presentation (acute or chronic) and symptoms is usual.

Treatment of frontal sinus fractures

Treatment aims

1. Restoration of forehead continuity and prevention of long-term deformity.

2. Surgical access to assess and repair any dural tear, to prevent the long-term risk of intracranial complications.
3. Access to the frontal sinus so that sinus obliteration can be carried out and deliberate blockage of the nasofrontal duct communication can be undertaken. This prevents long-term frontal mucocoele and reduces the risk of CSF leak through the nasal roof.
4. Note that if process 3 is not part of the overall treatment plan (e.g. when the posterior wall is intact and there is little evidence of frontal sinus lining damage and dysfunction), the essential step is to maintain ventilation of the sinus by a patent nasofrontal duct. This may require intervention ranging from minimal treatment (inhaled nasal decongestants for a week) to maximal conservative intervention (functional endoscopic sinus surgery).

Preoperative consent

Warn the patient about the coronal incision and the small risk of alopecia and temporal hollowing. The patient's sense of smell may be further altered. Postoperative drains will be present.

Fracture repair

Access is via a coronal flap, which exposes the frontal bone, orbital roof, medial orbital wall and nasal bones. If the frontal bone is minimally displaced it is reasonable to reposition the fragments and fixate by microplating. In the case of missing frontal bone the sinus can be directly examined for posterior wall fractures, CSF leak and mucosal damage. If the frontal bone fragments are displaced but not missing, it may be necessary to carry out a minicraniotomy of the frontal bone overlying the frontal sinus to examine the frontal sinus adequately. If the mucosa is significantly damaged, one school of thought is that it should be completely excised, the frontonasal duct obliterated and the sinus obliterated by bone graft. If the posterior sinus wall is involved, a popular neurosurgical technique is to remove the posterior wall, carry out dural repair and allow the brain to expand into the defect 'cranialization'. The most important issue is whether the sinus is maintained, in which case it must have adequate ventilation via the frontonasal duct as described earlier.

CSF leaks are uncommon and usually resolve without surgical intervention. Confirmation requires testing for the presence of beta-2 transferrin because glucose levels and the 'target sign' or 'ring test' are not reliable. Antibiotics are not recommended because of acquired resistance. Initially leaks are observed for 7 to 10 days, followed by CSF direction (lumbar drain) for 5 to 7 days. If repair is required, high-resolution CT or intrathecal fluorescein is needed to identify the site of leakage.

Repair of the frontal bone defect can be accomplished with inner table from the cranial vault, fracture fragments, outer table bone graft or free iliac bone. If there has been a substantial degree of bone loss, acrylic plates were popular as a custom made cover for the defect. Alternatively, titanium sheets can be used in the acute setting and cut to shape or fabricated based on CT scans. Several other cranioplasty materials have more recently become available (polyetheretherketone [PEEK]). Long-term follow-up involves monitoring for frontal mucocoele development, meningitis, frontal bone deformity, potential infection of the plates and CSF leak.

Indicators of favourable outcome

- Restoration of anatomy.
- Airway.
- Lacrimal function.
- Eye function.
- No meningitis.

Indicators of unfavourable outcome

- Facial deformity.
- Telecanthus.
- Eye problems.
- Retention cyst (mucocoele).
- Meningitis.
- Loss of sense of smell (anosmia).

Craniofacial fractures

These fractures are complex and require treatment by a multidisciplinary team. Defects in the skull vault can be replaced with autologous materials or recontoured with natural vault bone. It is imperative that the brain is covered to prevent further injury (Figure 16.38).

In cases of complex craniofacial trauma overlying soft tissue, skull and brain may be lost (Figure 16.39). Rotational flaps, free tissue transfers or tissue expansion may be needed to provide soft tissue coverage and a healthy environment for the rigid protection for the injured brain.

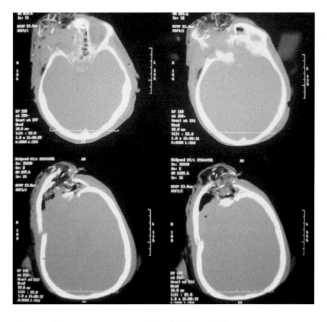

Figure 16.38 Combined craniofacial injuries create hard tissue defects.

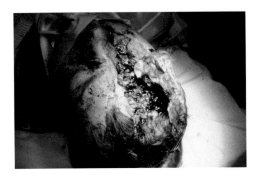

Figure 16.39 Craniofacial injuries with associated brain and soft tissue loss.

Craniofacial injuries may be associated with a significant head injury. The clinician must have a low threshold for further detailed imaging. The indications for a CT scan include the following (NICE guidelines, 2007):

1. Glasgow Coma Scale score lower than 13 when first assessed in emergency department.
2. Glasgow Coma Scale score lower than 15 when assessed in emergency department 2 hours after the injury.
3. Suspected open or depressed skull fracture.
4. Sign of fracture at skull base (haemotympanum, 'panda' eyes, CSF leak from ears or nose, Battle's sign).
5. Post-traumatic seizure.
6. Focal neurological deficit.
7. More than one episode of vomiting.
8. Amnesia of events more than 30 minutes before impact.

Injuries to the cervical spine

Traditionally plain radiographs are the initial investigations of choice to detect cervical spine injuries. Three views of sufficient quality are needed for reliable interpretation. With rapid access spiral CT used much more frequently in major trauma centres, plain radiography of the cervical spine, although described in ATLS, has become less common. Definitive interpretation of ligamentous injury requires magnetic resonance imaging.

FURTHER READING

Greaves I, Porter K, Ryan J. *Trauma care manual.* London: Arnold, 2001.
Chapter 12 has a nice overview of the primary treatment of maxillofacial trauma by well-recognized UK authorities.
Rowe N, Williams J. *Maxillofacial injuries,* vols 1 and 2. Edinburgh: Churchill Livingstone, 1985.
Although quite an old text and inevitably out of date in many areas, this was for many years the definitive text on maxillofacial trauma.
Yaremchuk M, Gruss J, Manson P. *Rigid fixation of the craniomaxillofacial skeleton.* London: Butterworth-Heinemann, 1992.
This text contains much of what is said in the Rowe and Williams book but from an American perspective.
Specific literature includes the following:
Abdel-Galil K, Loukota R. Fractures of the mandibular condyle: evidence base and current concepts of management. *Br J Oral Maxillofac Surg* 2010;48:520–6.
Benson PD, Marshall MK, Engelstad ME, Kushner GM, Alpert B. The use of immediate bone grafting in reconstruction of clinically infected mandibular fractures: bone grafts in the presence of pus. *J Oral Maxillofac Surg* 2006;64:122–6.
Cobb AR, Jeelani NO, Ayliffe PR. Orbital fractures in children. *Br J Oral Maxillofac Surg* 2013;45:41–6.
Coletti D, Ord RA. Treatment rationale for pathological fractures of the mandible: a series of 44 fractures. *Int J Oral Maxillofac Surg* 2008;37:215–22.
Downie JJ, Devlin MF, Carton ATM, Hislop WS. Prospective study of morbidity associated with open reduction and internal fixation of the fractured condyle by the transparotid approach. *Br J Oral Maxillofac Surg* 2009;47:370–3.
Drage NA, Sivarajasingam V. The use of cone beam computed tomography in the management of isolated orbital floor fractures. *Br J Oral Maxillofac Surg* 2009;47:65–6.
Eckelt U, Schneider M, Erasmus F, Gerlach KL, Kuhlisch E, Loukota R, Rasse M, Schubert J, Terheyden H. Open versus closed treatment of fractures of the mandibular

condylar process: a prospective randomised multi-centre study. *J Craniomaxillofac Surg* 2006;34:306–14.

Ellis E, 3rd. Treatment methods for fractures of the mandibular angle. *Int J Oral Maxillofac Surg* 1999;28:243–52.

Ellis E, 3rd, McFadden D, Simon P, Throckmorton G. Surgical complications with open treatment of mandibular condylar process fractures. *J Oral Maxillofac Surg* 2000;58:950–8.

Evans BT, Webb AAC. Post-traumatic orbital reconstruction: anatomical landmarks and the concept of the deep orbit. *Br J Oral Maxillofac Surg* 2007;45:183–9.

Gear AJL, Apasova E, Schmitz JP, Schubert W. Treatment modalities for mandibular angle fractures. *J Oral Maxillofac Surg* 2005;63:655–3.

Loukota RA, Eckelt U, De Bont L, Rasse M. Subclassification of fractures of the condylar process of the mandible. *Br J Oral Maxillofac Surg* 2005;43:72–3.

Luhr HG, Reidick T, Merten HA. Results of treatment of fractures of the atrophic edentulous mandible by compression plating: a retrospective evaluation of 84 consecutive cases. *J Oral Maxillofac Surg* 1996;54:250–4.

Mehra P, Van Heukelom E, Cottrell DA. Rigid internal fixation of infected mandibular fractures. *J Oral Maxillofac Surg* 2009;67:1046–51.

Mitchell DA. A multicentre audit of unilateral fractures of the mandibular condyle. *Br J Oral Maxillofac Surg* 1997;35:230–236.

National Collaborating Centre for Acute Care. *Head injury: triage, assessment, investigation and early management of head injury in infants, children and adults.* National Institute for Health and Clinical Excellence (NICE) clinical guideline 56. London: National Collaborating Centre for Acute Care, 2007.

Perry M. Maxillofacial trauma: developments, innovations and controversies. *Injury* 2009;40:1252–9.

Zide MF, Kent JN. Indications for open reduction of mandibular condyle fractures. *J Oral Maxillofac Surg* 1983;41:89–98.

17

Maxillofacial trauma – soft tissue

Contents

Aims and learning outcomes

For undergraduates:

- To be able to describe common facial soft tissue injuries.
- To be able to outline the principles of their management.

For postgraduates:

- To be able to discuss the common mechanisms of injury of facial soft tissue injuries.
- To be able to demonstrate an understanding of the importance of these injuries
- To be able to describe individual techniques in managing facial soft tissue injuries.

Primary management of facial soft tissue injuries

As with all trauma, adopt the ABC principles described under Advanced Trauma Life Support (see Chapter 16).

Types of soft tissue injury

Soft tissue injuries may be divided into several types, roughly indicative of the mechanism of injury. There may be some overlap among types of soft tissue injury, or they may be found in combination (Figure 17.1). Wounds may be categorized as described in the following paragraph.

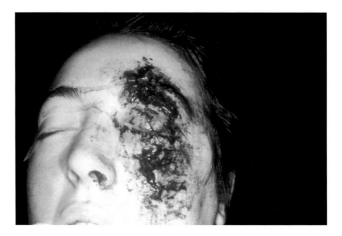

Figure 17.1 Combination of abrasions, incised wounds, lacerations and implanted foreign bodies caused by a high-speed collision with a windscreen.

Abrasions

Abrasions are caused by the force of an object rubbing on the surface of the skin. This results in detachment of the epidermis and a 'raw', flat wound. The epidermis may be partially detached, heaping toward one side of the wound (following the direction of the blunt force), or it may be totally detached, leaving a raw surface. Most abrasions scab over and reepithelialize with minimal scarring provided there is no superinfection.

Contusions

Contusions are bruises caused by rupture of blood vessels subcutaneously or deeper within tissue. The vessels rupture as a result of blunt trauma, and they release small to large amounts of blood into the tissues. The area of bruising is invariably larger than the area of contact with the object causing the trauma. There may also be abrasion or laceration of the skin at the site of bruising. Contusions tend to resolve over a varying course from weeks to months, depending mainly on the extent of release of blood into the tissues. This is obviously influenced by drugs or conditions promoting bleeding.

Lacerations

Lacerations are splits in the skin and underlying tissues caused by blunt impact that crushes the tissues over a site of bony prominence. The blunt trauma causes tearing of the skin, subcutaneous and deeper tissues, whereas blood vessels and nerves deeper in the wound may stay intact (Figure 17.2).

There may be associated abrasion and contusion injuries at the site of laceration.

Incised wounds

These wounds are 'clean' incisions through the skin and deeper tissues that are caused by a sharp instrument or object such as a knife or broken glass. Nerves and blood vessels within incised wounds risk being partially or completely severed. Often these wounds are the result of an alleged assault, although some neck wounds may be self-inflicted. Although it is common to misuse the

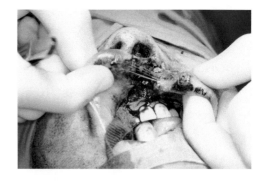

Figure 17.2 Lip laceration demonstrating preservation of nerves across the wound.

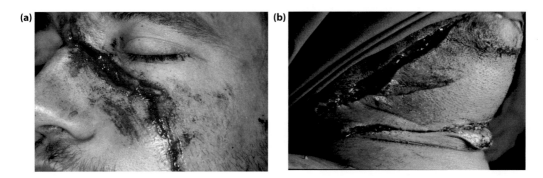

Figure 17.3 (a) Sharp facial wound made with a bladed weapon. (b) Beware underlying injuries.

terms 'laceration' and 'incised wound', it is important to understand the practical difference between incised wounds and lacerations because of the increased risk of injury to underlying vital structures (Figure 17.3 (a) and (b)).

Avulsions

In an avulsion injury, tissue at the wound site may be displaced from the underlying tissue layers yet still be partially attached (avulsion flap or 'partial' avulsion; Figure 17.4), or it may be totally detached from the wound site (complete avulsion).

Haematomas

A haematoma is a collection of blood within the soft tissues. A volume of blood released into the tissue, with no 'break' in the tissue to allow

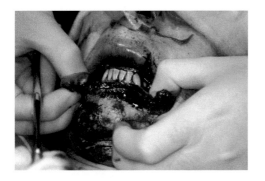

Figure 17.4 Even avulsion-type injuries on the face can be viable as long as a vascular pedicle can be maintained.

further escape, may collect to form a haematoma. In trauma this usually occurs when a blunt force ruptures one or more veins, which release blood into the tissue spaces. The blood release tends to be self-limiting because, with no escape route, the tissue is limited in its capacity to expand; the result is an increase in pressure within the collection. The pressure increase may reach the point where it compresses the vessel and resists further blood release (tamponade). Evacuation of a haematoma therefore may carry the risk of recommenced haemorrhage. Haematomas may also form in areas where the tissue layers have been separated, thus creating 'dead spaces' for blood to pool. Haematomas, being stagnant collections of blood, are at high risk of infection.

High-velocity missile injuries

Injuries caused by a high-velocity object, such as a bullet or shrapnel (which may include biological – human – body parts), may produce any combination of the foregoing wounds. In some cases the damage superficially may appear minimal, whereas deeper structures have sustained much more damage. In other cases, such as a shotgun wound at close proximity, large quantities of tissue may have been completely avulsed. In missile injuries the degree of damage depends on the energy expenditure at impact. Small pellets from a distance at low speed penetrate the skin but cause little underlying damage and are often impossible to recover (Figures 17.5 and 17.6).

Larger pellets (e.g. high-velocity airguns) can penetrate significant distance and present an

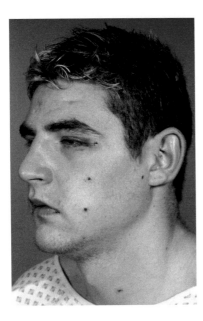

Figure 17.5 Clinical appearance of shotgun pellets impacting at low velocity.

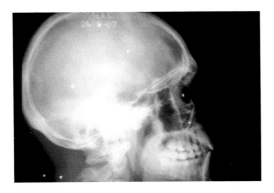

Figure 17.6 Radiographic appearance of the patient in Figure 17.5.

infection risk. Bullets create damage directly related to the degree of energy transfer and are usually associated with composite tissue loss. Contaminated shrapnel containing body parts (e.g. that produced by suicide bombers) may also create the risk of microbial contamination, particularly hepatitis B virus (HBV), hepatitis C virus (HCV), human immunodeficiency virus (HIV) or prions. High-velocity wounds may be self-sterilized at the point of departure from the weapon but can introduce virulent and unusual contaminants from victims' clothing, which can

be contaminated to varying degrees (battlefield in comparison with civilian). In general, bullets cause tissue damage by laceration or crushing, shock waves and cavitation. The principles of management include:

- Early aggressive débridement.
- Packing of deep wounds with iodine swabs.
- Waiting until the area of damage declares itself.
- Serial débridement until vitality is observed in wound margins.
- Administration of a single dose of broad-spectrum intravenous antibiotics.

Assessment of wounds

History

The following key questions must be answered.

How and where did it happen?

The cause of the wound must be identified. For example, if it was caused by a sharp object, deeper structures within the wound are more likely to be injured. If a weapon was used, obtain as much information about the weapon as possible (including whether it broke in use). If the wound was caused by broken glass, there should be suspicion that the wound may contain fragments of glass (Figures 17.7 and 17.8). Human or animal bites indicate a high risk of wound infection or, indeed, systemic infection (e.g. hepatitis B or C, HIV infection, rabies).

The location of the traumatic event is also important because it may provide further information. A wound sustained by a cyclist in a road traffic accident may contain gravel. A wound contaminated by soil carries an increased risk of tetanus.

When did it happen?

The older the wound, the more likely it is to become infected. Wounds that are more than 6 hours old are often assumed to be infected.

What is relevant in the medical history?

The medical history influences how the patient is treated (see Chapter 5). Whereas a healthy young patient may be treated uneventfully, a patient who

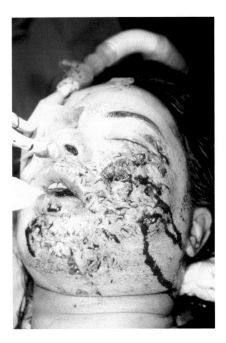

Figure 17.7 Typical windscreen laceration injury. The patient sustained fractures of the zygoma and mandible.

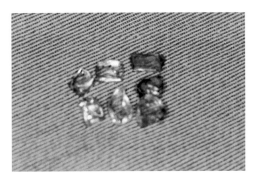

Figure 17.8 Fragments of windscreen glass removed from the patient in Figure 17.7.

is taking warfarin will have an increased bleeding time, and a patient who is immunocompromised may require antibiotic prophylaxis.

Important points raised in the medical history include:

- **Allergies** – Latex, dressings, antibiotics, anaesthetics, and so forth.
- **Current medications** – Anticoagulants, antibiotics, steroids, and so forth.

- **Complicating medical conditions** – Diabetes, haemophilia, HIV infection, and so forth.

Tetanus status

Wounds considered to be prone to tetanus include:

- Those wounds with evidence of infection.
- Puncture wounds or stab wounds.
- Wounds contaminated by dirt or soil.
- Old wounds (>6 hours).
- Wounds with necrotic tissue.

Immunization with tetanus toxoid (with or without tetanus immunoglobulin) is required if the patient has not received a tetanus booster within 10 years or has never been immunized.

Special investigations

For the most part these are limited to plain radiographs, to exclude either underlying **bony injury** (see Chapter 16) or **foreign body**. Swabs for culture and sensitivity of contaminated or frankly infected wounds are probably worthwhile even though treatment will be with 'best guess' antibiotics (Co-amoxiclav [amoxycillin and clavulanic acid] in patients with bite wounds).

Clinical examination

Notes should be made of

- The site and type of wound.
- The size, shape and depth of wound.
- Any tissue loss or avulsion.
- The state of deep structures within the wound (e.g. nerves, vessels).
- The condition of the wound (e.g. clean, dirty, infected, areas of necrosis).
- The presence or suspected presence of foreign bodies.

It is advisable to use a photograph or diagram to illustrate the type and location of wounds; once the wound is photographed it should be covered with a sterile dressing and not further exposed until formal closure can be performed.

Exploration of wounds

- **Do not explore a gaping penetrating wound of the neck (deep to the platysma) outside the operating theatre environment** (Figure 17.9).
- Blood vessels – Identify bleeding vessels (often those only partially transected) and those in spasm (often completely transected). As a damaged vessel is seen – Ligate, use diathermy or, if it is a vital vessel, repair using synthetic monofilament suture on a round body needle.

Methods of treating haemorrhage

- Direct pressure (all types of bleeding).
- Vasoconstrictors (e.g. adrenaline – this has a temporary and reversible effect).
- Haemostatic agents, either topical (e.g. fibrin-based products) or systemic (e.g. tranexamic acid) (see Chapter 6).
- Diathermy, cautery or coblation.
- Ligation (small vessels).
- Vascular repair (large or major vessels).
- Nerves.

The patient is assessed before anaesthesia when possible. Nerves that have been partially or completely divided may require microsurgical repair. Preoperative clinical assessment and in-theatre microscopic identification of the proximal and distal ends allow repair primarily or by grafting.

Other structures and organs

In the face, the eyes (Figure 17.10), ears or salivary glands may also be involved in a wound. Failure to note damage and failure to repair such structures are significant omissions that could result in long-term morbidity. A scalp laceration may overlie a skull fracture, a black eye may overlie an orbital or zygomatic fracture and a facial laceration may overlie a parotid duct laceration, facial nerve laceration or underlying fracture.

Other investigations

Foreign bodies

If the mechanism of injury suggests a foreign body (tooth, glass, dirt, projectile), radiograph the area of injury in two planes for localization (Figure 17.11). Some foreign bodies may be more obvious (Figure 17.12). Note that some foreign bodies may not be demonstrated on imaging – organic structures such as wood can be confusing and thin, hollow plastic objects may resemble air pockets on computed tomography.

Depending on size, location, nature and toxicity, most foreign bodies require removal, although

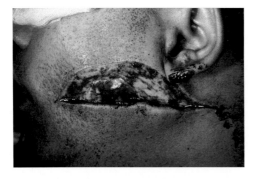

Figure 17.9 The marginal mandibular branch of the facial nerve and the mandible were damaged in this meat cleaver injury.

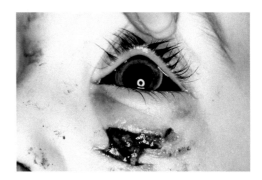

Figure 17.10 Penetrating facial skin injury with underlying globe damage.

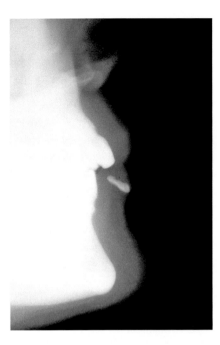

Figure 17.11 Fractured tooth fragment in the upper lip localized by radiographs. Such foreign bodies must be removed because they will always cause persisting severe infection. They can, however, be difficult to find.

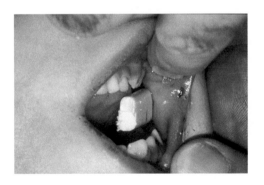

Figure 17.12 In contrast to fractured tooth fragments (see Figure 17.11), this toothbrush injury was obvious to all concerned.

in certain circumstances, it may be acceptable to leave inaccessible or innocuous objects.

Infection

Swabs for culture and sensitivity provide baseline information but rarely actually influence management. Most patients with traumatic soft tissue wounds should have the bacterial contamination treated by surface cleansing and should be given a broad-spectrum antistaphylococcal antibiotic

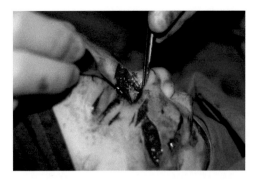

Figure 17.13 Multiple lacerations in children (e.g. this dog bite) should be addressed in theatre.

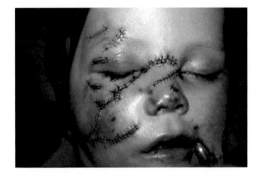

Figure 17.14 The patient in Figure 17.13 after repair.

(flucloxacillin, Co-amoxyclav or co-fluampicil [flucloxacillin and ampicillin]).

Large complicated or deeply contaminated wounds are best treated while the patient is under general anaesthesia. Most wounds and all complex wounds in children are best treated using general anaesthesia (Figures 17.13 and 17.14).

Frankly infected wounds or wounds with a high likelihood of infection are sometimes best left dressed with an antiseptic dressing; antibiotics are administered, and the wounds are closed once clean.

Cleansing and débridement

Cleaning the wounds is the most important stage in reducing the risk of infection and in preventing possible 'tattooing' of the tissues by debris (e.g. gravel) that may have become impacted in or around the wound. **Do not compromise adequate cleaning of the wound just to avoid general anaesthesia.**

There are a variety of cleansing solutions available, including:

- Normal saline.
- Chlorhexidine 0.5% (aqueous).
- Chlorhexidine 0.5% (alcohol based).
- Iodine (povidone iodine) 1% (aqueous).
- Iodine (povidone iodine) 1% (alcohol based).

Normal saline has little antiseptic effect but is the least irritating to the tissues. It makes an excellent solution for irrigation ('lavage') of wounds during exploration and cleansing. Chlorhexidine is an effective antiseptic that is less of an irritant to the tissues than iodine. However, iodine is a more effective antiseptic.

Alcohol-based solutions are generally more effective antiseptics than their aqueous counterparts, but alcohol-based solutions are also more irritating to the tissues and carry a flammability risk. Therefore, although alcohol-based solutions make better surface antiseptics, aqueous solutions are the only preparations used for facial wound disinfection.

Direct irrigation of deep, obviously infected puncture wounds with a 20% solution of hydrogen peroxide followed by saline irrigation is a useful occasional technique and an effective haemostatic manoeuvre.

Method of cleansing

- Aseptic scrub.
- The antiseptic solution is applied to a sterile gauze swab, which is held in forceps.
- The swab is applied to the skin closest to the wound and is used to clean the periphery of the wound in an increasing radius. The swab is then discarded.
- Any impacted material can be removed by surgical forceps or with a surgical scrubbing brush dipped in antiseptic.
- The wound is explored again for further foreign material and tissue damage.
- Any small areas of necrotic tissue or tags of ischaemic tissue are trimmed with sharp scissors or a scalpel.
- The wound can then be irrigated with normal saline and is ready for closure.

Hair-covered epidermis may pose a problem when exploring and closing wounds, particularly when a wound is complex. For simpler wounds, provided that access is good and cleansing and débridement are easily achievable, it may be acceptable to leave hair in cosmetic areas alone or to trim it. However, where the presence of hair is likely to make cleansing, débridement or closure difficult or when hair is likely to become trapped in a wound, the hair around the wound should be shaved before cleansing. There is, however, evidence to suggest that wound infection rates increase significantly if the wound area is shaved in elective surgery. A pragmatic compromise is needed, so be guided by experience and common sense.

Wound closure

Wound closure should always be performed in a good light and preferably with assistance (it often requires the hands of more than one operator). The patient should be positioned supine, even when he or she is under local anaesthesia, to minimize the risk of a faint.

Choice of materials

- Adhesive paper strips (Steri-Strips, Suture Strips).
- Tissue glue (Dermabond, Tisseel, and Histoacryl).
- Sutures – Resorbable.
- Sutures – Nonresorbable.
- Staples – These are rarely if ever used on the face.

Adhesive paper strips

These are paper or material strips which come in varying sizes. They are most useful for closing small wounds in areas where skin tension is not excessive. Adhesive paper strips are sometimes used to close wounds temporarily before further treatment and to close wounds that have been closely apposed by a deeper layer of sutures.

Tissue glue

Glues have been used to close superficial, uncomplicated skin wounds in areas where skin tension permits. They require no anaesthesia but are technically demanding to use well. They are popular for children because no anaesthesia for placement or removal of sutures is needed.

Sutures

There are many types of suture material available for use. Sutures are available in a variety of sizes and may be resorbable or nonresorbable. Different materials also have different tensile strengths and handling properties, and they react with the tissues in different ways. Sutures may be biological or synthetic, monofilament or multifilament, braided or twisted, coated or uncoated (see Chapter 3).

Chose a suture material and strength to match the defect you aim to close. Tight immobile wounds require thicker sutures (higher breaking strength 2-0 or 3-0). Delicate, lax areas require fine stitches (5-0 or 6-0) (Figure 17.15).

Resorbable sutures

These sutures may occasionally be used to close skin wounds in children in whom suture removal at a later date would necessitate another anaesthetic. Resorbable sutures are used in deep layer closure routinely and in inaccessible sites. They can play a useful role in subcuticular closure techniques.

Removal of sutures

All sutures, being foreign bodies, cause irritation to the tissues and hence have the potential to cause scarring. Skin sutures are removed as soon as tissue healing allows, preventing further irritation of the tissues and avoiding bind of the sutures to the tissues as they heal.

As a rough guide, nonresorbable sutures are best removed from the face 5 or 6 days after placement, when sufficient healing has usually taken place to allow function of the tissue without reopening of the wound. Tissues such as the scalp may require a longer period (e.g. 7 to 10 days) because tension within certain tissues is higher and the wound may not be strong enough at the 5-day stage to withstand the tension.

Staples

Staple placement can be used as an effective method of closure of the skin surface in simple larger wounds. Staples are removed using a staple remover, which is often less uncomfortable than removing sutures.

Wound closure with sutures

Where there has been little or no tissue loss and the margins of the wound consist of viable tissue, primary closure can usually be achieved.

Commonly used suture techniques

Interrupted sutures – These are the simplest type of suture but also tend to be the most time consuming. Individual interrupted sutures can be used to close points of apposition in wounds until the entire length of the wound is closed (Figure 17.16). They are most useful for closing wounds of irregular contour and have the advantage that the closure of the entire wound does not depend on just one suture (Figures 17.17 and 17.18). The mattress suture is a modification of the interrupted suture that can give strong and accurate apposition of tissues. The vertical mattress suture is very

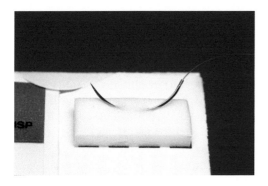

Figure 17.15 Typical monofilament nylon suture.

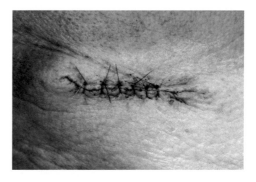

Figure 17.16 Closure of a simple linear incision with interrupted sutures.

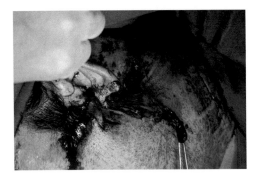

Figure 17.17 Complex facial laceration caused by multiple slashes.

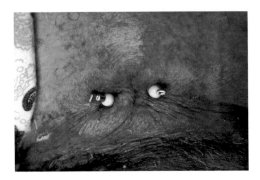

Figure 17.19 An example of continuous subcuticular suture to close a simple linear wound.

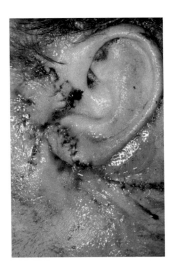

Figure 17.18 The patient in Figure 17.17 after repair of the wounds.

effective at wound edge eversion. The horizontal mattress suture is a good haemostatic suture.

Continuous sutures – Continuous sutures are useful for closing straight wounds where tissue apposition is easy to achieve with accuracy (Figure 17.19). There is no interruption to the course of the suture, thus giving the suture the advantage of being less time consuming and possibly creating a more evenly balanced force of closure on the tissues. However, continuous sutures have the disadvantage that the whole layer of wound closure depends on just one suture, and therefore failure may mean resuturing of the entire wound. Continuous

sutures also tend to be useful only for closure of straight wounds.

Technique for interrupted sutures

A basic technique for closure of a wound with interrupted sutures is described here.

Following cleansing and débridement, the appropriate suture for the tissue is selected. The wound margins are accurately opposed such that when closed they will align in the correct position. If there are no clues (e.g. skin creases or angles in the wound), straight wounds may be brought together by means of skin hooks at either end of the wound, which create apposition under gentle tension. The suture needle is held with the needle holder positioned at least one third away from the end of suture attachment – this reduces the chance of bending or breakage of the needle in the wound. A 'bite' of skin is taken at a landmarked site; the size of the bite depends on the depth of the wound (the deeper the wound, the farther the bite from the wound edge). The suture needle is advanced to the depth of the wound margin and then out through the wound opening. The needle is next inserted via the depth of the wound and is rotated up through the opposite skin margin and the landmarked site for apposition of the wound. The breadth of bite of skin by the suture on either side of the wound should be the same. If the bites are inconsistent, 'stepping' of the skin will occur when the suture is knotted, and ultimately scarring will result.

If the suture is correctly placed and approximates the wound margins accurately, the knot should be tied in the suture to bring the margins together, such that the skin edge is slightly everted. Inverted skin margins will heal with a poor aesthetic result. Once the correct suture position is achieved, the suture should be 'locked' with a further knot or series of knots.

Layered closure

Wounds that involve only the skin are often best closed with a single layer of interrupted sutures. Where wounds are deep, tissue should be closed in layers to remove dead space and confer strength to the wound.

The technique for layered closure involves closing the deeper tissues first, usually with a continuous suture or 'buried' interrupted sutures, and then closing the skin with interrupted sutures (or occasionally adhesive strips) as described earlier.

Augmenting suture lines

Some surgeons advocate the use of paper strips or adhesive dressings over a closed skin wound. In the torso, abdomen and limbs, this approach is probably useful. On the face, neck and scalp, it is less so. A thin layer of sterile petroleum jelly (conveniently found in antibiotic eye ointment) keeps the wound moisturized and clean and minimizes crusting, thus making suture removal easier. In wounds under high tension or muscular activity, intramuscular botulinum-alpha toxin injected on either side of the wound to remove temporarily the activity creating stretching forces on the scar can help.

Reasons for failure of sutures

- Breakage – the tensile strength of the suture material is too low or the suture is too small.
- Cutting out – too fine a suture material is used or the suture is placed in friable tissue.
- Knot slippage – knot tying is inadequate. Every material other than silk benefits from an extra throw on the conventional surgeon's knot.
- Extruded suture – this occurs in combination with infection.
- Resorption that is too rapid – nonabsorbable or more slowly absorbable suture should have been used.
- Removal too early – suture is removed before sufficient healing.

Drains

Deep or extensive wounds may require the insertion of a drain, which lies along the length of the depth of the wound. The purpose of a drain is to remove excessive inflammatory exudate and 'oozed' blood from the wound to prevent it from collecting as a focus of infection. A drain placed in a wound is usually exited via an area of intact skin and subcutaneous tissue and may cause a small scar at that point following removal. Drains are usually made from plastic tubing that is perforated along the section lying within the wound to allow inflow of fluid. The outer portion of tubing remains intact and can be attached to a container (usually vacuumed) to collect the outflowing fluid.

Wounds with tissue loss

In wounds with tissue loss, occasionally the surrounding tissues are sufficiently elastic to allow them to be advanced into the area of defect and achieve functional and aesthetic closure. Where a substantial amount of tissue loss has occurred such that closure of the defect without excessive tension on the tissues cannot be achieved or would cause disfigurement, there are several options available for treatment, as described here.

Undermining of the skin

When tissue loss is not extensive and mainly involves skin, a small border of skin on either side of the wound may be carefully separated from the underlying fat. This allows advancement of the released elastic skin across the wound. Specific areas of the face are suitable for this technique (see Chapter 18).

Partial closure or granulation

This involves suturing the wound such that it is partially closed and not under excessive tension. The resulting defect is then allowed to heal by granulation. This technique is suitable for smaller defects but tends to increase the level of scarring;

therefore, it is usually inappropriate for facial wounds.

Skin grafting

Skin grafting is used mainly when large areas of skin have been lost. It is often possible to harvest skin from a donor site elsewhere in the body for placement over the wounded area. Skin can be taken in a partial-thickness or full-thickness graft from a site such as the inner thigh or arm (split-thickness graft) or the supraclavicular, preauricular or post-auricular region (full-thickness graft). The donated skin may be meshed (multiply punctured to allow stretching of the skin over a wider area, with the epithelium spreading into the small resulting defects as healing occurs). Skin colour varies across the body, and therefore care must be taken to ensure that the donor site is a reasonable match with the recipient site (Figure 17.20) (see Chapter 18).

Local flap repair

It may be possible to use skin from an area local to the defect by means of raising a flap of skin and repositioning it to cover the defect. This requires some 'give' in the skin at the donor site and therefore may require wide undermining of the skin in areas where the skin and underlying tissues are under tension or are tightly bound to underlying structures (e.g. the scalp). Common designs of flap for repair of defects include rotation and advancement flaps (see Chapter 18). Local tissue can be augmented by local tissue expansion (Figures 17.21 and 17.22). This procedure takes time but creates a large amount of surplus local tissue for wound repair that gives close to the ideal colour and texture match.

Distant flap repair

This procedure involves removing donor tissue, including vasculature from a distant site, and anastomosing the vessels to the vasculature of the recipient site before repair (see Chapter 23). There is a (~5%) risk that the circulation in the 'free flap' will fail (usually from thrombosis in the venous system), and this is generally a time-consuming and complex operation. This method should be reserved for areas of extensive tissue loss where local flap repair would not suffice.

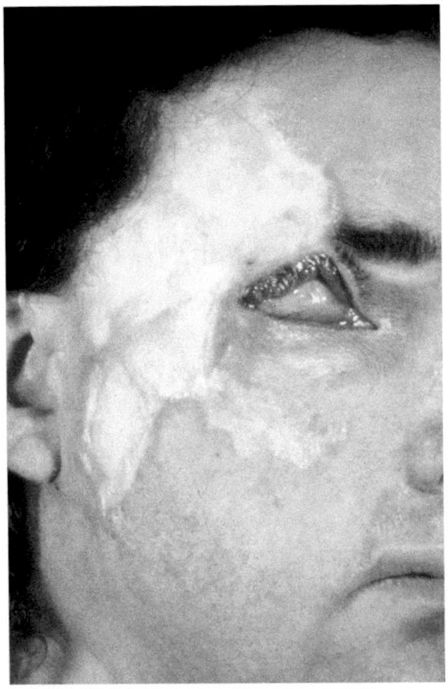

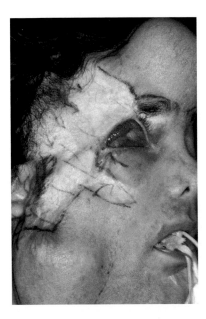

Figure 17.20 Split-thickness skin grafting seldom produces a good aesthetic result in the face but does allow coverage and initial wound healing.

Figure 17.21 Tissue expansion in the patient in Figure 17.20 to use healthy local tissue for closure.

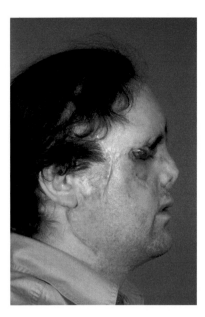

Figure 17.22 After excision of skin graft and movement of local flaps.

Wound healing

Following tissue trauma, there is an initial acute inflammatory response. Protein-rich exudate is released into the wound. Coagulation of blood occurs as fibrinogen is converted to fibrin. White blood cells – lymphocytes and phagocytes – migrate to the wound. Capillaries and lymphatic vessels infiltrate the wound to form granulation tissue, and epithelial cells multiply from the margins of intact skin and begin to grow across the surface of the wound. Fibroblasts and collagen fibres begin to appear within the wound as the tissue becomes organized. Contracture of the wound occurs as healing continues and the blood vessels become less obvious. The fibrous tissue in the wound eventually matures to form a 'scar'.

Factors affecting wound healing

1. Site of the wound (e.g. tissue, blood perfusion, movement).
2. Timing of treatment.
3. Nature of treatment (correct or incorrect technique).
4. Infection.
5. Systemic factors (e.g. age, health, nutrition, steroids).

Postoperative wound care

Care of wounds postoperatively is key in preventing infection and in minimizing scarring. Wounds that are kept relatively moist (not wet) tend to heal faster than dry wounds. However, moisture is a good breeding environment for bacteria. Exposure to a dirty environment should be avoided during the initial healing phase because of this high risk of infection in 'raw' tissue.

Dressings

Various dressing materials are available, including dry, nonadherent dressings and moist dressings (see Chapter 3). Some materials are impregnated with bactericidal compounds to reduce infection risk. It may be desirable to apply dressings to certain wounds.

All dressings must be changed regularly to allow air circulation and reduce the risk of adherence of the dressing to the wound and the risk of infection.

Closed wounds

Although most closed wounds do not usually benefit from dressing, when it cannot be guaranteed that the wound will not be exposed to a dirty environment, and to ease suture removal, an antibiotic ointment is helpful.

Open and granulating wounds

Such areas benefit from a moist environment to prevent drying of the healing tissue and encourage new growth and epithelialization. Such wounds usually do well with a moist dressing such as paraffin-impregnated gauze (e.g. Jelonet). Paraffin-impregnated gauze has antiseptic properties and resists colonization with bacteria. This can be improved by using dressings soaked in iodine-based antiseptics.

Healing wounds

It may be desirable to keep epithelializing wounds and closed wounds moisturized to encourage healing. In the later stages of healing, good moisturization of the area tends to assist in softening of any scar tissue, thus allowing for a minimal scar. In a healing wound, a standard moisturizer may provide this effect; however, in the early stages of healing, an antibiotic-based preparation (e.g. chloramphenicol or bacitracin ointment) may be safer and more convenient.

Wound infections

Wounds may become infected at any stage. Wounds that are frankly infected preoperatively or have failed to heal because of postoperative infection should not normally be closed until the infection has been eradicated. Once the infection has been treated *and* resolved, it may be appropriate to débride and close the wound or to allow the wound to heal by granulation. Primary closure is usually delayed in contaminated wounds where there has been a delay in treatment. The wound is usually dressed and remains open for up to 5 days to ensure that infection has not taken hold before further débridement and closure are performed.

The infecting organisms may come from a variety of sources – either endogenous or exogenous. Most wounds encountered, other than clean surgical wounds, must be considered contaminated and therefore require antibiotic treatment. Although an 'informed guess' may often be made about the most likely causative organism and antimicrobial therapy may be commenced on that basis, it is important to take swabs of the wound and send them for culture and sensitivity analysis, to ensure that the appropriate drug regimen is in place.

Reasons for infection

Common reasons for infection include preoperative and postoperative factors.

Preoperatively

- Wound contamination with organisms at the time of trauma.
- Delay in treatment.

Postoperatively

- Contamination at the time of injury.
- Poor cleansing/wound débridement or poor aseptic operative technique.
- Poor closure of the wound.
- Failure to administer appropriate prophylactic antibiotics.
- Host susceptibility.

Common infecting organisms

See also Chapter 10.

Staphylococcus aureus

Staphylococcus aureus is the most frequent cause of wound infection. It is commonly found in the commensal skin flora of around 30% of the population. *S. aureus* has a variety of strains, which vary in their virulence. Although multiple antibiotic resistance is on the increase, the more common stains of *S. aureus* still tend to be sensitive to flucloxacillin and similar antibiotics.

Streptococcus pyogenes

Streptococcus pyogenes, albeit far less common than *S. aureus,* is still found in many wound infections. It is usually sensitive to penicillin.

S. aureus and *S. pyogenes* are the most likely causes of infection in most facial wounds where other sources of contamination have been ruled out. Therefore initial treatment of wound infections with flucloxacillin, co-fluampicil or Co-amoxyclav is effective in most cases. Clarithromycin, clindamycin and doxycycline are the alternatives of choice in such infections when the patient is penicillin allergic. It is worth bearing in mind that the cross-reactivity between penicillins and cephalosporins has probably been overstated in the past.

Other organisms

Depending on the source of contamination, wounds may be infected with enterococci, other streptococci or staphylococci or *Clostridium* species, or they may be mixed infections.

Most aerobes are sensitive to penicillin, flucloxacillin, a cephalosporin or erythromycin; for anaerobes, metronidazole is the drug of choice.

Methicillin-resistant *S. aureus* (MRSA) is a meticillin (multiply)–resistant strain of *S. aureus*. It is difficult to treat because it is resistant to most antibiotics. Intravenous vancomycin is one of the few treatments that is effective in most cases. Cross-infection control must be put in place to prevent this organism from being spread among patients.

Clostridium species include *Clostridium tetani,* the agent of tetanus (discussed previously). The importance of checking the patient's tetanus immunization status cannot be overemphasized. *Clostridium* species are also responsible for 'gas gangrene' whereby infection causes rapid tissue necrosis via bacterial toxins, and gases are produced. 'Synergistic gangrene' may be caused by a mixed infection of aerobes and anaerobes and also results in tissue necrosis. Both forms of gangrene can be rapidly fatal and require urgent treatment with broad-spectrum antibiotics, wide margin excision of the wound and lavage with hydrogen peroxide.

Streptococcus milleri is the head and neck organism most frequently found in serious necrosis-producing head and neck infections. Radical débridement with the appropriate antibiotics as early as possible is the appropriate tactic.

Scarring

Almost every injury involving a breach of the skin results in a degree of scarring. In many circumstances, scars are in areas where they will not readily be noticed by other people and therefore are of little or no consequence. Indeed, even in clearly visible areas, scars are often so fine as to be barely noticeable, or they may be disguised within the natural skin creases or relaxed skin tension lines or 'Langer's lines'. Elective incisions for surgery are designed such that they respect the relaxed skin tension lines and thus produce as minimal scarring as possible. However, trauma has no respect for aesthetics, and therefore the scar produced by a wound may prove to be particularly unsightly (Figure 17.23). Linear wounds tend to develop more obvious scarring than do irregular wounds unless a linear repair such as vermillion border or eyebrow has been mismatched (Figure 17.24). Good wound care, early suture removal, moisturization and massage all help to reduce scarring.

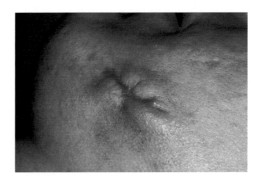

Figure 17.23 A typical hypertrophic scar.

Nonsurgical techniques to improve scars include silicone-based gels for self-application, silicon pressure dressings, intralesional steroids and steroid-impregnated tape.

If a scar is particularly aesthetically disturbing to a patient, it may be possible to perform 'scar revision' (i.e. surgical modification of the scar such that it is reduced or is aesthetically disguised). Various techniques are employed to revise scars, and the choice of technique depends on the size, shape and alignment of scar tissue. It must be borne in mind that all these techniques require further surgical incisions and as such produce scarring themselves, albeit in a (hopefully) more desirable position. Techniques include, among others, scar excision, Z-plasty, multiple Z-plasties, V-Y plasty and advancement and rotation flaps.

If surgery is to be performed, it should be appropriately timed. A scar tends to reach maturation approximately 18 months following closure of the wound, and hence surgery should not be performed

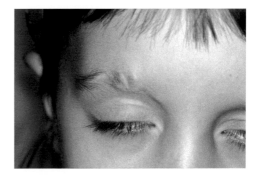

Figure 17.24 A mismatch of natural facial features (in this case the eyebrow) produces a poor aesthetic appearance.

before this point; this is an area where the patient's choice can radically influence treatment. In a medically led environment, waiting 18 months for scar maturity is optimal; however, few patients are able to accept that length of time. A 6-month waiting period may be an acceptable compromise.

FURTHER READING

Edlich RE, Kenney JG. Soft tissue injuries of the face. In Dudley H, Carter D, Russell RCG, editors. *Rob & Smiths operative surgery, 4th ed, vol 1.* London: Butterworth, 1989.

A standard text.

Managing bites from humans and other mammals. *Drug Ther Bull* 2004;42:67–70.

Stone C. *Plastic surgery: facts.* London: Greenwich Medical Media, 2001.

Lots of useful but very superficial information; although it covers the entire (some would say absurd) scope of plastic surgery, it contains useful and relevant sections throughout. Worth dipping into for postgraduates.

Wardrope JP, Smith AR. *The management of wounds and burns.* Oxford: Oxford University Press, 1990.

Old but classic text.

Specific literature includes the following:

Allonby-Neve CL, Okereke CD. Current management of facial wounds in UK accident and emergency departments. *Ann R Coll Surg Engl* 2006;88:144–50.

Ardeshirpour F, Shaye DA, Hilger PA. Improving posttraumatic facial scars. *Otolaryngol Clin North Am* 2013;46:867–81.

Barker DA, Bowers DT, Hughley B, Chance EW, Klembczyk KJ, Brayman KL, Park SS, Botchwey EA. Multilayer cell-seeded polymer nanofiber constructs for soft-tissue reconstruction. *JAMA Otolaryngol Head Neck Surg* 2013;139:914–22.

Favia G, Mariggio MA, Maiorano F, Cassano A, Capodiferro S, Ribatti D. Accelerated wound healing of oral soft tissues and angiogenic effect induced by a pool of amino acids combined to sodium hyaluronate (AMINOGAM). *J Biol Regul Homeost Agents* 2008;22:109–16.

Rieck KL, Fillmore WJ, Ettinger KS. Late revision or correction of facial trauma-related soft tissue deformities. *Oral Maxillofac Surg Clin North Am* 2013;25:697–713.

18

Facial skin cancer

Contents

Aims

At the end of reading and understanding this chapter, you will be able clinically to recognize the three common facial skin cancers and be in a position to discuss surgical treatment modalities to the degree relevant to your seniority.

Learning outcomes

For undergraduates:

- To be able to describe the common features of the three major skin cancer types.
- To be able to list the more common treatments of facial skin cancer.
- To be able to describe the principles of treatment of the common facial skin cancers.

For postgraduates:

- To be able to describe the steps involved in diagnosis of common facial skin cancers.
- To be able to discuss the treatment of common facial skin cancers.
- To be able to describe the steps in surgical excision of facial skin cancers.
- To be able to describe the steps of common local flap closure of skin defects.

Introduction

The three most common skin cancers affecting the head and neck region are basal cell carcinoma (BCC), squamous cell carcinoma (SCC) and malignant melanoma. Exposure to ultraviolet (UV) light on a cumulative basis is the major risk factor for BCC and SCC, and therefore, unsurprisingly, these lesions are most commonly found on the sun-exposed skin (e.g. face, scalp, hands and arms of the white-skinned population in sunny climates).

Changing patterns of sun exposure for social reasons has led to the increasing incidence of BCC in the United Kingdom.

Basal cell carcinoma

Numerous types of BCC are described clinically and pathologically (nodular, cystic, pigmented, morphoeic and ulcerated), but the most important feature is that of margin definition. The distinction is between clearly defined margins and ill-defined margins. BCCs with ill-defined margins are more clinically dangerous because infiltration can extend far beyond the visible margins (Figures 18.1 and 18.2).

BCCs very rarely metastasize, but they will progressively cause local damage if neglected. These tumours are called 'rodent ulcers' because of the progressive gnawing away of tissue; their rate of growth is slow and is measured in months and years

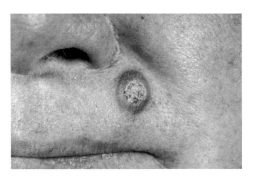

Figure 18.1 Basal cell carcinoma with well-defined edges on the upper lip.

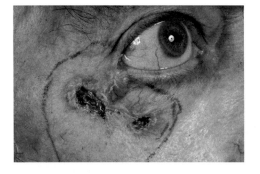

Figure 18.2 Basal cell carcinoma with ill-defined edges that requires a wider margin of excision.

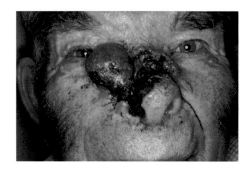

Figure 18.3 Neglected extensive basal cell carcinoma of the nose and paranasal sinuses. This patient refused treatment for 18 years.

(Figure 18.3). BCC is a slow-growing, locally invasive malignant epidermal skin tumour predominately affecting white-skinned people. Perivascular invasion and perineural invasion are features associated with the most aggressive lesions. BCC is the most common cancer in Europe. The strongest aetiological factors appear to be genetic predisposition and UV radiation. Increasing age, male sex, fair skin types I and II, immunosuppression, high-fat diet and arsenic exposure are other factors. Multiple BCCs are a feature of basal cell naevus (Gorlin's) syndrome. The use of imaging techniques such as computed tomography (CT) or magnetic resonance imaging (MRI) is indicated when bony involvement is suspected or where the tumour may have invaded major nerves, the orbit or the parotid gland. Broadly, the available treatments for BCC can be divided into surgical and nonsurgical, and surgical techniques can be subdivided into excision and destruction.

Squamous cell carcinoma

SCCs usually arise in sun-damaged skin, especially of the scalp and ear, and manifest as a raised nodule, as an ulcer with raised everted edges or as a fleshy, fungating lesion (Figure 18.4).

Clinical differentiation between SCC and BCC is not always easy, but with SCC metastasis to the regional lymph nodes occurs much more frequently, and the rate of growth of SCC is greater (Figure 18.5).

Primary cutaneous SCC is a malignant tumour that may arise from the keratinizing cells of the epidermis or its appendages. It is locally invasive and has the potential to metastasize to other organs

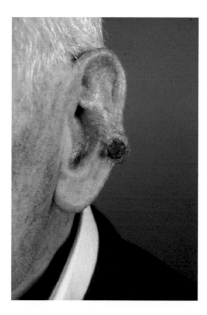

Figure 18.4 Squamous cell carcinoma of the ear showing a typical appearance.

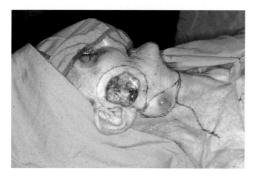

Figure 18.5 Squamous cell carcinoma of the cheek. Some skin cancers such as this spread to the cervical lymph nodes and require the kind of major ablative and reconstructive treatment commonly seen in mucosal cancer of the head and neck.

of the body. SCC is the second most common skin cancer. Its occurrence is usually related to long-term UV light exposure and is therefore especially common in people with sun-damaged skin, fair skin, albinism and xeroderma pigmentosum.

Others causes include:

- Ionizing radiation.
- Arsenic.
- Preexisting lesions such as Bowen's disease.
- Immunosuppressive drugs (e.g. transplant recipients, patients with inflammatory conditions).
- Lymphoma or leukaemia.
- Human papillomavirus (HPV).

Factors that influence **metastatic potential** include anatomical site, size, tumour thickness, level of invasion, rate of growth, aetiology, degree of histological differentiation and host immunosuppression. Topical agents such as imiquimod may have a role in preventing the development of skin dysplasia in high-risk renal transplant recipients. In patients with multiple, frequent or high-risk SCCs, consider the prophylactic use of systemic retinoids.

Keratoacanthoma is a self-resolving but rapidly developing skin lesion that can mimic SCC because it produces a dome-like or volcano-like lesion with central ulceration. Although keratoacanthoma spontaneously resolves, the diagnosis is often very difficult, and concern over this means that accurate histological diagnosis is needed and excision is often advisable.

Malignant melanoma

The incidence of malignant melanoma, a more serious skin cancer, is doubling each decade in the United Kingdom, where it affects a younger age range and carries a mortality of around 40%. It is more common elsewhere on the body (in men, the back; in women, the leg), but it does appear on the face and is classified as follows:

- Superficial spreading melanoma – the most common type.
- Nodular melanoma – the most aggressive type (Figure 18.6).
- Lentigo maligna melanoma – the type most like to affect the face of elderly patients.
- Acral lentiginous melanoma.
- Amelanotic melanoma.

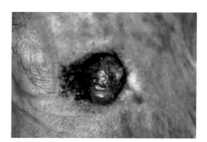

Figure 18.6 Example of nodular malignant melanoma.

Lentigo maligna is a pigmented patch on the face that progressively enlarges, shows atypia of the melanocytes histologically and has the potential to develop into lentigo maligna melanoma. Early surgical excision is advised.

Diagnosis

Diagnosis of all skin tumours is by clinical recognition, biopsy or both. Because of the difficulty of clinical diagnosis, a close liaison between dermatologists and surgeons is vital in the management of skin cancer. Histological confirmation of the diagnosis is essential if extensive surgery, as opposed to simple excision, is necessary for any individual case.

Treatment

Simple treatment of skin cancer is often undertaken by dermatologists or by general practitioners/primary care physicians with suitable training. Techniques such as cryotherapy, curettage and cautery, photodynamic therapy and local excision treat the majority of skin tumours successfully, leaving a smaller percentage requiring formal surgical excision and reconstruction. The evidence base for best-choice curative treatment does, however, support surgery.

Both BCC and SCC can be successfully treated by radiotherapy or surgery, but the overwhelming preference is for surgery for a variety of reasons – aesthetics, speed, tumour bulk and histopathological evidence of clearance of the tumour. Radiotherapy (particularly electron beam) is used as adjuvant therapy after surgery and when surgery is inappropriate either for technical reasons or because the patient is not a suitable surgical candidate.

Surgical excision

BCCs are excised with a margin of 4 to 5 mm, although tumours with poorly defined margins are more difficult to judge and may need a wider margin. Mohs' micrographic surgery can be useful in certain anatomical sites to determine clearance while minimizing the extent of resection. Mohs' surgery involves excision with chemical cautery and multiple repeat biopsies of the specimen until the margins are tumour free. Popular in the United States, this procedure is time consuming and costly, but it does offer advantages in patients with ill-defined morphoeic BCCs and with BCCs encroaching free margins in the nasal and eye regions. Various modifications of this technique using frozen section or conventional histology have been used to fit local resources. For example, in difficult cases, a two-stage approach can be used, leaving the wound dressed until the histopathology report is available. The final pathology report, looking carefully at the resection margins, can be reviewed before reconstruction because additional marginal resections may be necessary.

In more straightforward cases, frozen section can be used to assess completion of resection. In these cases the resection and reconstruction can be performed as a one-stage procedure using the common clinical margin and reconstruction techniques described.

The **indications for Mohs' surgery** include:

- Specific tumour sites (especially central face, around the eyes, nose, lips, ear).
- Large tumour size (>2 cm).
- Specific histological subtypes (especially morphoeic, infiltrative, micronodular, basosquamous subtypes).
- Poor clinical definition of tumour margins.
- Recurrent lesions.
- Perineural or perivascular involvement.

For **incompletely excised BCCs,** there are various prospective and retrospective reviews that suggest that **not all** these tumours will recur. Tumours that have been incompletely excised, especially lesions incompletely excised at the deep margin, are all at high risk of recurrence.

SCCs and melanomas are excised more widely. The margin for excision for melanomas has decreased over the years as prospective trials have shown no disadvantage in the outcome with smaller margins. Current guidelines indicate margins of 1 to 3 cm, depending on the depth and size of melanoma and even less than 1 cm in important anatomical regions such as the face.

Excision of all skin cancers involves the deeper tissues as well as peripheral skin around the lesion, and this is of great significance in the head and neck region. Deep excision on the trunk or legs is straightforward because the subcutaneous layer of fat is considerable and allows excision margins to be easily achieved without involving important nearby structures. This is not the case on the face, scalp or neck, where margins of excisions are affected by the close proximity of vital structures. These include the facial nerve, the eye and free margins (e.g. the eyelids), the lips and the alar rim of the nose. Another limitation is the limited depth of tissues available for excision (e.g. on the scalp). Achieving an adequate margin of clearance around and beneath a tumour on the face may involve a smaller than recommended margin (in millimetres) to preserve important structures and minimize aesthetic damage. It is, however, **not** sensible to plan an excision that will leave a macroscopically positive margin.

The majority of patients with skin cancers on the head and neck may be surgically treated using local anaesthesia with or without sedation (see Chapter 4). A smaller group of patients (about 30% in major units) will require a general anaesthetic for the surgery and reconstruction.

Reconstruction of cutaneous surgical defects

There are a number of options in healing cutaneous surgical defects (see Chapter 17). These include healing by secondary intention, primary closure, skin grafting, local tissue transfer with random pattern or axial flaps and free flaps. The choice is based on the individual patient's needs including the defect, the patient's comorbidity and wishes and the resources available. A particular reconstructive technique may offer a clearly superior result, but if not the simplest choice is usually the best one.

No repair

It has been shown that healing by secondary intention can give excellent functional and cosmetic results, particularly if it is used for small defects in concave regions. This technique may also be useful in larger areas in some patients in whom contraction of the wound during healing is not cosmetically or functionally important. The longer healing time, increased wound care and poorer cosmesis must be taken into account when judging the appropriateness of this technique (Figure 18.7 (a) and (b)).

Primary closure allows quick reconstruction, rapid healing and a linear scar and is often the simplest reconstructive approach. If the technique can be accomplished without significant tension across the wound and with the suture line lying in the lines of relaxed skin tension or favourable skin line with no dog ears, then this approach may well be the best available. Any distortion of free margins or an anatomical subunit within the face, as well

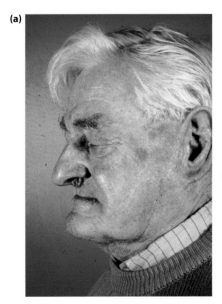

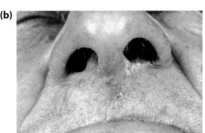

Figure 18.7 Basal cell carcinoma of the nasal base (a) treated by excision, with healing by secondary intention (b).

Table 18.1 Phases of scar healing

Red phase	First 2–3 months following surgery, the scar becomes red, raised, tight and itchy and increasingly becomes more visible.
Pink phase	Slow settlement of the scar occurs, with fewer symptoms and a progressively less visible appearance.
White phase	The scar becomes pale, soft and flat and blends into the facial lines.

The process is complete at approximately 1 year.

as the creation of long linear lines of poor aesthetic appearance, would be an indication to consider another reconstructive option.

With these and other techniques it is important that an explanation to the individual patient be given of the stages of wound healing and the physical changes that will occur with time after the surgery. This will help patients understand the slow improvement that will occur and will explain the variety of symptoms they may experience following the surgery as the wounds heal and the scars develop and mature (Table 18.1).

Skin grafts

Skin grafts may be the treatment of choice in certain defects, but equally they may be the only option because of a lack of adjacent tissue or the size of defect. Three types of grafts are commonly used (full-thickness, split-thickness and composite) but the full-thickness skin graft is the most useful for facial reconstruction. Commonly used as the treatment of choice for the nasal tip and the lower eyelid, it is useful for defects of the nasal alae (Figure 18.8 (a), (b) and (c)) and the ear, as well as for larger defects of the temple and forehead. Suitable donor sites are the postauricular region and the supraclavicular area of the neck.

The perichondrial cutaneous graft is more substantial and three-dimensionally stable than normal full-thickness grafts. It is harvested from the conchal bowl of the ear by taking both skin and perichondrium for grafting of the nose or eyelids. This donor site defect is reconstructed with an island flap ('flip flop flap') from the postauricular sulcus.

Split-thickness grafts are harvested from the inner thigh (Figure 18.9 (a)) or arm either manually or with an electric dermatome and are useful for large defects, particularly of the scalp (Figure 18.9 (b)). Because these grafts allow more contraction than full-thickness grafts, they must be used with care on the face and close to free margins and are usually the last reconstructive choice in these areas.

For all skin grafts there must be sufficient vascular tissue in the defect bed to support the graft, to allow initial diffusion of oxygen and nutrients to the graft (osmotic imbibition), followed by

(a) (b) (c)

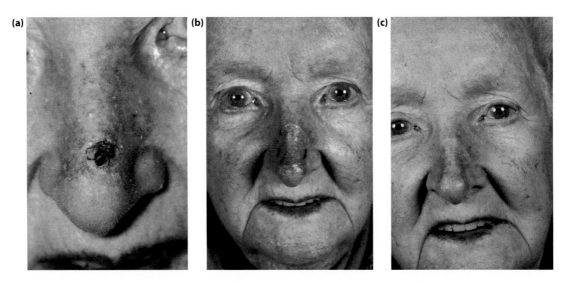

Figure 18.8 Basal cell carcinoma of the nose treated by excision and full-thickness skin graft before (a), during (b) and after (c) long-term results of healing.

(a)

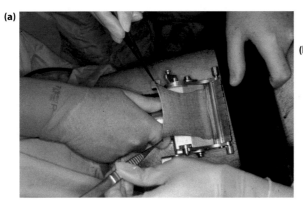

(b)

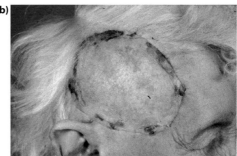

Figure 18.9 (a) Harvesting a split-thickness skin graft from the thigh. (b) Split-thickness skin grafting of the right scalp and temple.

revascularization around the fourth to the seventh day. Bare bone, tendon or cartilage will not allow grafts to take, and other reconstructive options must be employed. Following skin grafting to a defect site, the avoidance of movement or shear of the graft on the vascular bed during the healing phase is vital and necessitates careful stabilization of the graft with sutures and appropriate dressings such as a tie-over pack (Figure 18.10) or negative pressure splinting (Vac-Pac) for up to 10 days. Infection and the development of a haematoma between the graft and the defect bed are the two other major causes of graft failure.

When properly chosen, skin grafts are often functionally and aesthetically successful. The disadvantages are that the colour, texture and physical bulk may not match the original tissue and may be inferior to the result that could be achieved with a local flap. Occasionally hypopigmentation or hyperpigmentation can occur in the skin graft, and it is cosmetically detrimental.

Local flaps

The movement of local tissue from an area of surplus into the surgical defect that still allows closure of the donor site offers significant advantages in facial reconstruction. The disadvantages are that flaps require additional incisions, and tissue movements can distort skin and may lead to increased complications. These flaps certainly require greater surgical skill, knowledge and practice.

THE ADVANTAGES OF LOCAL FLAPS

- They can cover bare bone, tendon and cartilage.
- Tissue bulk can be restored and with similar tissue.
- Distortion of free margins within the cosmetic subunits can be avoided.
- They can frequently be aesthetically superior.

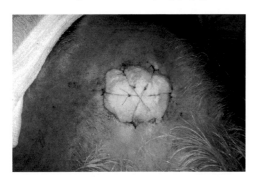

Figure 18.10 Stabilization of skin grafts is necessary. Proflavine-soaked packs and sponges are commonly used.

When assessing skin cancer for repair, the site and the resulting defect that will occur following its excision have to be thought through. The surgeon draws on the patient with a skin marker pen (before any local anaesthetic is given – it distorts the tissues), to show first the visible extent of the tumour margin and then the surgical excision margins outside this visible tumour margin; this drawing gives both the surgeon and the patient a visual impression of the defect and clarity regarding the procedure. Visual aids such as diagrams and before and after photographs of similar lesions that show the progress of healing and the maturation of scars over a year are very useful for counselling the patient and for developing the patient's understanding and tolerance of the surgery and its likely reasonable functional and aesthetic results.

The design of local flaps should take into account the natural facial lines, the junction lines between cosmetic units and the lines of relaxed skin tension, for placing the resultant scars in these lines to achieve camouflage wherever possible. An irregular pattern of scars is often less noticeable than a long linear scar, and local flaps allow reconstruction with adjacent tissue of similar colour, texture and thickness.

The diagrams represent the concepts of reservoirs of facial spare tissue (Figure 18.11), the lines of relaxed skin tension and the facial cosmetic units and subunits (Figure 18.12). The judgement involved in flap surgery is to assess how much tissue can safely be moved from one site to another while allowing closure of the donor site, preferably in a line of relaxed skin tension. Each individual varies, but the temple, cheeks, jowl, nasolabial area and glabella are characteristic reservoirs of excess tissue. Cosmetic or aesthetic units can be further divided into subunits; examples are the nose, eyelids, cheeks and temples. From a surgical viewpoint,

the importance lies in trying to reconstruct defects in those units with tissue from within the same unit and wherever possible avoiding moving tissue across a well-defined junction line from one unit to another.

The junction lines represent the areas between the cosmetic units and, along with the visible wrinkle lines of the individual patient and those lines seen in facial expression, allow scar placement with maximum disguise. However, relaxed skin tension lines are not always visible and may not always coincide with the patient's visible lines. These lines indicate the directional pull that exists in relaxed skin, and surgical incisions should be parallel to these lines.

Tissue movement with flaps

Classically there are three types of tissue movement in flap surgery:

- Advancement.
- Rotation.
- Transposition.

Frequently the flaps show combinations of these movements. When tissue is moved from one site to another, as well as the primary movement of the flap itself, there is a secondary movement of adjacent tissue to which it is sewn as the flap pulls that tissue

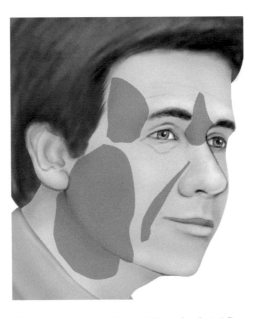

Figure 18.11 The reservoirs of 'lax' tissue that can be mobilized for facial flaps.

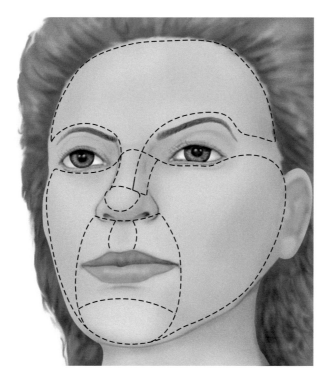

Figure 18.12 The cosmetic units of the face.

toward it. The consequences of this pull and secondary movement are particularly important when the flaps are close to free or distortable margins, such as the eyelids (Figure 18.13), lips or the nasal rim, so that this pull does not cause anatomical distortion.

The three types of flap are illustrated in the following section.

Reconstruction of anatomical structures

Scalp

The scalp is a relatively inelastic structure because of the presence of the galea aponeurotica, and large flaps are required to reconstruct small defects. Should flaps be required to reconstruct large defects or maintain hairlines, then tissue expansion before flap surgery (Figure 18.14 (a), (b) and (c)), or a decision to use very large flaps bilaterally to allow sufficient laxity for closure (Figure 18.15 (a) and (b)), is needed. Many scalp

lesions are treated with surgical excision below the galea layer. In this instance the pericranium should be preserved to allow reconstruction with skin grafts. If this is not possible, grafting onto bone can be successful if the dense cortical bone is removed and the graft is placed in contact with diploe. Generally this would be an indication for a flap. Full-thickness grafts are appropriate for smaller lesions (Figure 18.16 (a), (b) and (c)), whereas large areas often require split-thickness grafting.

Forehead

The forehead has characteristics of both the face and the scalp. In general, primary closure or a local flap is preferred in the management of defects here. Because the skin is relatively tight, forehead laxity should be assessed before flaps are designed, given the significant interpatient variation. Skin grafts on the upper forehead are acceptable, but flaps designed to match the horizontal lines of

(a) **(b)**

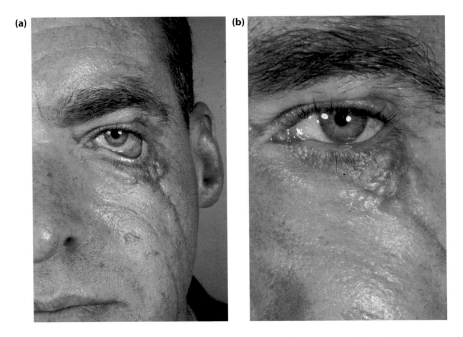

Figure 18.13 (a) Special areas such as the eyelid can be distorted following excision of tumour or trauma. (b) Distortion is corrected using a perichondral cutaneous skin graft.

(a) **(b)** **(c)**

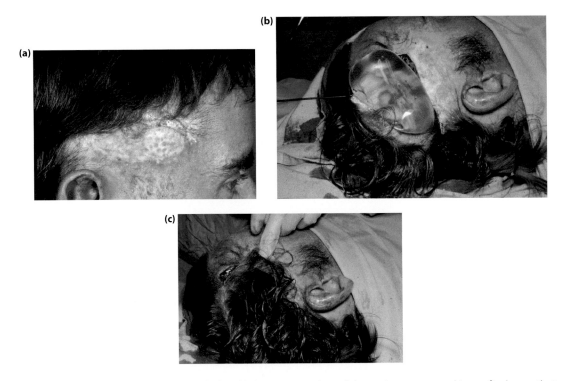

Figure 18.14 Before (a), during (b) and after (c) tissue expansion of the scalp to cover a skin grafted area that was unaesthetic following trauma.

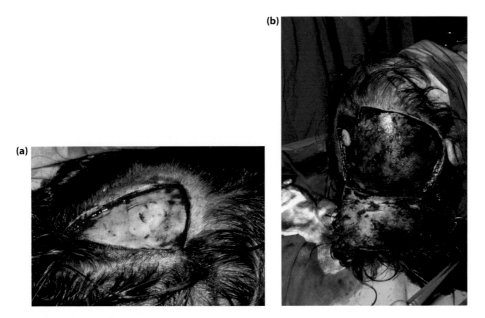

Figure 18.15 (a) and (b) The large flaps that must be raised to close excision defects in the scalp because of the relatively limited mobility of the tightly adherent scalp.

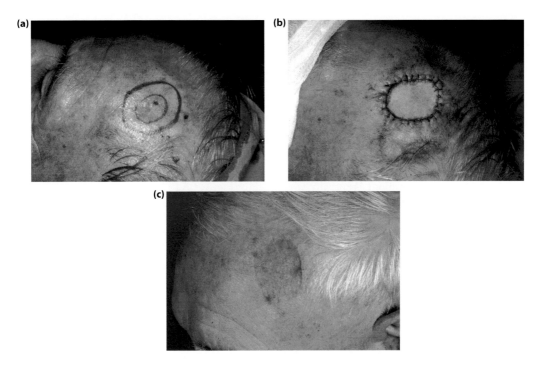

Figure 18.16 The results of a full-thickness skin graft into a small excision defect of the scalp (a) and (b) and its result at 2 months (c).

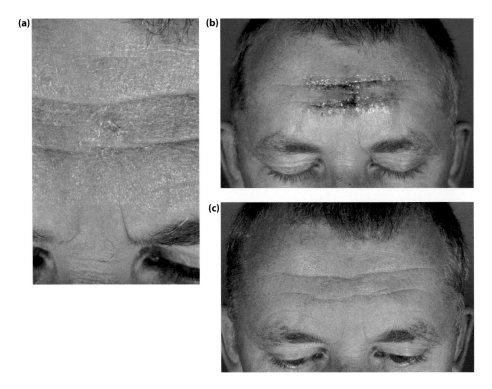

Figure 18.17 All lesions of the middle of the forehead can be closed by bilateral advancement flaps resting into vertical resting skin tension lines, as shown in the before (a), during (b) and after (c) sequence.

the forehead or the vertical lines that originate from the glabella region often give best results. Advancement flaps make maximal use of the horizontal creases and blend in to give a good aesthetic result (Figure 18.17 (a), (b) and (c)).

The anatomical position of the branches of the facial nerve can usually be predicted throughout the face, so this nerve can be spared whenever possible. Although it is acceptable to sacrifice the nerve if it is involved by tumour (generally when it is not working) when the patient is appropriately informed and counselled, it is not acceptable for this nerve to be damaged during flap surgery. Detailed knowledge of the locations where the facial nerve branches lie in relation to musculature, the superficial musculoaponeurotic system layer and the other fascial structures of the face is vital. It is also good practice to lift facial flaps in the layers above those containing sensory branches of the trigeminal nerve, so as not to create areas of anaesthesia beyond the surgical wounds.

If the facial nerve is damaged in the resection of the tumour, then the predicted deformity resulting from a lack of muscle action can in part be corrected by careful design of the flap and/or suspension of the tissues with permanent, buried periosteal sutures.

Temple

As seen in the diagram of areas of excess tissue on the face, the temple often has sufficient spare tissue for local flaps, such as the rhomboid flap (Figure 18.18 (a) and (b)). Larger lesions may require skin grafting. The use of the round block suture for larger lesions, particularly those that involve the hairline, can minimize the defect. This circumferential suture acts like a purse string in reducing the defect significantly when the suture is tightened (Figure 18.19 (a) and (b)). Depending on tissue laxity, it can completely close the defect or it can be used to reduce the defect by 50% to 60%, thus allowing a smaller skin graft to be used centrally. It has the advantage of pulling the hairline into a more anatomically correct position. The significant cutaneous deformities that result initially from this stitch gradually disappear as the skin relaxes. The stitch is usually retained for at

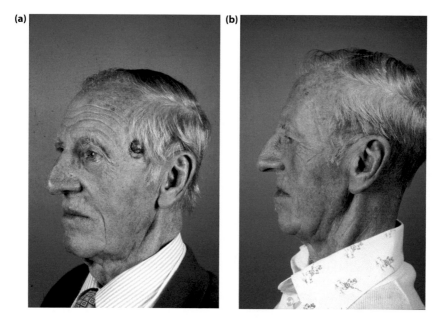

Figure 18.18 (a) and (b) The outline of the rhomboid flap and its use in treating basal cell cancer of the temple.

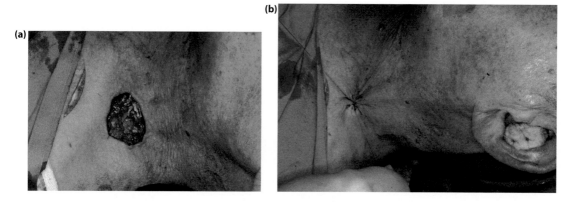

Figure 18.19 The perioperative (a) and postoperative (b) results of the round the block purse-string suture technique.

least 2 weeks if a skin graft is used or for 4 weeks and more if complete closure is the desired result. This method of closure is a simple procedure that is particularly applicable in the temple, cheeks and neck in elderly patients with lax skin.

Cheek

The cheek is a relatively safe area in which to practice cutaneous surgery because the skin is lax, with favourable lines, particularly the junction lines, which hide scars well. These include the nasofacial, nasolabial and preauricular areas. Treatment of midcheek lesions has to take advantage of resting skin tension lines to minimize the aesthetic impact, and this is particularly important in the younger cheek, which has fewer lines in which to hide the surgical incisions and resultant scars.

The cheek is frequently considered in three subunits – the preauricular cheek, the medial cheek

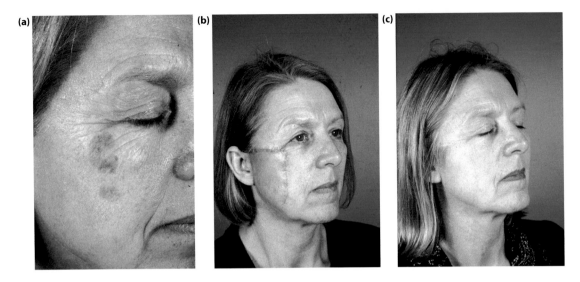

Figure 18.20 The preoperative (a), short-term postoperative (b) and long-term postoperative (c) results of a large cheek rotation flap on the right cheek.

and the midcheek. Reconstructive options vary according to these sites.

In general the cheek has a significant amount of subcutaneous fat, which makes surgery relatively safe. The inherent elasticity of the cheek allows all forms of flaps to be undertaken, limited only by individual patient-related factors. The flaps are based on the vascular perfusion pressures of those vessels present within the flap base extending to its tip and not on a simple length versus width formula (Figure 18.20 (a), (b) and (c)).

The medial cheek, as it meets the nose, is a common site for BBCs, and the subcutaneously based triangular advancement flap is frequently useful (Figure 18.21 (a), (b) and (c)). This flap has the skin cut in a triangular fashion but with its deep connections via the subcutaneous fat left intact. The laxity of the base allows advancement based

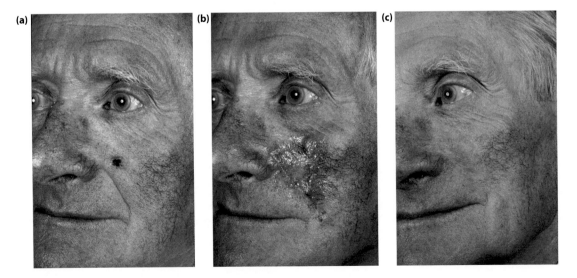

Figure 18.21 The preoperative (a) short-term postoperative (b) and long-term postoperative (c) results with the subcutaneously based triangular advancement flap.

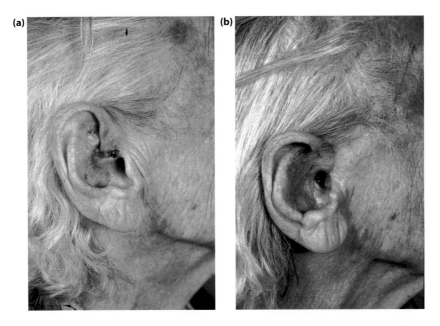

Figure 18.22 The preoperative (a) and postoperative (b) results of excision of a squamous cell carcinoma and the underlying cartilage of the ear with a full-thickness skin graft repair.

on the subcutaneous pedicle and careful closure in a V-Y fashion.

Transposition flaps are frequently used on the cheek, and careful assessment of where the scars will lie needs to be made to maximize the number of scars that will lie within the lines of relaxed skin tension.

Flaps in the region of the eyelid may need periosteal suspension sutures, which take up the tension within the flap to prevent excessive pull on the lax tissue of the eyelid that can result in ectropion.

Ear

The ear is morphologically complex, composed of skin and underlying cartilage, both of which are important for function and cosmesis. Significant tissue loss at the margins is particularly noticeable. Surprisingly, if the structure and shape of the ear can be maintained, a reduction in size can often pass unnoticed.

Central defects of the ear should be repaired with full-thickness skin grafting because it provides a simple and effective reconstruction so long as the support for the margins is maintained.

A prerequisite for this procedure is that the skin on one side of the cartilage and the cartilage itself are removed. This allows the grafting to take place on the perichondrium of the other side for its vascular support (Figure 18.22 (a) and (b)).

Wedge excision of defects of the rim (helix) of the ear can be successful, but this procedure should be used only for small defects that allow tension-free closure and no cupping or shape distortion of the ear resulting from tension within the cartilage. Larger defects of the helix and other tissues of the ear are best addressed with rim or chondrocutaneous advancement flaps, with an intact posterior skin pedicle providing the vascularity (Figure 18.23 (a), (b), (c) and (d)). This procedure allows reconstruction of the ear with a relatively normal shape, albeit somewhat smaller. One of the primary functions of the external ear is to act as a support for the individual's glasses – do not forget how important this is to the patient.

Pedicle flaps from areas of lax tissue in the postauricular sulcus or the neck are possible and can reconstruct larger defects of the rim in two-stage techniques if rim advancements are not possible.

Reconstruction of the whole ear is a major undertaking and can be addressed by a multistage surgical technique involving cartilage from another source

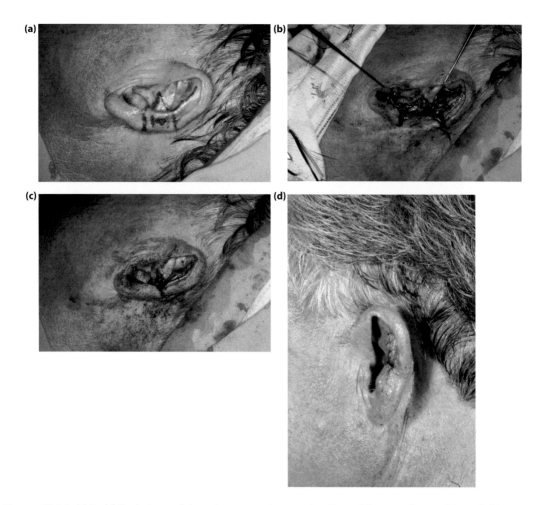

Figure 18.23 (a) to (d) Technique of rim advancement reconstruction of the ear after excision of skin cancer.

(e.g. the rib), followed by soft tissue cover obtained from the temporoparietal region. This specialist service requires experience and is undertaken in only a few centres. Osseointegrated implant-borne prosthetic reconstruction of the ear is frequently successful and is a cheaper and easier option.

Nose

The nose is one of the most challenging areas of the face to reconstruct. A variety of flaps may be used according to the site and extent of the tumour and depending on which cosmetic subunits are involved in the tumour and the respective repair. Reconstruction should consider not only the skin of the nose, but also the underlying structures including bone, cartilage and muscle, which are crucial for the maintenance of nasal respiratory function. Full-thickness defects of the nose must involve internal and external reconstruction.

Mobile skin is at a premium on the nose, with little available toward the tip because of its fibrosebaceous nature and a relative absence of subcutaneous fat. The upper two thirds of the nose has slightly more mobile skin that may be used for primary closure or local flaps. Interpersonal variability in the amount of lax skin is common, and every patient should be assessed by the simple method of pinching the skin to see what is potentially available. It is vital to maintain the free margins of the nose, particularly the alar rims, so that elevation or distortion does not occur. Despite the limited tissue available for local flaps, reconstruction of nasal defects is best undertaken with these procedures because they allow the return of normal contour, colour and texture. If a local flap is not feasible full-thickness skin grafts are used.

Bilobed flaps and dorsal nasal rotation flaps are useful (Figure 18.24 (a), (b), (c) and (d)), but they must be designed not to transgress the junction lines of the face or obtund the natural creases and hollows. The face, particularly around the nose and its junction with the cheeks, is a series of hills and valleys, and flaps that cross the valleys, from one cosmetic unit to another, have the potential disadvantage of leaving a bridge across a sulcus that immediately catches the eye and appears abnormal in comparison with the unaffected side.

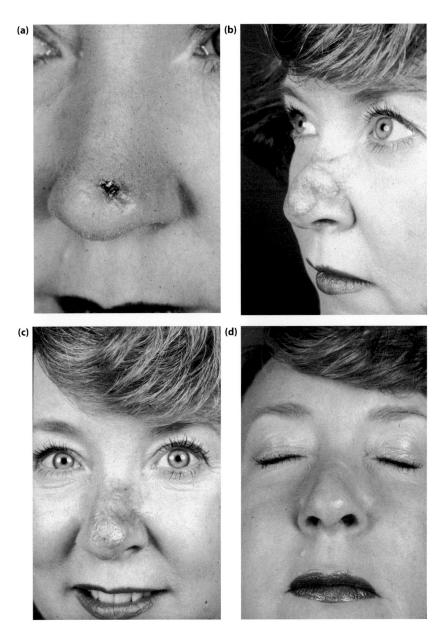

Figure 18.24 (a) to (d) Use of the bilobe flap to repair nasal defects following excision of basal cell carcinoma in a young woman.

Large or structurally complex defects that cannot be reconstructed by grafts or local flaps call for a transfer of tissue from a nearby cosmetic unit by means of a two-stage technique in which the tissue is transferred on a pedicle and is allowed to regain a blood supply at the recipient site for several weeks before second-stage division and insetting of the flap. The intervening pedicle is sacrificed, and the site of donation of tissue is either closed primarily or is closed with a skin graft.

This concept is illustrated very clearly by the paramedian forehead flap based on the supratrochlear artery, which is the flap of choice for reconstruction of large and complex nasal defects following cancer surgery (Figure 18.25 (a), (b), (c) and (d)).

Cartilaginous grafts can be inset within the layers of the flap to give structural support to the nose, and if a full-thickness defect has been created, the inner aspect of the flap can be skin grafted or have a mucosal flap placed on it from within the nose to complete the reconstruction. Division at 3 to 5 weeks occurs when the revascularization process has completed. The longer you leave it, the safer the sculpting of the flap will be. Alar rim reconstruction frequently requires a third stage for the in-turned flap that reconstructs the curved alar rim (Figure 18.26). This often needs delayed tertiary trimming, which cannot be undertaken at the second stage because of the risk to the vascularity of the flap.

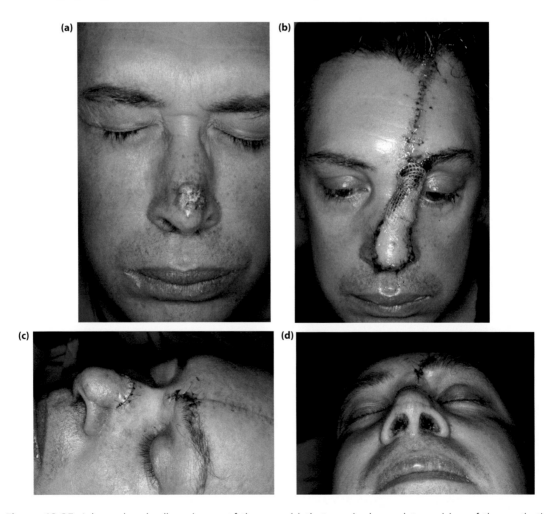

Figure 18.25 A larger basal cell carcinoma of the nose (a) that required complete excision of the aesthetic lobules and reconstruction with the two-stage paramedian forehead flap (b), (c) and (d).

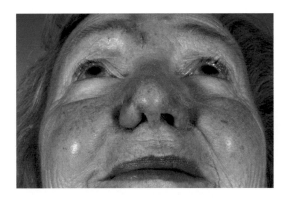

Figure 18.26 When reconstructing the alar rim with the paramedian forehead flap, a third stage is required to thin the flap and sculpt the alar rim aesthetically.

Medial canthal or lateral nasal bridge defects can be reconstructed using transposition flaps from the glabella region, which are designed to adapt to the concave area of the lateral nose and the medial canthal region. The use of thermoplastic nasal splints to hold the flap into position until suture removal improves the appearance.

As with the ear, an implant-retained prosthesis following rhinectomy can have very satisfactory results and may obviate the need for complex two-flap surgery.

Lip and chin

Cancers of the oral lip are discussed in Chapter 22. Both lips are free margins; therefore avoidance of distortion presents the greatest challenge. Many landmarks exist on the lips that, if altered, may cause disfigurement. Wedge excision with primary closure minimizes deformity when possible. Similarly, facial grooves and folds (nasolabial, melolabial) can be blunted by otherwise effective and useful flaps (Figure 18.27 (a) and (b)). This effect may be minimized by periosteal sutures to try to create a new groove.

Cutaneous defects are often treated with advancement flaps in the upper lip, such as bilateral advancement flaps or the subcutaneous triangular advancement flap (Figure 18.28 (a), (b) and (c)), which is particularly useful for lateral upper lip lesions that lie close to the nasolabial or meliolabial fold. For centrally placed defects in the lip, the best option is the perialar crescentic advancement flap, which can be used both

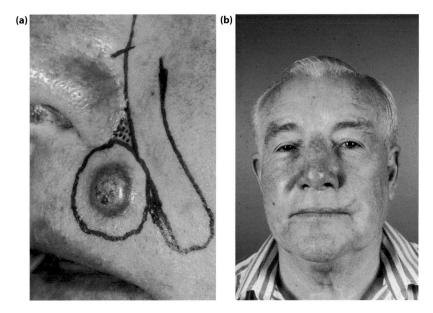

(a)   (b)

Figure 18.27 (a) and (b) The superiorly based nasolabial flap while filling the defect created blunts the nasolabial fold.

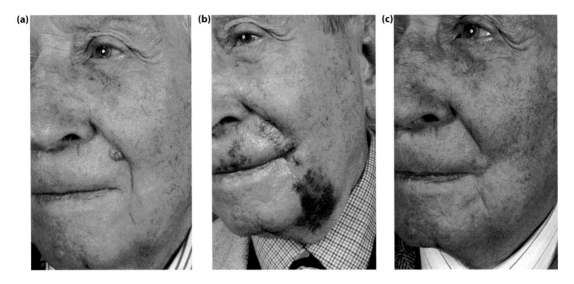

Figure 18.28 The subcutaneous island advancement flap for upper lip reconstruction (a) and (b) with a 3-month result (c).

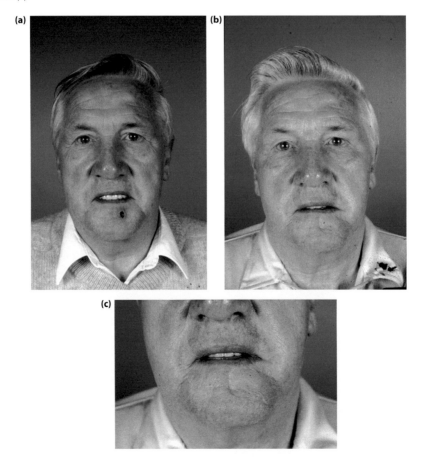

Figure 18.29 (a) to (c) Excision of a basal cell carcinoma of the chin and lower lip with flap repair maximizing the use of natural skin creases.

unilaterally and bilaterally to reconstruct difficult larger defects.

The lower lip has the same problems and reconstructive considerations as the upper lip, and any advancement flap should take note of the mentolabial crease in the design of advancement and rotation flaps.

The chin is a separate cosmetic unit. Flap design must take into account the interrelationship between chin and lower lip, so that repair of one does not compromise the other (Figure 18.29 (a), (b) and (c)). Rotation flaps using the mentolabial crease or flaps using the crease at the cheek-chin junction offer the best results in this difficult and inelastic area. Design of the flaps must be considered carefully and often increased in size to diminish any vertical tension.

Summary

Various reconstructive options for the face are available, and the overriding idea should be to replace lost tissue with tissue of the same size, elasticity, pigmentation and skin characteristics. This ideal cannot always be achieved without significant damage to other adjacent areas, thus necessitating the use of a variety of other reconstructive options ranging from skin grafts to importation of distant tissue using multistage techniques. Consideration of the patient should be uppermost in the surgeon's mind, both from the standpoint of physical reconstruction and in view of the psychological effect of this treatment on the patient. The face is the structure with which we present ourselves to the world, and its loss or damage is more keenly felt than damage to any other structure.

FURTHER READING

Bath-Hextall F, Bong J, Perkins W, Williams H. Interventions for basal cell carcinoma of the skin: systematic review. *BMJ* 2004;329: 705–8.

Gurney B, Newlands, C. Management of regional metastatic disease in head and neck cutaneous malignancy. 1. Cutaneous squamous cell carcinoma. *Br J Oral Maxillofac Surg* 2014;52:294–300.

Main BG, Coyle MJ, Godden A, Godden DR. The metastatic potential of head and neck cutaneous malignant melanoma: is sentinel node biopsy useful? *Br J Oral Maxillofac Surg* 2014;52:340–3.

Marsden RJ, Newton-Bishop JA, Burrows L, Cook M, Corrie PG, Cox NH, Gore ME, Lorigan P, Mackie R. Nathan P, Peach H, Powell B, Walker C. Revised U.K. guidelines for the management of cutaneous melanoma 2010. *Br J Dermatol* 2010;163:238–256.

Motley RJ, Preston PW, Lawrence CM. Multiprofessional guidelines for the management of the patient with primary cutaneous squamous cell carcinoma. British Association of Dermatology (BAD); 2009. www.bad.org.uk/library-media/documents/SCC_2009.pdf: 2–21.

Newlands C, Gurney, B. Management of regional metastatic disease in head and neck cutaneous malignancy. 2. Cutaneous malignant melanoma. *Br J Oral Maxillofac Surg* 2014;52:301–7.

Telfer NR, Colver GB, Morton CA. Guidelines for the management of basal cell carcinoma. *Br J Dermatol* 2008;159:35–48.

Wong CS, Strange RC, Lear JT. Basal cell carcinoma. *BMJ* 2003;327;794–8.

19

Orthognathic surgery

Contents

Aims

For both undergraduates and postgraduates:

- To be able to outline the principles of orthognathic treatment.
- To be able to discuss the scope and limitations of orthognathic treatment.

Learning outcomes

For both undergraduates and postgraduates:

- To be able to describe the principles of combined care and planning.
- To be able to demonstrate basic assessment of common facial anomaly patterns.
- To describe the steps of common orthognathic surgical procedures and demonstrate an ability to obtain informed consent.

- To describe preoperative and postoperative management.
- To discuss the stability of surgical procedures.

Introduction

Orthognathic treatment, which has evolved over the years, is concerned with the correction of certain aspects of dentofacial deformity. It requires a team approach and is not just about an operation. Members of the team include an orthodontist, a maxillofacial surgeon, anesthetists, nursing staff, hygienists, clinical psychologists, psychiatrists, dieticians, speech and language therapists and general dental practitioners. Obviously, it may not be possible or desirable to incorporate all these disciplines in the multidisciplinary clinics, but access to the various specialties should be available.

Indications

Orthognathic treatment can improve patients' function (e.g. mastication in patients with a large anterior open bite), appearance or both. It has a major facial and dental aesthetic component. It may be the only viable option for those patients with a skeletal or dental discrepancy outside the limits of that achievable with orthodontic treatment alone. Masking of the skeletal discrepancy may be possible orthodontically, but this will essentially address the dental problem only and may lead to an unsatisfactory facial aesthetic result. Orthognathic treatment is required in those selected patients whose skeletal discrepancy would not be addressed by orthodontic camouflage. Examples include:

- Severe class II malocclusions.
- Severe class III malocclusions.
- Anterior open bite.
- Skeletal asymmetry.
- Significant vertical discrepancies.
- Markedly increased overbite in adults.

General assessment

History

A prime reason for taking a history is to identify the patient's perception of the problem. Occasionally a cause (e.g. a family trait, congenital deformity, or trauma in infancy) is identified, although usually there is no obvious aetiological factor.

The history is also used to assess the patient's fitness for surgery. This is entirely elective surgery; therefore, it is even more essential that any risks to the patient be kept to a minimum.

Patients present with various complaints. Most patients are concerned about their appearance; they may also be concerned about their ability to chew, bite or speak. Occasionally patients are referred in the belief that their temporomandibular joint (TMJ) dysfunction may be helped by surgery. There is little evidence that the correction of malocclusion can improve TMJ pain or dysfunction. It is inadvisable to promote orthognathic treatment as a treatment for TMJ conditions. During the consent process patients should

be advised that preexisting TMJ symptoms may worsen, persist or improve because the effect of orthognathic treatment on the TMJ is entirely unpredictable.

When assessing patients, one must always be mindful of those patients with unrealistic expectations. Some patients have excessive concern for minor or imperceptible abnormalities and may produce diagrams or photographs showing how they would like to appear. Some believe that an operation would improve their relationships or job prospects and would thus provide an instant solution to their problems. These patients may react unfavourably postoperatively. It is, however, true that in carefully selected patients with realistic expectations, surgical correction can bring about great satisfaction and improved social confidence.

Clinical examination

The clinic examination should consist of a systematic approach to both the soft and hard tissues.

Profile

The patient should be sitting comfortably with the Frankfort plane horizontal. It is useful here to consider the concept that the face is divided into thirds – upper, middle and lower. The lower third is itself divided into thirds; the upper lip is one third compared with the lower two thirds, which extend from the lower lip margin (stomion) to the chin margin (menton). Facial aesthetics is maintained when the lower face height is about 50% to 55% of the total face height when measured from nasion to menton. The relationship of the maxilla with mandible is noted (skeletal classification). In the maxilla, prognathism or retrognathism can be diagnosed because the face will appear more convex or concave, respectively. In addition, look at the shape and size of the nose.

The nasolabial angle is normally about 90°. Retraction of the upper incisors may open this angle, thereby leading to poorer aesthetics by potentially causing dishing of the lower face and making the nose more prominent (Figure 19.1).

The important horizontal relationship of the maxilla with the mandible can be assessed.

The most common problems are mandibular prognathism and retrognathism. By examining the

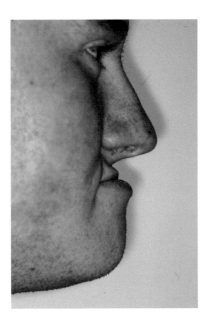

Figure 19.1 Patient with a class III skeletal relationship, showing an acute nasolabial angle.

maxilla first, apparent mandibular prognathism caused by a hypoplastic maxilla can be ruled out (Figure 19.2). Some clinicians place cotton wool under the patient's upper lip to mimic maxillary advancement. Similarly, the surgical correction of

a retrognathic mandible can be visualized by asking the patient to posture the mandible forward the desired amount.

Some points to consider at the planning stage include:

1. Advancement of the maxilla increases upper incisor show.
2. The alar base cinch suture:
   - Controls the transverse dimension of the alar base.
   - Improves tip projection.
   - Maintains the thickness of the upper lip.
   - Decreases shortening of the upper lip.
3. Nasal tip relative to A point moves in a ratio of approximately:
   - 1:3 for Le Fort I osteotomies.
   - 1:2 for Le Fort II osteotomies.
   - 1:1 for Le Fort III osteotomies.
4. Chin:
   Soft tissue-pogonion movements – 1:1 with either mandibular advance or setback.
5. Lower lip:
   - 85% of the skeletal movement in advancement.
   - 60% in setback.

The data in Table 19.1 can be used as a guide.

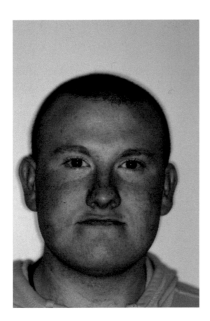

Figure 19.2 Full-face view showing paranasal hollowing indicating maxillary hypoplasia.

Table 19.1 Measurements used in orthognathic assessment

Anatomical area	Measurement
Intercanthal width	34 ± 4 mm
Alar base width	34 ± 4 mm
Interpupillary distance	65 ± 4 mm
Upper lip length	22 mm (male), 20 mm (female)
Lower lip length	33 mm (male), 30 mm (female)
Upper incisor show	0–3 mm (at rest), 7–10 mm (smiling)
Nasolabial angle	90°–120°
Labiomental angle	115°–135°
Lower face height	66 mm (male), 60 mm (female)
Midface height	66 mm (male), 60 mm (female)

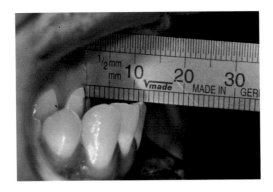

Figure 19.3 Patient with a reverse overjet of approximately 12 mm.

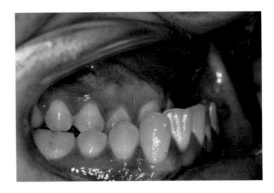

Figure 19.5 Intraoral view showing a class III incisal relationship.

Full face

Examine any asymmetry of the face, including the level of the eyes. This is the time to compare facial and dental midlines, which can then be transferred to the study casts. Any cant in the occlusal plane can be confirmed by placing a wooden spatula transversely between the teeth. Lip seal and incisor show both at rest and during smiling should be measured. Overjet can be measured directly (Figure 19.3). This allows assessment of any excessive incisor or gingival show, an important baseline in surgical planning.

Intraoral examination

The molar and incisal relationships are examined visually and are formally documented by photographs (Figures 19.4, 19.5 and 19.6) and study models.

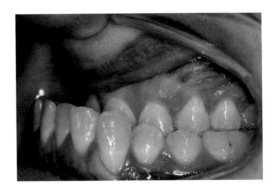

Figure 19.6 Intraoral view showing a class III incisal relationship.

A thorough dental examination should take place, especially noting oral hygiene and carious teeth. Routine dental care must be completed, and the patient should be referred back to the general dental practitioner for this care.

Temporomandibular joints

Patients are often referred to orthognathic clinics either for the management of TMJ dysfunction or with coincident symptoms and signs. Therefore a thorough history and examination must be performed. The problem should be managed conservatively and the patient counseled with regard to the effects of surgery on the condition. TMJ dysfunction has a multifactorial aetiology (see Chapter 14).

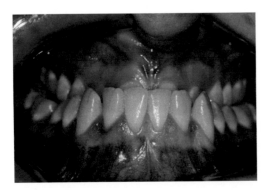

Figure 19.4 Intraoral view showing a class III incisal relationship.

ORTHOGNATHIC EXAMINATION – BRIEF GUIDANCE FOR CLINICAL USE

1. Introduction.
   - Thank you for being here today.
   - This is what I am going to do:
     - I will ask you a few questions (Name, age, past medical history, social history).
     - I will look at you from all angles.
     - I will take down some notes.
     - I will discuss with you the available options.
2. Position the patient:
   - Aim for neutral head position.
   - Bring the patient to your level.
   - Bring the patient's head off the headrest.
   - Ensure that the Frankfort plane (porion to orbitale) is parallel to the floor.
3. Look from the side:
   - Anteroposterior relationship. ⟨ Maxilla / Mandible
   - Vertical relationship. ⟨ One thirds. / Frankfurt mandibular plane angle (FMPA).
   - Nasolabial angle.

4. Look from the front:
   - Symmetry (transverse relationship).
   - Alar base.
   - Upper lip length.
   - Lip competency.
   - Upper incisor show.
5. Lay the patient flat for an intraoral examination:
   - Centre line.
   - Occlusal cant.
   - Overjet.
   - Overbite.
   - Incisor relationship.
   - Canine relationship.
   - Molar relationship.
   - Cross bites.
   - Alignment or crowding.
6. Examine the temporomandibular joint.

Radiographic examination

Series of standardized radiographs are studied as part of the assessment.

Dental panoramic tomogram (DPT) – this reveals caries and periodontal disease, unerupted or impacted teeth (Figure 19.7) and the presence of coincidental pathology (e.g. cysts).

Lateral cephalogram – all orthognathic patients require this view to supplement clinical analysis with cephalometric analysis (Figure 19.8).

Intraoral radiographs – these are obtained as needed.

Upper anterior occlusal view – there are various intraoral films, but the upper anterior occlusal is the most commonly used. This view is essential for the assessment of unerupted canine teeth.

Cephalometric analysis – this is, in essence, the measurement of the skull and facial bones by using agreed angulations and linear distances to aid in determining the underlying aetiology of a particular problem (Figures 19.9 and 19.10). Many analyses exist, with varying degrees of complexity. Some have a specific set of indications for use. However, most clinicians favour a few analyses with which they are familiar.

The Bolton standard is a widely used analysis. This is a composite tracing that contains average measurements with each year of age. This analysis is based on a small number of the white population of the United States of either sex.

It is important to remember that a patient is being treated, and not a radiograph, so whichever analysis is used, it is only a guide. Table 19.2 shows

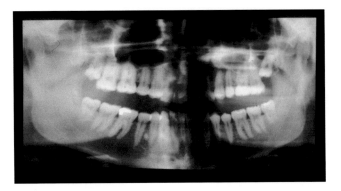

Figure 19.7 A dental panoramic tomogram of a patient showing wisdom teeth destined for removal in an otherwise 'dentally fit' person.

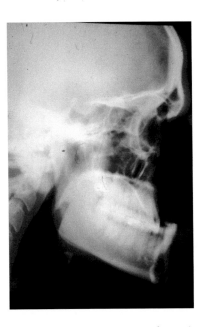

Figure 19.8 A lateral cephalogram of a patient with a class III malocclusion.

some commonly used values. See the later section on the German perspective.

Photographs

These usually consist of a standardized set of photographs. Extraoral photographs consist of full face at rest and smiling, right and left three-quarter face views and right and left profiles. Intraoral views should show anterior and buccal teeth in occlusion.

Some clinicians like to construct a montage using the lateral cephalogram and profile photograph in a 1:1 ratio. This tries to mimic postsurgical soft tissue movement. This technique, like computer-generated programmes that purport to simulate the variable impact of surgical movement of the jaws, has limitations, and one must be careful not to mislead the patient or impart unrealistic expectations.

Study models

Records are taken at various stages of treatment, usually before and after orthodontic treatment, before and after surgical intervention and at review appointments at yearly intervals for up to 5 years after treatment. These records are combined with a record of the occlusion in the form of a wax squash bite (Figure 19.11). The models are trimmed in a standardized manner. On the models, markings can be made with the patient present (e.g. the facial midline in relation to the dental midline). Models can be taken at various stages of treatment and are used for differing reasons (e.g. clinical records, orthodontic planning and model surgery).

Before orthognathic surgery, the patient has a face-bow recording (Figure 19.12), and the most recent study models are mounted on a semiadjustable or fully adjustable anatomical articulator (Figures 19.13 and 19.14). These models are duplicated for the fabrication of occlusal wafers, which are essential for perioperative localization of the maxilla in bimaxillary procedures.

Model surgery is performed to gauge whether a satisfactory occlusion is attainable, and it also gives

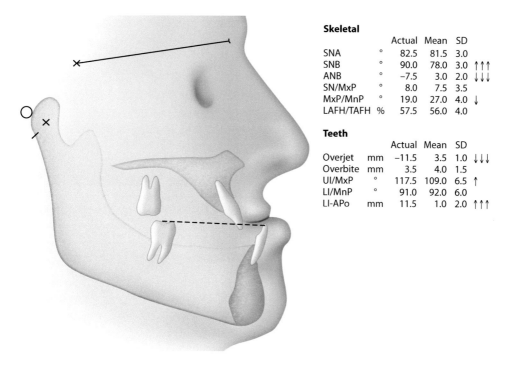

Skeletal

		Actual	Mean	SD	
SNA	°	82.5	81.5	3.0	
SNB	°	90.0	78.0	3.0	↑↑↑
ANB	°	−7.5	3.0	2.0	↓↓↓
SN/MxP	°	8.0	7.5	3.5	
MxP/MnP	°	19.0	27.0	4.0	↓
LAFH/TAFH	%	57.5	56.0	4.0	

Teeth

		Actual	Mean	SD	
Overjet	mm	−11.5	3.5	1.0	↓↓↓
Overbite	mm	3.5	4.0	1.5	
UI/MxP	°	117.5	109.0	6.5	↑
LI/MnP	°	91.0	92.0	6.0	
LI-APo	mm	11.5	1.0	2.0	↑↑↑

Figure 19.9 Computerized traced cephalometric analysis. ANB, A point, nasion, B point; Apo, A point, pogonion; LAFH, lower anterior facial height; LI, lower incisor; MnP, mandibular plane; MxP, maxillary plane; SD, standard deviation; SN, sella, nasion; SNA, sella, nasion, A point; SNB, sella, nasion, B point; TAFH, total anterior facial height; UI; upper incisor.

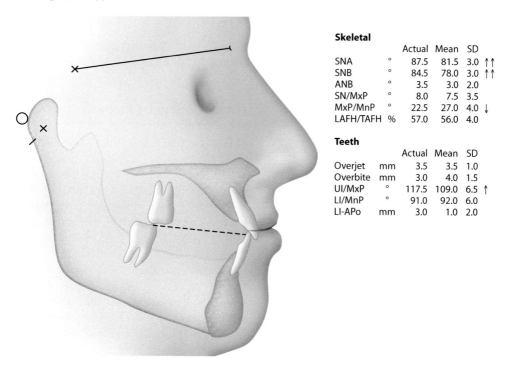

Skeletal

		Actual	Mean	SD	
SNA	°	87.5	81.5	3.0	↑↑
SNB	°	84.5	78.0	3.0	↑↑
ANB	°	3.5	3.0	2.0	
SN/MxP	°	8.0	7.5	3.5	
MxP/MnP	°	22.5	27.0	4.0	↓
LAFH/TAFH	%	57.0	56.0	4.0	

Teeth

		Actual	Mean	SD	
Overjet	mm	3.5	3.5	1.0	
Overbite	mm	3.0	4.0	1.5	
UI/MxP	°	117.5	109.0	6.5	↑
LI/MnP	°	91.0	92.0	6.0	
LI-APo	mm	3.0	1.0	2.0	

Figure 19.10 Computerized predictive analysis (Opal). Abbreviations are as in Figure 19.9.

Table 19.2 Mean angular cephalometric values

Measurement	Mean angle (°) ± SD
SNA	81 ± 3
SNB	78 ± 3
ANB	3 ± 2
SN/maxillary plane	8 ± 3
SN/mandibular plane	35 ± 4
Maxillary/mandibular plane	27 ± 4
Upper incisor/maxillary plane	109 ± 6
Interincisal angle	130 ± 6
Lower incisor/mandibular plane	93 ± 6

ANB, A point, nasion, B point; SD, standard deviation; SN, sella nasion; SNA, sella, nasion, A point; SNB, sella, nasion, B point.

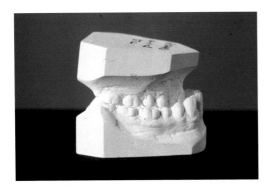

Figure 19.11 Trimmed study models.

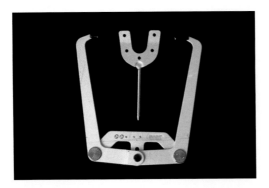

Figure 19.12 A face bow for recording the relative positions of the jaws and fixed cranial and facial reference points.

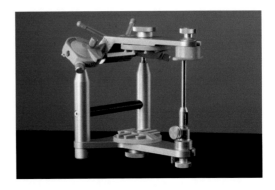

Figure 19.13 Semiadjustable articulator (clinical).

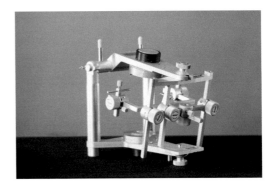

Figure 19.14 Semiadjustable articulator (laboratory).

a measure of the required surgical movements (Figure 19.15 (a) and (b)).

Orthodontic treatment

The presurgical orthodontic phase is designed to place the teeth in their correct position over the dental bases before surgery. This treatment involves the correction of dental alignment (Figure 19.16), arch leveling, decompensation of teeth in all three planes of space and arch coordination.

It is essential that both the patient and the orthodontic and surgical team are clear about this phase because orthodontic decompensation before surgery will make the occlusal relationships significantly worse. The presurgical orthodontic phase can last between 12 and 18 months (Figure 19.17), and it would be utterly inappropriate for the patient then to decide that he or she did not want surgery because all the preceding treatment would have been moving the teeth in

(a) 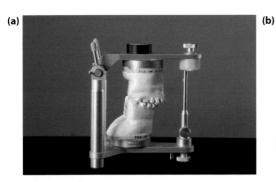 **(b)**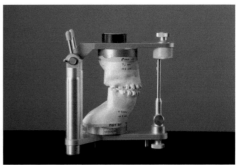

Figure 19.15 Model surgery: (a) preoperative view; (b) postoperative appearance.

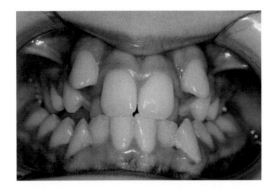

Figure 19.16 Dental crowding that will require preoperative orthodontic correction.

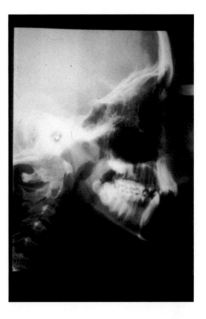

Figure 19.18 A lateral cephalogram of a patient with a class II division 1 malocclusion before orthodontic treatment.

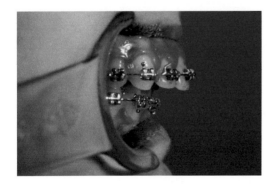

Figure 19.17 Intraoral view of a patient with a class II division 1 malocclusion who is undergoing treatment.

the opposite way from that used by orthodontic camouflage (Figures 19.18 and 19.19).

Postsurgical orthodontic treatment involves final detailing of the occlusion and should be kept as brief as possible.

Common surgical procedures

It is a prerequisite that the patient should be adequately assessed and prepared for surgery. This includes the preoperative, intraoperative and postoperative phases (see Chapter 5). The removal of third molars before orthognathic surgery is commonly performed to avoid poor splits. The presence of third molars during sagittal split osteotomies is not associated with an increased frequency of unfavourable fractures. Concomitant third molar removal in sagittal split osteotomies also decreases

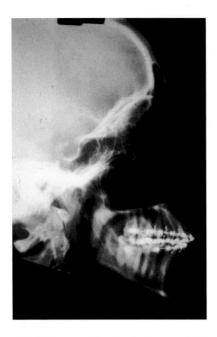

Figure 19.19 Same patient as in Figure 19.18 undergoing orthodontic decompensation.

proximal segment inferior alveolar nerve entrapment but only slightly increases operating time (Doucet et al. 2012).

Mandibular procedures

Ramus surgery

Bilateral sagittal split osteotomy

Bilateral sagittal split osteotomy (BSSO) is one of the most commonly performed and versatile mandibular procedures (Figure 19.20 (a), (b) and (c)). It can be used for backward or forward correction of the mandible in isolation or in combination with a maxillary osteotomy. It is usually performed while the patient is under general anaesthesia. It was originally described by Trauner and Obwegeser in 1957. The procedure has since undergone numerous modifications, including those by Dalpont, Hunsuck, Bell and Epker.

Even when there are large advancements, bone grafting is rarely required because of the long bony

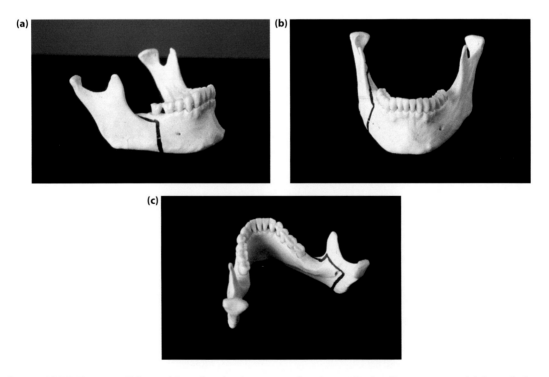

Figure 19.20 Dry mandible markings for the bone cuts for the sagittal split osteotomy: (a) buccal view; (b) anterior view; (c) lingual view.

interface between the two fragments. Indications for BSSO include mandibular advancement, setback and correction of asymmetry. It is contraindicated in ramus hypoplasia, narrow lateral to medial ramus thickness and severe asymmetries.

BSSO has several advantages and disadvantages.

Advantages
- The mandible can be advanced, set back or rotated in an axial plane to allow correction of asymmetry.
- Rigid fixation can be employed to allow early mobilization of the mandible and easier management of the airway.
- Healing is rapid, with predictable bony union.
- It has good stability.

Disadvantages
- There is an incidence of inferior alveolar nerve damage that can lead to altered sensation of the lower lip. Although this is usually temporary, permanent loss can occur. Interestingly, lingual nerve problems are rarely encountered.
- Unfavorable mandibular splitting may occur such that rigid fixation is impossible.

Vertical subsigmoid osteotomy

Vertical subsigmoid osteotomy (VSS) is a relatively simple and rapid osteotomy (Figure 19.21). It can be approached either extraorally or intraorally. However, for intraoral VSS specialized equipment is required, although this is not unusual in most centres in the developed world. The procedure involves making a vertical cut from the sigmoid notch to the angle of the mandible/antegonial notch. In essence, a condylotomy is performed to allow the mandible to be set back. The main indication for VSS is for mandibular setback when the movements are small. It can be a good alternative to BSSO. Larger movements may require coronoidectomies. VSS can be used to correct asymmetries where the mandible is set back on both sides. It cannot be used for mandibular advancements unless bone grafting is also used.

Advantages
- The procedure is rapid and easy to perform.
- It is excellent for small setbacks.

Disadvantages
- In units without the specialist equipment for intraoral rigid fixation (right-angle drills and screwdriver), intermaxillary fixation is required for about 6 weeks.
- It is difficult to control the condylar position.
- The extraoral approach (which does allow fixation) leaves visible scars.
- Bony union may take longer to achieve.
- In correcting asymmetries, if one fragment needs advancement when it was anticipated, it would require a setback, and a VSS has no flexibility.

Inverted-L osteotomy

This is a relatively rare operation in most practices (Figure 19.22). It is very similar to VSS in its approaches, indications, contraindications, advantages and disadvantages. It is said that ramus elongation or advancement can occur if the inverted-L

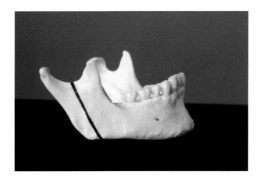

Figure 19.21 Bone cuts for the vertical subsigmoid osteotomy.

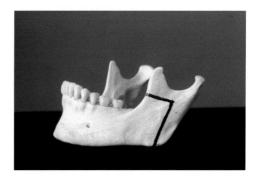

Figure 19.22 Bone cuts for the inverted-L osteotomy.

osteotomy is used in conjunction with a bone graft. Occasionally rigid fixation is possible.

Complications of ramus surgery
General complications
- Bleeding.
- Infections.
- Nonunion or delayed union.
- Malunion.

Specific complications
- Nerve damage.
- Unfavorable splitting.
- Condylar sag.
- Relapse, both early and late.
- TMJ dysfunction, oedema, haemarthrosis.
- Tooth extrusion.
- Periodontal problems.

Mandibular segmental procedures

These operations are designed to alter dentoalveolar segments. The indications for these operations are probably diminishing because orthodontic treatment can manage most problems.

Anterior subapical osteotomy (Köle procedure)

This procedure is performed anterior to the mental foramina, usually from canine to canine (Figure 19.23). Vertical osteotomies are placed interdentally and are joined by a horizontal cut below the apices of the teeth. An obvious prerequisite is space between the teeth to allow instrumentation without damage.

Posterior subapical osteotomy and total subapical osteotomy

These are very difficult procedures with very few indications. The inferior alveolar nerve and vessels are at great risk, along with the tenuous blood supply and risk to the tooth root apices. These procedures have little to recommend them.

Genioplasty

Genioplasty procedures are used to move the chin. The chin can be moved forward or backward, rotated or reduced or increased in height (Figure 19.24). Genioplasty can be performed with a mandibular procedure or secondarily. These operations are not without risks (e.g. mental nerve damage), which must be borne in mind, especially when genioplasty is combined with BSSO. If genioplasty is combined with sagittal split osteotomy, the genioplasty is performed after BSSO. It is easier if the patient is left in intermaxillary fixation (IMF) while the genioplasty is carried out.

Alloplastic augmentation is advocated because of its simplicity and lesser degree of postoperative pain, oedema and ecchymoses that leads to a faster recovery. Occasionally, patients who present for aesthetic chin surgery do not have a severe dentofacial deformity and have class I occlusion and retrogenia. These patients desire an increase in chin projection, which can be accomplished with an alloplastic implant or sliding osseous genioplasty. Implants are suited for small advancements on the order of 4 to 5 mm, usually as part of a face lift procedure. The sliding osseous genioplasty can be used for shorter as well as longer advancements and is

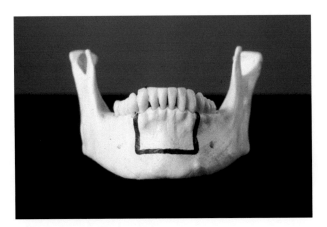

Figure 19.23 Bone cuts for the Köle subapical osteotomy.

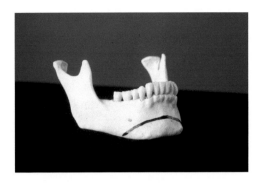

Figure 19.24 Bone cuts for genioplasty.

especially suited for vertical height alterations. The implants are susceptible to infection, more so than the hardware used in osseous genioplasty. Migration and deep bony erosion are complications unique to implants. Erosion can be limited by placing the implant low over the thicker cortex of the inferior mandible, with at least 9 cm of surface area of the base of the implant to disperse pressure, and by placing at a minimum the central position of the implant superficial to the periosteum.

Maxillary procedures

Maxillary deformities will occur in anteroposterior, transverse and vertical planes. The maxillary Le Fort I osteotomy is a versatile procedure that can address all these problems. Thus once mobilized, the maxilla can be repositioned in any plane. The stability of these moves is variably predictable.

The maxilla can also be segmented allowing levelling, narrowing or widening of the upper arch.

The approach is via a horseshoe buccal vestibular incision. Preservation of the palatine vessels is thought by some surgeons to be essential, but many operators ligate these vessels or use diathermy if required, with no apparent compromise to the vascularity of the maxilla.

Le Fort I osteotomy

The bony cuts are a straight line starting a few millimetres above the floor of the pyriform aperture and continuing backward just above the tooth root apices to the zygomatic buttress and back to where they contact the pterygoid plates (Figure 19.25 (a) and (b)). This design tends to slope downward from front to back; thus in moving the maxilla forward, it tends to move it upward as well. Similar cuts are made along the lateral nasal walls (medial wall of maxillary sinus), and the nasal septum is freed from the nasal surface of the palate (nasal floor). Pterygoid disjunction is finally performed before down fracture of the maxilla. Modifications of these cuts are described, but they are essentially variations on a theme. Some operators step the lateral cuts in the buttress region with a vertical cut (5 to 10 mm in length), with the horizontal cut then continuing backward to the pterygoid region. This is done in an attempt to prevent the unwanted upward movement. The step also gives a vertical reference point in forward repositioning. The heights of the bony cuts are limited only by the position of the infraorbital nerve. If this is carefully preserved, then even the infraorbital rims can be advanced (Kufner's modification).

Another variation is the horseshoe osteotomy, which can be done as part of a standard Le Fort I

(a)

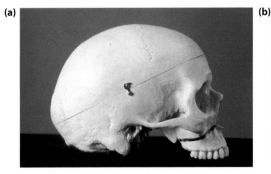

(b)

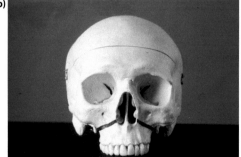

Figure 19.25 Skull showing approximate level of bony cuts for a Le Fort I osteotomy: (a) lateral view; (b) anterior view.

procedure or as a definitive osteotomy. It is indicated in superior movements, especially when attempting to gain a large impaction.

With the advent of modern orthodontic techniques, segmental surgery is seldom indicated.

Complications
General complication
- Bleeding – this can be a major problem in maxillary surgery.
- Infection.
- Nonunion.

Specific complications
- Relapse – this is more likely to occur with downward movements.
- Maxillary settling – this results from inadequate stabilization and is a posterior or vertical movement.
- Condylar distraction (sometimes called condylar sag).
- Avascular necrosis – this is an unmitigated disaster!
- Nerve injury – this is nearly always temporary and affects the infraorbital nerves.

Segmental procedures

These procedures are employed when one or more teeth, in addition, of course, to the supporting alveolus, must be moved and orthodontic correction cannot (for whatever reason) be achieved. Tunnelled approaches via limited incisions to preserve blood supply to the tooth or bone segments are used. This technique makes visualization and fixation difficult.

The Wassmund-Wunderer procedure allows movement of the upper anterior teeth *en bloc*. This can reduce an increased overjet, close a small anterior open bite and increase or decrease incisor show.

Schuchardt described a posterior segmental osteotomy based on similar principles.

The maxilla can be segmented as part of a Le Fort I osteotomy. The posterior segments can be similarly mobilized as described by Schuchardt.

Surgically assisted rapid palatal expansion

Surgically assisted rapid palatal expansion (SARPE) is a useful adjunct to either orthognathic surgery or orthodontics alone for maxillary expansion. If the maxilla is significantly hypoplastic in a lateral dimension, it is not possible to expand it orthodontically to correct a buccal crossbite. In nongrowing patients, one option is SARPE. This procedure involves making osteotomy cuts (but not fracture and mobilization) to allow orthodontic expansion by a fixed rapid maxillary expansion (RME) appliance. The extent of the bone cuts varies but should involve the lateral wall of the maxilla and often a midpalatal split. Separation of the pterygoid plates may sometimes be performed. The fixed RME is expanded at a rate of 0.25 mm twice per day.

Soft tissue procedures

- Alar base cinch suture – this is performed to control the alar base width, which nearly always increases.
- V-Y closure – this is used to reduce lip shortening.
- Inferior turbinectomy – reduction of these structures allows impaction of the maxilla and may prevent postoperative nasal obstruction.

Relapse

Relapse can be defined as movement of osteotomized fragments back to their original positions. Many of the factors that are associated with post-treatment relapse can be anticipated in advance. Good planning and an experienced team can minimize problems and take steps to avoid or limit relapse.

The University of North Carolina followed up almost 1500 patients who received surgical repositioning of the jaws for a minimum of 1 year after surgery, and more than 500 of these patients were reviewed for at least 5 years (Proffit et al. 1996).

1. Highly stable procedures:
   - Maxilla upward.
   - Mandibular advancement.
   - Genioplasty.
2. Stable procedures:
   - Maxillary advancement.
   - Two-jaw surgery for the correction of class II (maxilla upward, mandible forward) and class III (maxilla forward, mandible set back) conditions.

3. Problematic procedures:
   - Isolated mandibular setback.
   - Maxilla downward.
   - Widening of the maxilla.

For ease of discussion, the factors involved can be broadly classified as surgical, orthodontic or patient-related factors.

Surgical factors

- Size of movement – movement of the mandible greater than 8 to 10 mm or of the maxilla 6 mm forward.
- Direction of the movement – the most stable movements are an advancement smaller than 6 mm in the mandible and impaction in the maxilla. The least stable in the mandible is thought to be a setback, and the least stable in the maxilla is either a setdown or an expansion.
- Inadequate fixation.
- Distraction of the condylar heads out of the glenoid fossa – this leads to immediate relapse. It should be corrected immediately unless of course the patient is placed into IMF postoperatively, in which case it will be recognized when the IMF is released, which may be too late!
- Poor planning.
- Movements that put the muscle attached to the fragments under tension – this can occur in large movements, and relapse tends to occur gradually.

Orthodontic factors

- Extrusion of teeth.
- Soft tissue forces (e.g. endogenous tongue thrust, which leads to recurrence of an anterior open bite).
- Tooth movement into a zone of muscle imbalance that leads to relapse on removal of the appliances.
- Poor planning.

Patient-related factors

- Poor compliance.
- Anterior open bite resulting from soft tissue factors (e.g. endogenous tongue thrust) – thus

the patient should be counselled on this possibility.
- Cleft lip and palate – it is often difficult to advance the maxilla more than 6 mm without using distraction techniques because of dense scar tissue from multiple surgical procedures, and relapse often occurs.

Surgery for obstructive sleep apnoea

Sleep-disordered breathing is increasingly recognized as a potential cause of medical morbidity. Obstructive sleep apnoea (OSA) is the most common form of sleep-disordered breathing. It is now appreciated that OSA occurs in a significant number of people, beyond the stereotypical patient with pickwickian syndrome. In simple terms OSA results in episodes of hypopnoea and apnoea during sleep that result from loss of muscle tone of the tongue and pharyngeal musculature, which leads to airway obstruction. Oxygen desaturation occurs as a result of this obstruction, and the consequent hypoxia stimulates breathing to correct this hypoxia (at the price of disrupting sleep). This cycle can be repeated literally hundreds of time a night in severe cases and can give rise to symptoms of excessive daytime sleepiness, which can lead to poor concentration and impaired performance. The cycles of hypoxia can have an adverse effect on many physiological functions and may contribute to the development of cardiovascular problems such as hypertension. The severity of sleep apnoea is classified by the numbers of episodes of apnoea and/or hypopnoea occurring per hour.

Hypopnea – a transient reduction (but not complete cessation) of breathing for more than 10 seconds.

Apnoea – complete cessation of breathing for more than 10 seconds.

Apnoea hypopnoea index (AHI) – the number of apnoea and hypopnoea episodes per hours of sleep.

These episodes are measured in a controlled manner during a sleep study known as polysomnography. This study also looks at the lowest oxygen saturation during hypopnoeic or apnoeic episodes and limb movements. The results are interpreted by a sleep medicine specialist.

Accepted criteria for severity of OSA based on AHI calculated during polysomnography are as follows:

Mild = AHI 5 to 14.
Moderate = AHI 15 to 29.
Severe = AHI 30 or greater.

The Epworth Sleepiness Scale (ESS) is a self-administered survey with which patients score their likelihood of dozing off during a number of daytime situations. This scale is used to assess the impact of sleepiness (which may be secondary to OSA) on daily life.

It is worth remembering that although many healthcare funders (including the UK National Health Service) exclude 'simple snoring' from treatment, even snoring without apnoeic events has a disruptive and potentially destructive effect on many relationships and sleeping arrangements. There is a demonstrated relationship between ESS scores and measures of relationship harmony.

Management of diagnosed OSA can be divided into medical and surgical management.

The mainstay of medical management is continuous positive airway pressure (CPAP). This involves the patient's wearing a special face mask during sleep through which air is provided at an adjustable pressure. CPAP provides a 'pneumatic splint' that overcomes the pharyngeal soft tissue collapse and keeps the airway patent. It is considered the standard against which other treatments for OSA are measured but is often poorly tolerated.

In cases of mild to moderate OSA, a mandibular positioning appliance can be made by a dentist to position the mandible forward. This has the effect of bringing the tongue muscle insertions forward and helps increase the resting muscle tone, thereby helping to relieve the obstruction.

Surgical management of OSA seeks to relieve obstructions at the level of the obstruction. The sites of obstruction were best described by Fujita and are nasopharyngeal, oropharyngeal and hypopharyngeal. Accurate determination of the site of obstruction may be challenging. Nasopharyngoscopy is typically used to look for the site of obstruction but is not fully diagnostic. Lateral cephalograms are also commonly used, but they provide a two-dimensional image of what is a four-dimensional situation.

Surgical management of OSA may be directed at either soft tissue or the facial skeleton. Surgery of the facial skeleton is based on the techniques of orthognathic surgery. The term *telegnathic* ('move the jaws a long way') surgery has been used to describe skeletal surgery for OSA. The common procedures used are genioplasty (genioglossal advancement), which is typically done in conjunction with another hard or soft tissue procedure, and maxillomandibular advancement (MMA), which is basically a bimaxillary advancement osteotomy, with or without genioplasty. MMA has been demonstrated to provide enlargement of the retrolingual airway and some advancement of the retropalatal airway. As such, MMA has the capacity to relieve obstructions at multiple levels. The surgery may be done without presurgical orthodontics in many cases, although in some cases orthodontic setup may allow for greater skeletal movement (the typical goal is to attain 10 mm more of mandibular advancement). There is a mounting body of evidence that MMA is effective and stable. It is increasingly used as first-line treatment for management of OSA in patients who are unable or unwilling to use CPAP.

German perspective

Although most aspects of orthognathic surgery are consistent internationally, there are some specifics that differ from the UK and US perspective.

Since the introduction of the lateral cephalogram, more than 100 different methods of analyses have been described. In Germany, measurements and average values according to Hasund (Hasund et al. 1973) and Schwarz (1958) have become widely accepted. Of course, very often combinations of different methods are used during daily routine.

Presurgical orthodontic treatment is designed for decompensation of teeth in all three planes of space and lasts on average between 12 and 18 months. To shorten this period, buccal alveolotomy for rapid movement of the aligned teeth can be performed.

In some patients the operation is performed as a first step to correct major skeletal deformity, followed by postsurgical orthodontic treatment to place the teeth in their correct position. This method is also popular in certain areas of the United States. The orthodontic tooth movement is certainly more rapid.

FURTHER READING

Doucet JC, Morrison AD, Davis BR, Gregoire CE, Goodday R, Precious DS. The presence of mandibular third molars during sagittal split osteotomies does not increase the risk of complications. *J Oral Maxillofac Surg* 2012;70:1935–43.

Epker BN. Modification in sagittal osteotomy of the mandible. *J Oral Surg* 1977;35:157–9.

A definitive paper on the final refinement of this very common and useful technique.

Epker BN, Stella JP, Fish LC. *Dentofacial deformities,* 2nd ed. St. Louis: Mosby, 1995.

An older text, but in its day this was the book everyone used to learn orthognathic surgery.

Mitchell L. *An introduction to orthodontics,* 4th ed. Oxford: Oxford University Press, 2013.

Good on orthodontic components with a useful section on orthognathic surgery.

Proffit WR, Turvey TA, Phillips C. Orthognathic surgery: a hierarchy of stability. *Int J Adult Orthodon Orthognath Surg* 1996;11: 191–204.

Ward Booth P, Schendel SA, Hausamen J-E, editors. *Maxillofacial surgery,* vol. 2. Edinburgh: Churchill Livingstone, 2007.

An extensive multiauthor text full of detail and wonderful obscurities, currently being rewritten.

20

Cleft and craniofacial anomaly surgery

Contents

Aims and learning outcomes

For undergraduates:

- To gain a general understanding of the nature of the common cleft and craniofacial anomalies and an outline of general management.
- To demonstrate this understanding by being able to list the common cleft anomalies and describe an outline of treatment from birth to adulthood.

For postgraduates:

- To be able to describe the stigmata and frequency of the common anomalies.
- To be able to describe the steps and sequence of interventions involved in their management.
- To be able to list and describe the role of individuals involved in treatment.
- To be able to describe the basic steps of surgical treatment.

Classification

Numerous classifications exist, but the most useful is to describe the actual deformity in words. These deformities have matching Read and International Classification of Diseases (ICD) codes. These include:

- Cleft lip and palate, unspecified – read code P9, ICD code 749.

- Cleft lip – read code P91, ICD code 749.1.
- Cleft palate – read code P90, ICD code 749.0.
- Cleft lip and palate – read code P92, ICD code 749.2.
- Unilateral complete cleft lip and palate – read code P921, ICD code 749.21.
- Bilateral complete cleft lip and palate – read code P923, ICD code 749.23 (Figure 20.1).

The advantage in describing the actual deformity is that it links both the prognosis and the treatment for the cleft. One of the disadvantages, however, is that the description may not be entirely accurate. Cleft palate can mean anything from a cleft uvula through a cleft soft palate to cleft of the soft and hard palate. A small cleft of the soft palate is a relatively simple surgical problem with an extremely good long-term prognosis in most instances, whereas a wide complete cleft of the palate may be both difficult to close, particularly in the junction of the hard palate and the soft palate, and it can result in significant speech impediment and long-term growth disturbance caused by scarring.

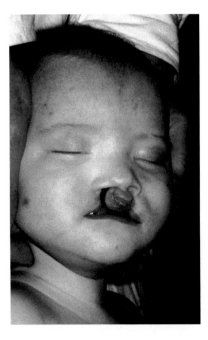

Figure 20.1 Complete bilateral cleft lip and palate showing unrestrained premaxillary growth.

Prevalence and incidence

Clefts of the lip and palate are the most common craniofacial malformations, and they comprise 65% of all anomalies affecting the head and neck. It is useful to distinguish between the two types of cleft anomaly – cleft lip with or without cleft palate and isolated cleft palate. There is a difference in the pathogenesis of the two types.

Cleft lip and palate

Among white populations, the incidence of cleft lip and palate is approximately 1 in 750 live births, with an increase in prevalence. In Germany, it is well accepted that the incidence is 1 in 500. The figure of 1 in 1000 has been used in international terms because the incidence varies among races and nationalities. The difficulty of accurate data collection in international terms has been discussed at length in specialist texts.

Family history can be found in around 40% of cases, although the actual genetic factors in cleft lip and palate are extremely complex. The commonly quoted statistic is that the risk that unaffected parents will have a second child with the anomaly is around 1 in 20. Clefts of lip and palate are more common in boys than in girls and more often affect the left side. The cleft is often more severe if it arises in the less common variant (i.e. in a girl and on the right side). The prevalence statistics for cleft lip and palate vary widely both geographically and among different racial groups (Asian populations, approximately 1 in 425 live births; Afro-Caribbean populations, 1 in 3000 live births).

Isolated cleft palate

This cleft occurs in around 1 in 2000 live births and is more common in girls than in boys (Figure 20.2). A genetic history is less clear in these patients; there is said to be a family history in approximately 20% of cases, and the risk to further children is around 1 in 80. Isolated cleft palate is often found in other syndromes such as Down's syndrome, Treacher–Collins syndrome, Pierre Robin sequence and Klippel-Feil syndrome.

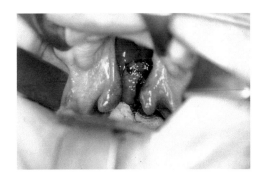

Figure 20.2 Isolated cleft of the hard and soft palates.

Aetiology

The aetiology of cleft anomalies is multifactorial. Some environmental factors, such as phenytoin taken in pregnancy, increase the risk of cleft lip and palate, and other drugs (e.g. retinoids), folate deficiency and the fetal alcohol syndrome also increase the incidence. Folic acid supplementation has been shown to reduce the incidence.

The mechanics of clefting are thought to be a failure of fusion of the embryological processes that comprise the upper lip at the sixth week of intrauterine life.

The hard and soft palates are formed by a different mechanism. The process described is 'flip up' of the palatal shelf from a vertical to a horizontal position followed by fusion to form the secondary palate around the eighth week *in utero*. This requires these embryological processes both to move into position by the process of flip up and to grow until they come into contact. Failure of growth, derangement of the flip up process or breakdown of the overlying epithelium to allow the flow of mesenchyme to create a solid structure can all result in clefting of the palate.

The terminology for this overall failure of normal development is that the formation of cleft lip and palate exhibits polygenic inheritance with a threshold.

One of the suggestions to explain why isolated cleft palate is more common in girls than in boys is that because the process of transposition of the palatal shelves occurs later in the female fetus than in the male fetus, a greater opportunity exists for environmental insult to affect successful flip up.

Defects caused by the clefting process

The disruption of the muscular sphincter of the mouth *(orbicularis oris)* may be partial, as in an incomplete cleft of the lip (Figure 20.3) or total, as in a complete cleft of the lip (Figure 20.4). This has a direct effect on the associated deformity. Patients with incomplete cleft lips often seem to have relatively normal alar bases and intra-alar widths. Patients with complete clefts have significant lateral and posterior migration of the alar base on the cleft side. A bulge around the region of the alar base is seen where the abnormal insertion of the orbicularis oris muscles are and a bulge is noted lateral to the alar base where the external nasal muscles are attached. In complete clefts, there is often a defect in the alveolus that may range from a slight notch to a complete cleft of the alveolus extending into the palate. In complete clefts of the lip, the nasal septum and columella are pulled to the side opposite the cleft by the contralateral,

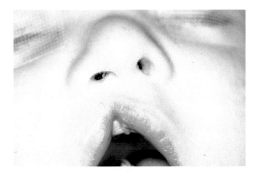

Figure 20.3 Incomplete unilateral cleft lip. Note the relative nasal symmetry.

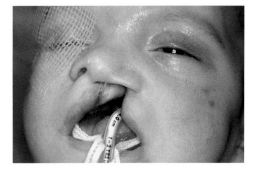

Figure 20.4 Complete unilateral cleft lip.

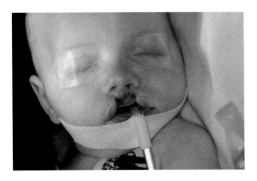

Figure 20.5 Incomplete bilateral cleft lip. Compare the relative symmetry with Figure 20.1.

normally attached musculature. This leads to a deviation of the tip of the nose and contributes to the classical appearance.

Patients with bilateral clefts may exhibit more apparent symmetry in both incomplete (Figure 20.5) and complete cases (see Figure 20.1). However, the main problem is that the premaxilla rotates forward because it contains no muscle and the orbicularis oris exerts no restraints on the forward growth of the premaxilla.

In clefts of the alveolus, whether bilateral or unilateral, the defect in the alveolus may be either simple notching, notching associated with congenital absence of the lateral incisor or the presence of supernumerary incisors, the presence of a rudimentary lateral incisor, or a complete oronasal fistula with a range of associated dental abnormalities.

If the defect extends between the lip and the palate, any combination of complete or incomplete, bilateral or unilateral clefts of the lip and alveolus may be associated with the cleft extending through the hard and soft palates. In unilateral cases, rotation and collapse of the segments of the maxilla in an inward and anterior direction are usually seen. These features are more marked on the side of the cleft. This part of the cleft maxilla is referred to as the lesser segment. In bilateral clefts, both the lateral segments are collapsed behind the prominent premaxilla.

Isolated clefts of the palate may affect the soft palate or the hard palate, or a combination of both or the uvula in isolation. There is also a condition known as submucous clefting in which the oral mucosa of the palate, and often the oral and nasal mucosa of the palate, are intact, but there is no underlying bone or muscle. This condition can be easily missed and may become obvious only once the child has had his or her adenoids removed and develops marked hyponasality in speech. The usual finding is a widening of the dental arch posteriorly, associated with the cleft, and significant eustachian tube dysfunction, which frequently results in otitis media and hearing impairment.

The common stigmata of cleft lip and palate therefore include problems with feeding because a communication between the mouth and the nasal cavity decreases the baby's ability to suck. This problem can be overcome by positional feeding and the use of appropriate bottles to deliver feedings.

Submucous clefts have been reported to be the most common clefts in the posterior palate – they occur in 1 in 1200 births. Common abnormalities include hypernasality, chronic otitis media and nasal regurgitation. The signs that may be indicative of a submucous cleft include bifid uvula, translucent palatal raphe area, palpable notch in the midline of the posterior hard palate and triangular muscle ridging on palatal elevation. The most common reason for treating a person with a submucous cleft palate is abnormal, nasal-sounding speech.

Problems with hearing

Eustachian tube dysfunction as a result of cleft palate inhibits adequate ventilation of the middle ear. The condition causes secretory otitis media (glue ear) and can result in deafness. This contributes to the child's difficulty in learning speech because hearing oneself talk is part of the natural biofeedback of learning to communicate.

Direct speech problems

In learning to speak, lip or alveolar defects, defects in the hard and soft palates and, in later life, dental anomalies have an obvious impact. These patients require early assessment and, if necessary, intervention by speech and language therapists.

The anatomical problems related to the nose can result in a poor nasal airway with resulting speech, breathing and sinus-related problems.

Issues in the management of cleft lip and palate

Approximately 20% of babies with clefts, particularly those with isolated cleft palates, will have associated congenital abnormalities, often of the heart or extremities.

Failure of growth and the preexisting cleft lead to clear aesthetic issues. The growth problems have also in the past been made remarkably worse by postsurgical scarring and distortion.

Concerns highlighted by the Eurocleft study around multiple interventions in children with cleft anomalies that were performed in a disjointed and discordant fashion, coupled with observations on the adequate growth patterns in individuals with unoperated clefts, raised concerns that in some instances postsurgical distortion resulting from scarring and inappropriately timed or performed surgery created defects to rival the clefts themselves.

In the United Kingdom, this problem was addressed by a national recommendation that the treatment of cleft lip and palate should be centralized to centres that could be adequately audited and consisted of a team comprising a cleft surgeon, an orthodontist, a speech and language therapist, an otorhinolaryngologist, specialized nursing, clinical genetics advice, paediatric intensive care facilities and the opportunity for neonatal counselling and specialist health visitors. Adequate access to paediatric dentistry and restorative dentistry was essential, as was access to appropriate psychological support. Within the United Kingdom, there has been a very gradual move toward coordinated teams such as these to manage all patients with cleft anomalies by geographic region, thus creating the opportunity for high-volume auditable outcomes. The opportunities for development of individual expertise and training become self-evident, as does the restriction of practice to a very limited number of people, with the inherent potential problems this could create.

In Germany, there are no regulations concerning treatment of cleft lip and palate. It is the patient (or parent) who has to make the decision where the child is to be treated. Of course, there are chatrooms, brochures and a lot of information, especially via the Internet. Usually these patients are treated at university hospitals or at least hospitals with major oral maxillofacial surgery units. Of course, there is competition among hospitals to treat these patients. Competition is believed to be one precondition for good results. Given the 'centralization' concept, now solidified into the UK National Health Service (NHS) system, that was based on the results of the Eurocleft study, it is fascinating to see how a major European country has responded.

In the United States, although degrees of specialization are widely accepted, it would be difficult to imagine the government's dictating to parents or patients where and how they or their child should be treated.

There are few areas of elective surgical practice that have been subjected to what is clearly a political differentiation, rather than one based on objective outcome criteria. One can see, at least in this instance, the common North American criticism of the UK NHS as 'socialized medicine'. What will be genuinely fascinating will be the long-term outcomes produced by such a process compared with similar centralized systems (e.g. in China) compared with outcomes from Germany and the United States, objectively and independently assessed.

Principles of management

In many centres, neonatal detection of cleft anomalies by ultrasound is possible because the shape of the face is detectable by the 14th week *in utero,* and the parents may well have been advised that their child will have a cleft. This knowledge does help parents come to terms with the shock of having a child with a cleft. However, parents commonly experience feelings of guilt and regret, and they often require time to grieve effectively for the loss of the anticipated 'normal' child. Parents may at this time be helped by taking photographs of the child with the cleft because this child effectively vanishes once the initial repair has been carried out.

At the point of diagnosis, home support by a specialist health visitor to assist with bonding between parents and child and to help with feeding is useful. Directed flow of milk into the mouth by using soft bottles and positioning the child will allow the child to be adequately nourished. A range of useful bottles and teats is available and can be obtained in the United Kingdom from the Cleft Lip and Palate Association, a cleft support group. At this stage a brief but positive explanation of the process by which the child's cleft will be repaired over time is essential.

Most centres in the United Kingdom have limited active intervention at this time; however, numerous presurgical orthopaedic techniques have been advocated worldwide at this point. Although practice varies throughout the world, these techniques are not currently in vogue in the United Kingdom.

In Germany, presurgical nasoalveolar moulding therapy is becoming increasingly popular. The first long-term results from New York look very promising. The practice in the United States varies considerably.

Timing of surgery

The precise details of the timing of surgery vary depending on the individual. A commonly used protocol includes the following:

- Lip with or without alveolus with or without soft palate repair at 3 to 6 months old.
- Repair of residual palatal defect at 9 to 12 months old.
- Audiology with or without myringotomy either at this time or as indicated by audiological assessment.
- Formal speech assessment around 2 years old.
- Pharyngeal surgery if indicated by speech and language therapy assessment at 4 to 5 years old.
- Alveolar bone grafting assessment at 8 years old, followed by actual alveolar bone grafting between 9 and 11 years old.
- Definitive orthodontics with or without orthognathic surgery between 15 and 18 years old.
- Definitive rhinoplasty plus definitive restorative dentistry at 18 years old or older.

Lip repair

In general neonatal lip repair (i.e. very early lip repair) has fallen into disrepute, and most surgeons undertake lip repair when the child is between 3 and 6 months old. The classical rule was the rule of

10, which is still referred to (the child is 10 weeks old, is 10 lb in weight, and has a haemoglobin value higher than 10 g/dl). In Germany, the rule is that the operation is not performed before the child is 3 months old and not if the child is less than 5 kg in weight. Usually at the age of 3 months, the babies are 7 or 8 kg in maximum weight.

Numerous different surgical techniques have been described. Perhaps the most important principles are reconstitution of the orbicularis musculature (Figure 20.6); repositioning, with the appropriate muscle attachments, of the alar base; restoration of the white role and vermilion border; and respecting the boundaries of labial skin, nasal skin and oral mucosa. Some of the main controversies in this area are whether release and advancement of the muscle, skin and mucosa should be achieved by subperiosteal undermining or by supraperiosteal undermining (Figure 20.7). The use of skin lengthening cuts by geometric design that transgress the actual skin boundaries or the allowance of the reimposed muscle to stretch the skin within the natural skin boundaries is another area of controversy (Figure 20.8). Dissection of the alar cartilage should be carried out to allow its repositioning, but there is

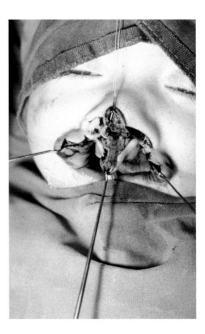

Figure 20.6 Wide exposure for orbicularis oris muscle repositioning in a Delaire-type repair of a bilateral cleft lip.

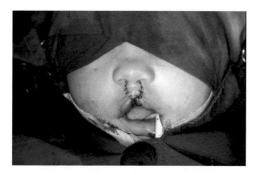

Figure 20.7 The patient in Figure 20.6 at surgical closure. Note the puckering of the lip caused by muscle reattachment after wide subperiosteal undermining. This rapidly settles with muscle function.

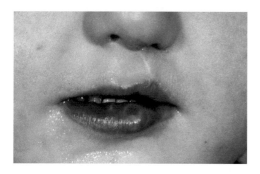

Figure 20.8 Geometric designs can produce good nasal symmetry and lip length.

controversy over the extent of cartilaginous dissection and so-called primary rhinoplasty, and some controversy remains over the use of a mucosal flap from the vomer to reinforce the floor of the nasal cavity.

The technique popularized by Delaire includes soft palate repair at the same time as lip repair to allow functional moulding of the residual cleft in the hard palate; this technique may or may not be practised, depending on the centre in which the child undergoes operation. Primary bone grafting of the alveolus has generally fallen into disrepute.

Palate repair

Closure of the palate in the United Kingdom is generally performed relatively early. The principle is to attempt to close the palate before the development of speech and a hypernasal speech pattern. In some European countries, closure of the hard palate is delayed to minimize the unwanted effects of early surgery on growth. This delay may improve transverse growth of the maxilla, but there is an obvious compromise in terms of speech development. In Germany, there are also many different concepts concerning sequence and timing of the operation. The common opinion is that the palate should be closed at the age of 2 years at the latest.

Palatal closure

Palatal closure (Figure 20.9), by common consensus, is now carried out using techniques that leave minimum stripped palatal mucoperiosteum and exposed bone in an attempt to decrease scarring and the unwanted effects on growth (Figure 20.10).

Primary dentition and speech assessment

The development of the primary dentition should be allowed to progress essentially naturally with good paediatric dentistry to maintain space. No orthodontic intervention in the primary dentition is warranted, but good preventive dentistry is. A joint ear, nose and throat and speech therapy assessment should be carried out to detect middle ear effusions and appropriate development of speech patterns. Hypernasal speech and/or glue

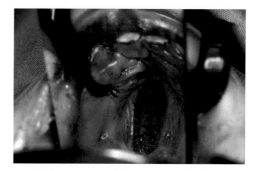

Figure 20.9 Second-stage closure of the cleft hard palate by using a double-layer technique; the first layer closes the nasal floor.

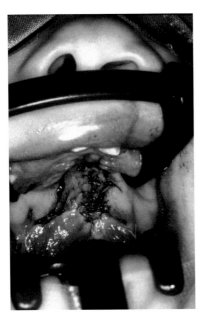

Figure 20.10 The second layer closes the oral mucosa and reinforces the first-layer repair.

ear should be addressed, either by therapy or surgery, such as pharyngoplasty or myringotomy (for glue ear).

Mixed dentition

At this stage the growth-retarding effects of initial surgery become more evident, seen predominately transversely in the upper arch and then anteroposteriorly as growth in this dimension predominates with age. The eruption of the permanent incisors demonstrates defects in enamel formation and position, and the upper incisors may erupt into lingual occlusion. Orthodontic preparation for alveolar bone grafting can usefully be combined with limited alignment of the incisors in the mixed dentition. Operation for alveolar bone grafting generally requires expansion of the maxillary arch and preferably alignment of the segments. There is an advantage to increasing the size of the alveolar defect. It allows adequate working space within the defect to recreate the nasal floor and oral mucosal layer, with cancellous bone sandwiched between the two layers and the anterior component closed by a sliding buccal mucosal flap (Figure 20.11).

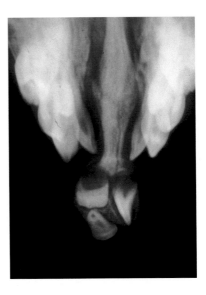

Figure 20.11 Anterior occlusal film of a bilateral cleft alveolus. Note the unrestrained premaxilla.

Alveolar bone grafting

Alveolar bone grafting provides bone through which a permanent canine and lateral incisor can erupt into the arch. This procedure unifies the maxilla and thus provides a stable intact arch, improves the alar base support, closes the residual oronasal fistula and provides a palatal base for later orthognathic surgery.

Initial assessment

Initial assessment should be carried out at the age of 8 years because, in rare instances, it may be possible to perform a graft procedure to allow an intact lateral incisor to erupt. More commonly the lateral incisor is rudimentary or missing or may have to be removed as part of the bone grafting procedure. In this instance the actual timing of the bone graft is predicated on the state of development of the canine tooth (Figure 20.12).

It is essential to work with the orthodontist on these cases, both in terms of timing of the bone graft and in terms of arch expansion and stabilization of the maxilla. Particularly in cases of bilateral alveolar bone grafting, the premaxilla should be stabilized with a heavy arch wire and either a trihelix or a quadhelix. This provides optimum stability

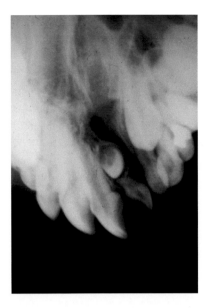

Figure 20.12 Preoperative radiograph before alveolar bone grafting.

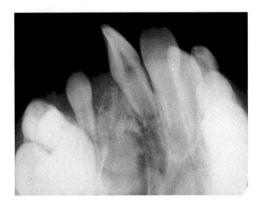

Figure 20.13 Postoperative radiograph showing good bony infill.

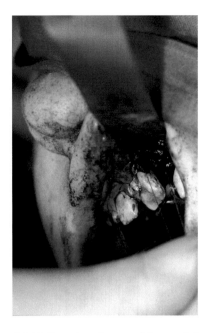

Figure 20.14 Suturing the nasal layer of the cleft alveolus repair.

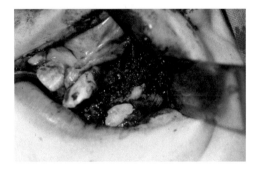

Figure 20.15 The periosteum and bone-lined defect are then packed with bone.

for the grafted bone (Figure 20.13). Preoperative removal of deciduous teeth and visible supernumerary teeth 6 weeks before alveolar bone grafting creates healthy attached gingivae and optimizes the flap design.

Surgical technique

A buccal lesser flap and major segment flaps are outlined. The flap in the major segment is a miniflap. Subperiosteal dissection exposes the cleft, and the lining of the oronasal fistula is incised to create two upper nasal flaps and two lower palatal flaps. These flaps are sutured (Figure 20.14) to create a pyramidal defect now lined by mucosa superiorly and inferiorly. This defect has either periosteum or bone on all its margins at this point, except for the base, which is the labial aspect. The defect is then packed with bone (Figure 20.15), which may be trephined or harvested by an open procedure from the iliac crest or the tibia. Skull and chin bone are popular in some centres. The bone used should be cancellous bone because this has the greatest propensity to become alveolar bone and allow migration of the canine through it. There is no good evidence to support the use of synthetic materials for this procedure. The periosteum of the lesser segment (larger) buccal flap is then incised and advanced to close the labial defect. It is important to remember that bone will not take against exposed cementum. Therefore, any obviously exposed root (e.g. from a supernumerary or residual lateral incisor) should result in removal of that tooth, rather than compromising the bone graft.

Prophylactic antistaphylococcal antibiotics (ampicillin/flucloxacillin or Co-Amoxyclav [amoxycillin and clavulanic acid]), topical antiseptics (chlorhexidine orally and nasally or mupirocin nasally) and local analgesia at donor and recipient sites improve both success and the patient's comfort.

Permanent dentition

The establishment of the permanent dentition, including guiding of the canines, which have to be exposed in about 15% of cases, is basically a decision on whether orthodontic camouflage or orthognathic surgery is indicated. If orthognathic surgery is indicated, standard orthodontic decompensation is carried out (Figure 20.16), and the osteotomies are relatively conservative anteroposterior movements. The chances of advancing a cleft maxilla farther than 7 mm without significant relapse is very small (Figure 20.17), and it is customary to balance the movements in the maxilla and the mandible (Figure 20.18), to achieve an optimum facial balance and occlusion (Figures 20.19 and 20.20).

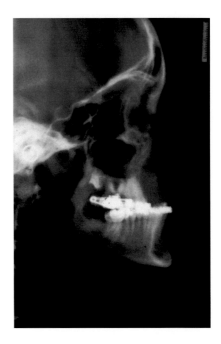

Figure 20.17 Lateral cephalogram obtained before cleft osteotomy. Note the extreme maxillary retrognathia.

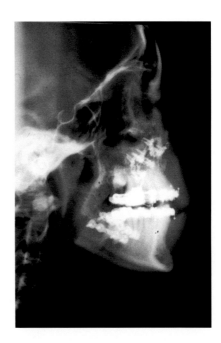

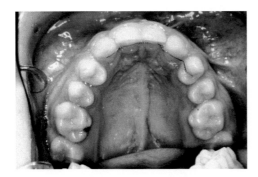

Figure 20.16 Surgery without orthodontics is a waste of time. Here the teeth have been aligned after palate and alveolus repair.

Figure 20.18 Lateral cephalogram obtained after cleft bimaxillary osteotomy shows a good balance of movements.

Once the maxilla is stabilized further completion surgery can be performed.

Rhinoplasty

Rhinoplasty should be performed at the end of treatment, rather than as an intermediary, because the final position of the nose can be predicted only once the maxilla is in a stable position (see Chapter 24). Open rhinoplasty techniques have been popularized in addressing the cleft nose principally because the dome of the nose, made up of alar cartilage, is frequently bifid and the columella is short. This allows access to the alar cartridges of the dome to allow primary refashioning and suturing.

Definitive restorative dentistry

Implant-borne permanent prosthesis or fixed-bridge prosthesis that can allow optimal oral hygiene should permit full and final rehabilitation of the patient with a cleft.

Noncleft craniofacial anomalies

Craniofacial surgery, sometimes known as cranio-maxillofacial surgery, is a subspecialty in its own right of both maxillofacial surgery and neurosurgery. Today, craniofacial teams essentially concentrate on paediatric craniofacial anomalies. The principal indications for paediatric craniofacial surgery, in the early months of life, are the craniosynostoses (Figure 20.21).

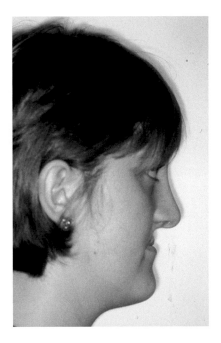

Figure 20.19 Clinical lateral view before osteotomy and rhinoplasty.

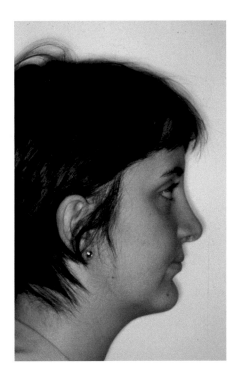

Figure 20.20 Clinical postoperative lateral view.

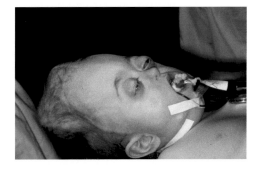

Figure 20.21 Complex craniosynostoses.

Craniosynostosis

Craniostenosis and craniosynostosis are the results of premature fusion of one or more of the sutures of the bone of the cranial base or vault. Effects depend on the site and extent of the premature fusion, and these anomalies can have significant effects on cranial and facial growth. Restriction of the growth of the skull vault can lead to a rise in intracranial pressure. This produces classical signs such as the 'beaten copper' skull of Crouzon's syndrome and Apert's syndrome. These patients require intervention early, both to relieve the raised intracranial pressure and to allow more normal skull and skull base growth (Figure 20.22). Single suture craniosynostosis results in classical skull deformities and may be released by simple strip craniectomy. Examples of single suture craniosynostoses are:

- Sagittal suture, resulting in scaphocephaly.
- Unilateral coronal suture, resulting in plagiocephaly.
- Metopic suture, resulting in trigonocephaly.
- Lambdoid suture, resulting in posterior plagiocephaly.

Multiple suture involvements tend to give rise to brachycephaly. The classical craniofacial synostosis syndromes include Crouzon's syndrome and a range of acrocephalosyndactyly syndromes, particularly Apert's syndrome, Saethre-Chotzen syndrome, Pfeiffer's syndrome and Carpenter's syndrome. These craniofacial synostoses may require both initial craniectomy (Figure 20.23) and subsequent craniofacial osteotomies in later life (Figure 20.24).

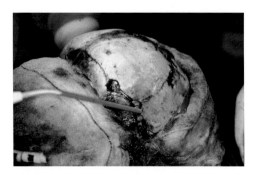

Figure 20.22 Coronal flap and burr holes for craniotomy.

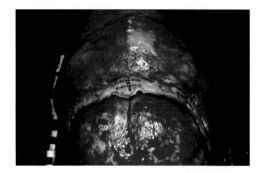

Figure 20.23 Operative view of brain (under reduced tension) with an osteotomized supraorbital bar.

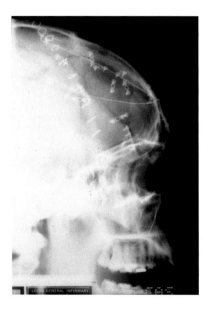

Figure 20.24 Postoperative radiograph. Titanium may be used less for the fixation in these cases if bioresorbable plates and screws become more accepted.

Craniofacial microsomia

This is the second most common craniofacial anomaly, with a prevalence of approximately 1 in 5000 births. It is a congenital defect characterized by lack of both hard and soft tissue on the affected side of the face, usually in the area of the mandibular ramus and external ear. Although this is usually a unilateral anomaly, 20% of craniofacial microsomias are bilateral. A wide spectrum of ear and cranial nerve deformities is found, and treatment is again multidisciplinary, although for these craniofacial syndromes, it seldom involves neurosurgeons. Patients with mild cases may be managed with hybrid orthodontic appliances. Patients with more significant defects, particularly those resulting in the complete absence or destruction of the temporomandibular joint, may require intervention with costochondral rib grafting between the ages of 5 and 8 years. Those patients with a functioning temporomandibular joint benefit from distraction osteogenesis around the time of the adolescent growth spurt (12 to 15 years old). Patients with milder cases, who are essentially considered to have asymmetric orthognathic problems, can be managed by conventional orthognathic techniques. An existing significant soft tissue defect can be managed by microvascular transfer of fat for bulking of the soft tissue.

Treacher–Collins syndrome

Also known as mandibulofacial dysostosis, this is a genetic deformity inherited as an autosomal dominant trait and shows the following bilateral features:

- Downward sloping palpebral fissures and colobomas – the downward sloping fissure is known as the antimongoloid slant, and the colobomas are a notched iris with a displaced pupil.
- Hypoplastic malar bones and mandibular retrognathia.
- Deformed ears, including both middle and inner ear deformities, which can result in deafness.
- Hypoplastic sinuses.
- Cleft palate in 30% of cases and completely normal intellectual function.

Pierre Robin association

The management is specific to the deformity. The Pierre Robin association is a syndrome causing retrognathia of the mandible, cleft palate and glossoptosis. It is probably a metabolic abnormality that results in a cleft palate by posturing of the tongue. There is significant catch-up growth in the Robin sequence, and maintenance of airway is the main initial requirement. Most children will catch up if they are nursed in an appropriate position.

Other rare craniofacial cleft conditions exist. These include the craniofacial clefts described by Paul Tessier, the Parisian doyen of craniofacial surgery, and the bizarre lesions induced by amniotic bands *in utero*. These cases are the province of the subspecialist.

FURTHER READING

Turvey TA, Vig KWL, Fonseca RJ, editors. *Facial clefts and craniosynostosis: principles and management*. Philadelphia: Saunders, 1996.
A massive, multiauthor tome but contains a vast array of erudite information from all around the world.
Specific literature includes the following:
Bianchi B, Ferri A, Ferrari S, Copelli C, Sesenna E. Myomucosal cheek flaps: applications in intraoral reconstruction using three different techniques. *Oral Surg Oral Med Oral Pathol Oral Radiol Endod* 2009;108:353–9.
De Jong T, Bannink N, Bredero-Boelhouwer HH et al. Long-term functional outcome in 167 patients with syndromic craniosynostosis; defining a syndrome-specific risk profile. *J Plast Reconstr Aesthet Surg* 2010;63:1635–41.
Kimonos V, Gold JA, Hoffman TL, Panchal J, Boyadjiev SA. Genetics of craniosynostosis. *Semin Pediatr Neurol* 2007;14:150–61.
Pattisapu JV, Gegg CA, Olavarria G, Johnson KK, Ruiz RL, Costello BJ. Craniosynostosis: diagnosis and surgical management. *Atlas Oral Maxillofacial Surg Clin North Am* 2010;18:77–91.
Rivera-Serrano CM, Oliver CL, Sok J et al. Pedicled facial buccinator (FAB) flap: a new flap for reconstruction of skull defects. *Laryngoscope* 2010;120:1922–30.
Van Lierop AC, Fagan JJ. Buccinator myomucosal flap: clinical results and review of anatomy, surgical technique and applications. *J Laryngol Otol* 2008;122:181–7.

21

Salivary glands

Contents

Aims

These are common for both undergraduates and postgraduates.

- To identify the signs and symptoms of common salivary gland disease.
- To outline the various treatments available.

Learning outcomes

These are principally for postgraduates.

- To be able to describe the differences between inflammatory, obstructive and neoplastic conditions.
- To describe some common diagnostic methods in salivary gland disease.
- To be able to demonstrate the ability to come to a clinical differential diagnosis.

- To list the indications for and appropriate investigations in salivary disease.
- To be able to initiate treatment in acute conditions.
- To describe the principles and main steps of surgical treatment.

Anatomy

The salivary tissue consists of three sets of paired major glands – parotid, submandibular and sublingual – and the minor glands, which are scattered submucosally throughout the mouth, oropharynx, palate and occasionally the nose.

The **parotid gland,** which consists almost entirely of serous acini, lies in the retromandibular fossa and has three surfaces. Its lateral surface is subcutaneous, enveloped in tight fascia closely related to the superficial musculoaponeurotic system (SMAS layer) with the greater auricular nerve branching anteriorly into the skin and to the posterior the lobe of the ear. Its anterior surface wraps around the posterior border of the ramus of the mandible and abuts the masseter and medial pterygoid muscles. The deep surface is complex and is related to the mastoid process, the posterior belly of the digastric muscle, the styloid process and its muscles and ligaments and the external carotid artery (Figures 21.1 and 21.2).

Within the parotid, the facial nerve ramifies, separating it into its superficial and deep lobes (Figure 21.3). There is no natural tissue plane here, and the nerve should be thought of as being embedded in the substance of the gland. Also within the gland are the retromandibular vein, the external carotid artery, lymph nodes and filaments from the auriculotemporal nerve.

The 5-cme parotid duct lies on the superficial surface of the masseter. It turns medially at the anterior border and pierces buccinator to open into the mouth at its papilla opposite the second upper molar tooth. It is also known as Stensen's duct. In about 50% of people a small accessory parotid gland lies between the duct and the zygomatic arch.

The *submandibular gland* is a mixed serous and mucinous gland. It is composed of a large superficial lobe and a smaller deep lobe, which is in continuity with the superficial lobe as it wraps around the posterior border of the mylohyoid

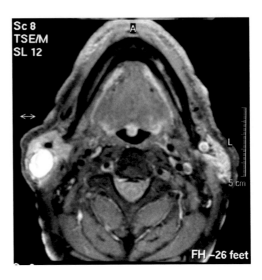

Figure 21.2 An axial view (magnetic resonance imaging) of the parotid gland. Note how the gland has been 'passed' into the area behind and around the ramus of the mandible.

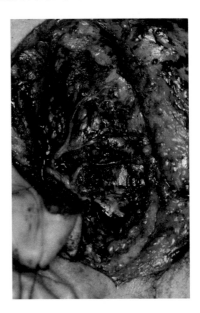

Figure 21.3 The facial nerve demonstrated here lies embedded in the parotid glandular tissue. Although it is said to separate the gland into 'deep' and 'superficial' lobes, there is no fascial compartmentalization.

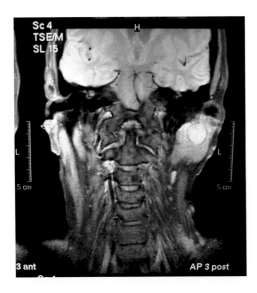

Figure 21.1 A coronal view (magnetic resonance imaging) of the parotid gland.

muscle. The gland is covered by a fibrous capsule (Figure 21.4).

The mandibular branch of the facial nerve is quoted to dip below the lower border of the mandible in 20% of people. The incision for

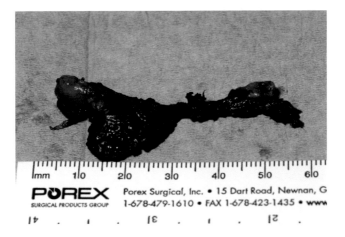

Figure 21.4 An excised submandibular gland. This gland has two components separated by the free edge of the mylohyoid muscle.

submandibulectomy is therefore placed at least 2 cm below the lower border of the mandible to avoid this nerve branch. The lingual nerve is intimately related to the submandibular duct (also known as Wharton's duct) as it makes an upward and anterior course into the floor of the mouth. The nerve is attached, by two rami, to the submandibular ganglion, which lies in the gland (Figure 21.5). The hypoglossal nerve lies deep to the gland and rarely (usually with more radical surgery) may be at risk of injury during gland excision.

The sublingual glands lie on the mylohyoid muscle and are covered superficially by the mucosa of the floor of the mouth. Rather than one duct, they have several small ducts that open directly into the mouth and also into the submandibular duct. Their intimate relationship with the lingual

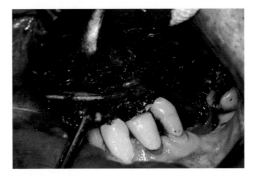

Figure 21.6 A visible lingual nerve after sublingual gland excision.

nerve and submandibular duct means that these structures are potentially at risk of injury during surgery (Figure 21.6).

Investigation of salivary gland disease

This investigation is straightforward. In patients with a history of preprandial swelling, including infection or obstructive symptoms, a plain radiograph (Figure 21.7), followed by a sialogram to image the architecture of the ductal system, is required after the acute episode has subsided. In patients with a lump, imaging to ascertain the nature of the lump is required. The best modality is magnetic resonance imaging. Ultrasound

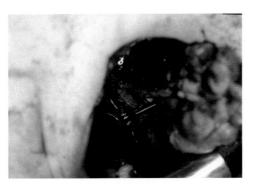

Figure 21.5 When removing a submandibular gland, the submandibular ganglion that attaches the gland to the lingual nerves must be divided.

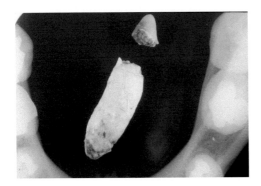

Figure 21.7 Calculus superimposed on a plain occlusal view of the anterior floor of the mouth.

in experienced hands can be quite satisfactory, as can computed tomography. Perhaps the most useful approach in requesting investigation is to ask yourself what you are trying to do. If it is simply to make a diagnosis with no real intention of progressing to surgery, the less invasive ultrasound is sensible. If there is a high likelihood of surgery, then an image that you can personally interpret as an adjunct to surgery is more logical.

Fine needle aspiration cytology (FNAC) is usually a simple (but often painful to the patient) procedure and may provide support to a provisional diagnosis if malignancy or a cystic lesion is suspected on imaging. Some surgeons do not carry out FNAC on parotid lumps routinely, particularly in the superficial lobe. Their argument is that the same operation will be performed regardless of the result, and outside specific centres, the specificity and sensitivity of FNAC on a typical superficial parotid lump are no better than chance (i.e. it will be a pleomorphic adenoma). Interestingly FNAC is also very controversial in Germany and is not regularly performed for this purpose.

Open or core biopsy of lumps of the major glands is not recommended because of the risk of seeding tumour. However, this view is increasingly questioned, and ultrasound-guided core biopsy of both salivary and cervical lumps carries the highest level of diagnostic accuracy under trial conditions. Whether that finding translates into routine clinical practice remains to be seen.

Examination of the constituents of saliva has no role in routine clinical practice.

Methods exist to measure salivary flow rates, but their interpretation is difficult, and the results, although used in research protocols, have little bearing on daily management of patients.

Developmental disorders

Significant developmental disorders of the salivary glands are rare. Agenesis of one or more glands has been described.

Heterotopic salivary tissue most commonly occurs in intraparotid and periparotid lymph nodes. It is of significance clinically when it manifests as a mass, a draining sinus or a neoplasm. Stafne's bone cavity occurs when heterotopic tissue indents the mandible and is seen as a well-corticated radiolucency at the angle of the mandible below the inferior alveolar canal.

Accessory salivary tissue adjacent to the glands is so common as to be normal.

Cystic disease may be developmental or acquired. The most common developmental cyst is the lymphoepithelial cyst of the parotid gland.

Obstructive disease

The ductal system of the major salivary glands may be blocked by calculi, mucus or strictures.

Approximately 80% of salivary calculi occur in the ductal system of the submandibular glands because of the greater length of the duct, its upward course and the thicker mucus. Patients give a history of painful, recurrent swelling in the submandibular region, particularly associated with eating or the anticipation of eating (preprandial swelling). Plain radiography usually demonstrates a calculus in the duct (see Figure 21.7), in the junction of the duct and gland or in the gland itself (Figure 21.8). In the duct a calculus is date shaped, at the junction of the duct and gland it is comma shaped and in the gland it is round. Should a calculus not be visible, a sialogram is required; it may demonstrate a radiolucent stone, a mucus plug or a stricture in the duct (Figure 21.9).

Alternatively, a patient with a history of less severe symptoms may have chronic obstruction, which can result in a fibrosed gland. In either case the patient may present acutely with an infected swollen gland. Treatment is with antibiotics, usually broad-spectrum penicillin, which is

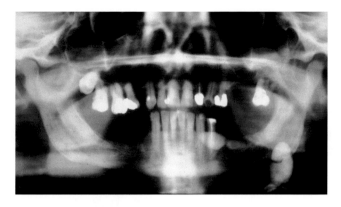

Figure 21.8 Calculi in the duct and submandibular gland.

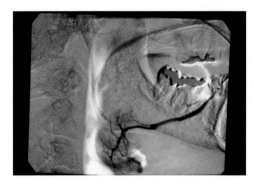

Figure 21.9 A sialogram. These images are useful diagnostically and therapeutically.

sometimes needed intravenously, and analgesia. Following cessation of the acute episode, removal of the calculus or the gland is required. It is often the case that the submandibular gland will have suffered irreversible damage and requires removal following a severe infective episode (Figure 21.10).

Of these calculi, 10% occur in the parotid duct. These are much less commonly radiopaque; only 10% are visible on plain radiographs. The substance obstructing the parotid may sometimes be thick, inspissated mucus rather than a frank calculus. It may pass out as a string of jelly-like material, followed by relief of the symptoms. The parotid gland survives acute infective episodes much better than the submandibular gland. Removal of the obstruction in a parotid gland usually results in recovery of normal function. Typically, the patient will report a sudden bad, often salty, taste in the mouth related to quite sudden relief of symptoms.

The remaining 10% of calculi occur in the sublingual and minor salivary glands.

Calculi may be dealt with in several ways. In the submandibular gland, if the calculus is visible

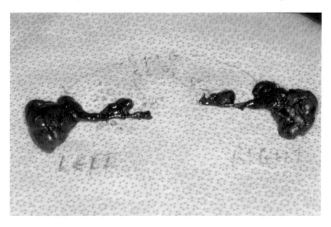

Figure 21.10 Excised bilateral submandibular and sublingual glands from a patient with recurrent aspiration pneumonias.

in the duct on an occlusal radiograph and is relatively anterior and palpable, it may be removed using local anaesthesia. The area is infiltrated with a local anaesthetic agent, and a stay suture is placed beneath the duct proximal to the palpable calculus. Traction is applied to the suture to tent up the tissues, and it also prevents the calculus from moving backward toward the gland (in fact, fibrosis around calculi and their irregular shape mean that they often do not move). A longitudinal incision is made over the calculus, thus exposing it. It can now be teased out of the duct. Mucosal closure is all that is needed; stenting the duct or duct repair does not improve the outcome. Anterior defects should be left open because this produces a wider meatus. Parotid calculi, when encountered, may be dealt with in a similar fashion. In either case the papilla should not be incised because it may form a stricture.

If the calculus is very proximal in the duct, at the junction of the duct and gland or within the gland, removal of the gland is usually indicated.

In certain cases calculi are amenable to other treatment modalities such as basket retrieval or lithotripsy. Strictures may be treatable with balloon dilatation. Sialoendoscopy and minimally invasive (cynics may say minimally effective) procedures have become popular in some areas but have yet to gain widespread acceptance.

Infections

Acute bacterial sialadenitis

Now relatively rare, this condition usually affects the parotid gland. It is microbiologically different from infected obstructive sialadenitis (usually seen in submandibular gland but also in the parotid gland). Classically it occurred in postoperative patients who were dehydrated. It still occurs in older patients who are dehydrated and debilitated, but underlying Sjögren's syndrome (SS) is a more frequent cause. The patient presents with a swollen, erythematous, painful gland and is often systemically unwell. *Staphylococcus aureus* is the usual organism, and initial antibiotic therapy should cover this. Streptococci and anaerobes are also frequently cultured (Figure 21.11).

Pus may be discharging from the papilla (Figure 21.12). If not, the gland should be milked to

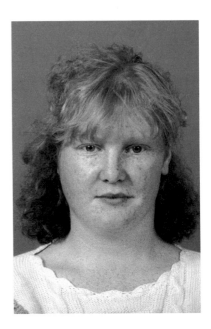

Figure 21.11 Patient with bacterial sialadenitis. These patients can become very unwell and often need intravenous fluid support and antibiotics.

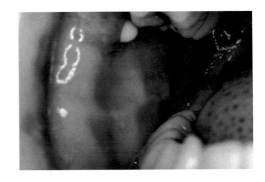

Figure 21.12 Pus at the parotid duct.

obtain pus for microbiology. Initial treatment involves antibiotics, rehydration and analgesia. Sialogogues (e.g. lemon drops) may be used to promote salivary flow. Abscess formation may be a sequela and may require incision and drainage. However, this complication is rare, and incision and drainage should be avoided if possible because the inevitable damage to the parotid may create a salivary fistula which can then necessitate excision of the gland.

Following recovery from the acute phase, a sialogram is required to investigate any underlying abnormality and often is therapeutic as a result of mechanical irrigation with an antiseptic (the contrast medium usually includes iodine).

Chronic bacterial sialadenitis

This condition tends to affect the submandibular glands, probably because of the more viscous secretion, which is more difficult to clear than that of the parotid gland, and the propensity for calculi to form in the submandibular duct (Figure 21.13). This infection usually occurs in a gland that has had a history of an acute infective or obstructive episode. Treatment is by removal of the offending gland. In the case of the parotid, a 'total' parotidectomy with facial nerve sparing and ligation of the duct will eradicate most cases. This involves morselization of the gland around the facial nerve and removal of most saliva-producing acini. Some surgeons attempt duct ligation alone, usually with some method of suppressing saliva production (e.g. propantheline [Pro-Banthine] and/or nasogastric feeding). The hope with this method is that the gland will undergo atrophy. Patients often have a very unpleasant initial few weeks, and the overall long-term success is questionable.

Viral sialadenitis

Several viruses can affect the salivary glands. By far the most common is the mumps virus (a paramyxovirus). Mumps is usually a disease of childhood. There is acute swelling of the salivary glands, particularly the parotid glands, which are involved in 70% of cases. The other glands may be affected

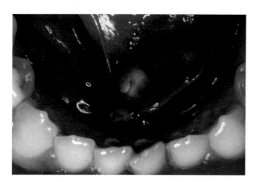

Figure 21.13 Calculus at the submandibular duct orifice.

less frequently. Mumps may occur in nonimmune adults, and in men the testes are involved in 20% of cases, resulting in sterility in 1%. Treatment is for symptomatic relief only. Immunity is lifelong.

Cytomegalovirus affects the salivary glands in congenital cytomegalic inclusion disease. The seriousness of the involvement of other organs overshadows any clinical impact of salivary involvement.

Sjögren's syndrome

SS is an autoimmune disease characterized by a dry mouth and dry eyes. It occurs most commonly in middle or old age, with women affected 10 times as often as men. When dryness of the mouth and eyes occurs in isolation, the condition it is termed *primary* SS (PSS). When this dryness occurs in combination with a connective tissue disease, it is termed *secondary* SS (SSS). It is of interest that the ocular and oral symptoms are usually more severe in PSS. The most commonly associated connective tissue diseases are rheumatoid arthritis and systemic lupus erythematosus. Of those patients with rheumatoid arthritis, 15% report symptoms consistent with SS, and of those with systemic lupus erythematosus, the figure is 30%.

Patients may present with a subjective feeling of a dry mouth before changes are clinically evident and may also, at this stage, have no ocular symptoms. Early ophthalmological assessment is indicated to check for the potentially sight-compromising keratoconjunctivitis sicca. As the salivary flow decreases, the mucosa takes on a dry and shiny appearance, with depapillation of the tongue. Diffuse nonpainful parotid swelling is uncommon at presentation, but 30% of patients will give a history of this swelling.

There are various diagnostic tests. History is important, and a convincing history in the presence of an established connective tissue disease makes further investigation unnecessary. The mainstay of investigation is detection of autoantibodies in the patient. Most clinicians would test for rheumatoid factor, anti-Ro and anti-La. If blood tests are unhelpful and further diagnostic information is required, then salivary gland biopsy may be performed. This entails removing five minor salivary glands from the lower labial region. The histological findings of periductal lymphocytic

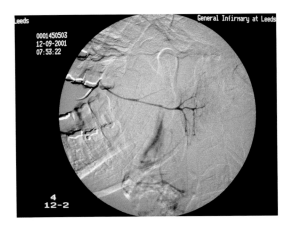

Figure 21.14 A sialogram showing mild 'snow-storm' appearance typical of sialectasis in Sjögren's syndrome.

infiltrate (T cells), duct ectasia and acinar atrophy are characteristic of SS. The lymphocytic infiltrate progresses with disease and eventually replaces the salivary tissue. Patients with SS are at increased risk of lymphoma formation, and this risk is greater in PSS.

In patients with a history of parotid swelling, a sialogram will show the characteristic 'snow-storm' appearance of punctate sialectasis in SS (Figure 21.14). Decreased tear secretion can be measured objectively by using small strips of paper placed in the lower eyelid.

Other causes of xerostomia are outlined in Table 21.1.

The criteria for diagnosing SS are outlined in Tables 21.2 and 21.3.

Table 21.1 Causes of xerostomia

- Fluid loss or deprivation including dehydration, haemorrhage.
- Radiotherapy and chemotherapy.
- Sjögren's syndrome.
- Diabetes mellitus.
- Sarcoidosis.
- Amyloid.
- Human immunodeficiency virus infection.
- Psychogenic conditions (e.g. stress, anxiety, depression)
- Drugs – antihistamines, antidepressants, anticholinergics, antihypertensives, antipsychotics, antiparkinsonian agents, diuretics.

The management of SS is largely directed toward symptom control. Involvement of a rheumatologist and ophthalmologist is often required. Relief of the symptoms of xerostomia is helped by frequent sips of water, artificial saliva preparations and measures such as chewing sugar-free gum. Pilocarpine, a cholinesterase inhibitor, helps in some cases, but the side effects (e.g. nausea and drowsiness) are often unacceptable.

The decreased salivary flow increases the risk of caries, and meticulous oral hygiene, regular dental attendance and fluoride supplements should be advised for all dentate patients. Edentulous patients may be more intolerant of dentures. All patients with xerostomia are at higher risk of candidiasis. This infection tends to exacerbate their discomfort and should be treated aggressively (often with a higher dose of fluconazole than normal with miconazole in recalcitrant cases because a few patients harbour fluconazole-resistant candida).

The lack of tears is treated with methyl cellulose eye drops.

The risk of lymphoma formation should be borne in mind when reviewing these patients should a lump develop in the parotid glands.

Salivary neoplasms

There is an extensive and bewildering range of salivary neoplasms (Table 21.4).

The more significant neoplasms are described here. The incidence of *malignant* salivary tumours in Europe is 1.2 per 100 000 population. Most salivary gland tumours (70% to 80%) are benign, and most of these are pleomorphic adenomas. The only established aetiology in some tumours is that of radiation (in nuclear bomb survivors). Most tumours have no clearly defined cause, although Warthin's tumour is associated with smoking.

Presentation of virtually all tumours is that of a slow-growing mass (Figure 21.15). In certain situations, one should have an increased suspicion of malignancy. Fast-growing lumps, pain and sensory or motor nerve symptoms all suggest that a lump may be malignant rather than benign. Site is also a risk factor for malignancy. In general the following apply:

Table 21.2 Revised international classification for Sjögren's syndrome

I. Ocular symptoms: a positive response to at least one of the following questions:
   1. Have you had daily, persistent, troublesome dry eyes for more than 3 months?
   2. Do you have a recurrent sensation of sand or gravel in the eyes?
   3. Do you use tear substitutes more than three times a day?
II. Oral symptoms: a positive response to at least one of the following questions:
   1. Have you had a daily feeling of dry mouth for more than 3 months?
   2. Have you had recurrent or persistently swollen salivary glands as an adult?
   3. Do you frequently drink liquids to aid swallowing dry food?
III. Ocular signs: objective evidence of ocular involvement defined as a positive result for at least one of the following two tests:
   1. Schirmer's I test, performed without anesthesia (≤5 mm in 5 minutes).
   2. Rose Bengal score or other ocular dye score (≥4 according to van Bijsterveld's scoring system).
IV. Histopathology: in minor salivary glands (obtained through normal-appearing mucosa) focal lymphocytic sialadenitis, evaluated by an expert histopathologist, with a focus score ≥1, defined as the number of lymphocytic foci (which are adjacent to normal-appearing mucous acini and contain >50 lymphocytes) per 4 mm² of glandular tissue.
V. Salivary gland involvement: objective evidence of salivary gland involvement defined by a positive result for at least one of the following diagnostic tests:
   1. Unstimulated whole salivary flow (≤1 mL in 5 minutes).
   2. Parotid sialography showing the presence of diffuse sialectasis (punctate, cavitary or destructive pattern), without evidence of obstruction of the major ducts.
   3. Salivary scintigraphy showing delayed uptake, reduced concentration and/or delayed excretion of tracer.
VI. Autoantibodies: presence in the serum of the following autoantibodies:
   1. Antibodies to Ro (SSA) or La (SSB) antigens or both.

Adapted from Vitali C, Bombardieri S, Jonsson R, Moutsopoulos HM, Alexander EL, Carsons SE, Daniels TE, Fox PC, Fox RI, Kassan SS, Pillemer SR, Talal N, Weisman MH, European Study Group on Classification Criteria for Sjögren's Syndrome. Classification criteria for Sjögren's syndrome: a revised version of the European criteria proposed by the American-European Consensus Group. *Ann Rheum Dis* 2002;61:554–8.

- 15% of parotid gland tumours are malignant.
- 35% of submandibular gland tumours are malignant.
- 50% of minor salivary gland tumours are malignant.
- 85% of sublingual gland tumours are malignant.

A parotid mass larger than 4 cm is said to have a higher risk of being malignant.

Benign tumours

Pleomorphic salivary adenoma (PSA) is the most common tumour of salivary glands; 75% of PSAs occur in the parotid gland, and most of those are in the superficial lobe. These tumours are thought to arise from duct and myoepithelial cells. They occur in equal proportion in men and women. The average age of presentation is around 40 years, but they may manifest over a wide age range. The pleomorphic epithet arises from the mixed fibrous, myxoid, cartilaginous and epithelial components. Although benign, the PSA is poorly encapsulated and requires excision with a margin of normal tissue. Therefore, superficial or total conservative parotidectomy has been the standard of care for many years. More recently, the use of magnification and the technique of extracapsular dissection have become popular at the ultraconservative end of treatment strategies. A more common approach is selective superficial parotidectomy, in which only the branches of the facial nerve above and below the tumour are

Table 21.3 Revised rules for classification of Sjögren's syndrome*

For primary SS

In patients without any potentially associated disease, primary SS may be defined as follows:
  a. The presence of any four of the six items is indicative of primary SS, as long as either item IV (histopathology) or VI (serology) is positive.
  b. The presence of any three of the four objective criteria (i.e. III, IV, V, VI).

For secondary SS

In patients with a potentially associated disease (e.g. another well-defined connective tissue disease), the presence of item I or item II plus any two from among the items III, IV and V may be considered as indicative of secondary SS.

Exclusion criteria

- Past head and neck radiation treatment.
- Hepatitis C.
- Acquired immunodeficiency syndrome.
- Preexisting lymphoma.
- Sarcoidosis.
- Graft versus host disease.
- Use of anticholinergic drugs (since a time shorter than fourfold the half-life of the drug).

Adapted from Vitali C, Bombardieri S, Jonsson R, Moutsopoulos HM, Alexander EL, Carsons SE, Daniels TE, Fox PC, Fox RI, Kassan SS, Pillemer SR, Talal N, Weisman MH, European Study Group on Classification Criteria for Sjögren's Syndrome. Classification criteria for Sjögren's syndrome: a revised version of the European criteria proposed by the American-European Consensus Group. *Ann Rheum Dis* 2002;61:554–8.
SS, Sjögren's syndrome.
* Roman numerals refer to the Revised international classification for Sjögren's syndrome (see Table 21.2).

dissected. In this procedure, the surgeon excises a segment of tumour and normal parotid gland under direct visual control of the facial nerve and leaves a greater or smaller portion of normal gland. There can be significant mucus-filled cystic areas in these tumours, which must be handled carefully at surgery because any spillage can produce recurrence. Tumour recurrence is often multifocal and very difficult to treat, with options ranging from total parotidectomy with radiotherapy to isolated removal of recurrence depending on individual circumstance.

There are many other benign tumours, most of which are uncommon. Of note is *adenolymphoma (Warthin's tumour)*, which can be bilateral in up to 10% of patients. This is the only salivary tumour with an association with smoking. It can sometimes vanish after FNAC, aspiration or enucleation despite being 'multifocal', a finding that raises questions about the true nature of this 'tumour'.

Malignant tumours

Adenoid cystic carcinoma represents 40% of all malignant salivary tumours. It is slow growing with local invasion. This tumour has a particular predilection for neural invasion and may produce 'skip' lesions such that there may be tumour left in nerves beyond a histologically clear resection margin. There is a slight female preponderance, and it manifests most frequently in patients in their 50s. The tumour has a characteristic 'Swiss cheese' pattern on histology, although there are several histological variants. Treatment is surgical, most often with adjuvant radiotherapy. Of patients with this tumour, 8% have cervical lymph node involvement at presentation and 30% will develop regional or distant metastases at some point, although this may be in the quite distant future. Pulmonary metastases are particularly frequent with this malignancy. Overall the prognosis is generally poor even with

Table 21.4 World Health Organization classification of salivary neoplasms

1. Adenomas.
   - Pleomorphic adenoma.
   - Myoepithelioma.
   - Basal cell adenoma.
   - Adenolymphoma (Warthin's).
   - Oncocytoma.
   - Canalicular adenoma.
   - Sebaceous adenoma.
   - Ductal papilloma.
   - Cystadenoma.
2. Carcinomas.
   - Acinic cell carcinoma.
   - Mucoepidermoid carcinoma.
   - Adenoid cystic carcinoma.
   - Polymorphous low grade adenocarcinoma.
   - Epithelial-myoepithelial carcinoma.
   - Basal cell adenocarcinoma.
   - Sebaceous carcinoma.
   - Papillary cystadenocarcinoma.
   - Mucinous adenocarcinoma.
   - Oncocytic carcinoma.
   - Salivary duct carcinoma.
   - Adenocarcinoma, not otherwise specified.
   - Myoepithelial carcinoma.
   - Carcinoma in pleomorphic adenoma.
   - Squamous cell carcinoma.
   - Small cell carcinoma.
   - Undifferentiated carcinoma.
   - Other carcinomas.
3. Nonepithelial tumours.
4. Malignant lymphomas.
5. Secondary tumours.
6. Unclassified tumours.
7. Tumour-like lesions.
   - Sialadenosis.
   - Oncocytosis.
   - Necrotizing sialometaplasia.
   - Benign lymphoepithelial lesion.
   - Salivary gland cysts.
   - Chronic sclerosing sialadenitis of submandibular gland.
   - Cystic lymphoid hyperplasia of acquired immunodeficiency syndrome.

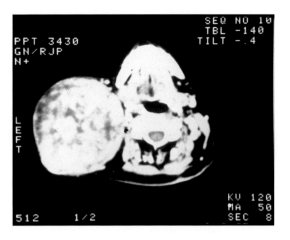

Figure 21.15 A massive parotid pleomorphic and adenoma on computed tomography.

Mucoepidermoid carcinomas account for up to 9% of salivary tumours. There is an equal sex ratio, presentation is in the third to fifth decades and most of these tumours occur in the parotid glands. They are malignant but tend to behave in either a relatively indolent way or an aggressively malignant way in which regional and distant metastases are common. Attempts to separate these behaviours on histological grounds have been the subject of controversy because 30% of tumours that look like low-grade lesions histologically behave aggressively, and 30% of those that appear to be high-grade lesions behave in the more benign fashion.

Acinic cell carcinomas account for 1% of all salivary tumours; 80% are relatively indolent and 20% are highly aggressive. Much more so than in mucoepidermoid carcinoma, the histological examiner struggles to predict the tumour's behaviour.

Carcinoma ex PSA is a highly malignant tumour that arises within a preexisting PSA that has usually been present for many years. After about 10 years, the incidence of malignancy in a PSA is about 1% per year. Sudden growth, pain or facial nerve weakness in a long-standing parotid lump is highly suggestive of malignant transformation. Features of this tumour are as follows:

- Rare, aggressive malignancy.
- The most common of three malignant mixed tumours of salivary glands. It is thought to arise from preexisting PSA.

maximally aggressive treatment, although the patients may coexist with the tumour for many years with relatively well-controlled symptoms.

- Male-to-female ratio of 2:1.
- Accounts for 3.6% of all salivary neoplasms.
- Occurs usually in older patients (sixth to eighth decade) who have had a PSA *in situ* for many years (typically 10 to 15 years). Patients experience rapid growth of a preexisting mass, often with painful facial nerve palsy from tumour infiltration.
- Overall 5-year survival of 30%.
- Regional metastasis developing in 50% of patients. Olsen and associates recommended selective neck dissection for all patients with high-grade tumours and also for those with high-grade tumours after operative therapy.
- A high rate of metastasis at the time of diagnosis (25% to 76%), typically to brain, bone, lung and local lymph nodes.

Other malignant diseases such as mesenchymal tumours or lymphoma may occur in the salivary glands. Secondary deposits can occur, and metastasis from a primary tumor of the skin to an intraparotid lymph node is the most frequent cause of a malignant parotid mass in areas of the world with a high incidence of cancer of the scalp. Polymorphous low grade adenocarcinoma is worth remembering because it is frequently difficult to distinguish histologically but is generally an indolent malignancy with a good prognosis. In addition, consideration should be given to malignant mixed salivary gland tumours of salivary glands. According to the World Health Organization, these are as follows: carcinoma ex PSA (already mentioned), which arises from preexisting PSA and is the most common; carcinosarcoma, which is a true malignant mixed tumour (99% also arise from preexisting PSAs) and is rare; and metastasizing pleomorphic adenoma, which remains something of a controversy.

Miscellaneous conditions

Necrotizing sialometaplasia is a nonmalignant condition of salivary gland tissue that clinically can appear to be a malignant tumour. It is a rare condition and occurs more commonly in men, usually in their 30s and 40s. The most common area is the palate, and it manifests as an ulcer. It has a short clinical course, with the ulcer appearing over up to 2 weeks or so. This short history is a clue to diagnosis. Biopsy is mandatory to exclude carcinoma. Biopsy results can be just as difficult to distinguish from cancer as the clinical appearance. The lesion heals by secondary intention in 2 to 3 months. More rapid healing can be obtained by excision with a small rim of normal mucosa and placement of a dressing plate with an obtundent dressing.

Drooling is almost never caused by excess saliva production (which itself is unusual) because saliva can simply be swallowed. It is usually caused by poor neuromuscular control of the lips or neck and head. Treatment is most commonly by removal of both sublingual glands and redirection of the submandibular ducts so they empty into the oropharynx. Careful preoperative assessment is required because not all patients may be suitable for the procedure. Treatment does not usually eliminate the problem completely, but it decreases it to become more manageable (less frequent bib changes). Intraglandular botulinum-alpha toxin can provide a temporary solution if reduction of 'resting' salivary flow (usually from the submandibular glands) is helpful. Aspiration of saliva is not helped by duct transposition, and the old-fashioned, but effective, remedy of bilateral sublingual and submandibular gland excision is more helpful.

Sialadenosis is enlargement of the salivary glands. It usually occurs in the parotid glands and may be idiopathic or associated with diabetes mellitus, alcoholism, drugs or pregnancy.

Sarcoidosis may affect the salivary glands, usually the parotids. If it is associated with lacrimal gland swelling, chorioretinitis and cranial nerve involvement, it is termed Heerfordt's disease.

Salivary gland surgery

Transoral sialolithotomy

Transoral sialolithotomy is simply the removal of a submandibular duct calculus. Local analgesia is obtained with a lingual block and local infiltration, a suture is passed behind the calculus (Figure 21.16) and the duct is approached by splitting the overlying mucosa and duct. The calculus is removed, and the mucosa is closed as described previously or is spatulated open.

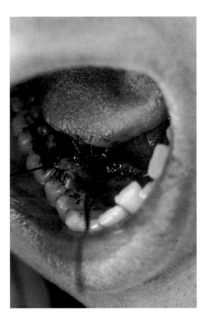

Figure 21.16 Silk suture passed behind a submandibular duct calculus.

Mucocele excision

Excision of mucocele is a very common procedure (Figure 21.17). It requires adequate local analgesia, usually via bilateral mental blocks. The secret to the dissection is complete excision of the cyst. This may be accomplished by performing a mucosal wedge excision that avoids resecting the vermilion border or by dissecting the cyst itself out submucosally. Most mucoceles are cured by mucosal wedge incision and removal of the associated damaged

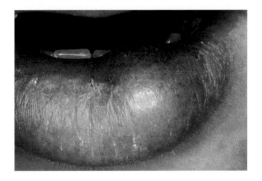

Figure 21.17 A mucocele of the lower lip – the most common site. A supposed 'mucocele' of the upper lip is usually a tumour.

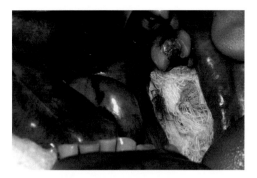

Figure 21.18 A ranula marked out for excision with the associated sublingual gland. The submandibular duct should be preserved.

minor salivary glands. Always warn patients about the small risk of recurrence.

Ranula and sublingual gland excision

Ranula is a mucous extravasation cyst and will reform if the sublingual gland is not removed (Figure 21.18). Consent should be obtained to include warnings regarding possible altered sensation of the anterior two thirds of the tongue and bleeding from the thin-walled veins that envelop the lingual nerve.

The sublingual gland lies in the anterior aspect of the floor of the mouth between the mucous membrane and the mylohyoid muscle. This gland can be difficult to approach because of the proximity of the anterior mandible, and if the patient is dentate any lingual inclination of the teeth can make the lateral aspect of the gland difficult to identify and visualize. The sublingual gland has numerous ducts and can open either directly into the overlying mucous membrane or into the terminal part of the submandibular duct.

Sublingual gland excision is performed in conjunction with excision of the ranula while the patient is under general anaesthesia. Haemostasis is helped by infiltrating 1:200 000 adrenaline solution and meticulous bipolar diathermy. The position of the submandibular duct can be found by identifying the opening of the duct, and a small cuff of mucosa around the opening should be incised both to identify and to allow mobilization of the duct (Figure 21.19). This procedure retains adequate drainage for the submandibular

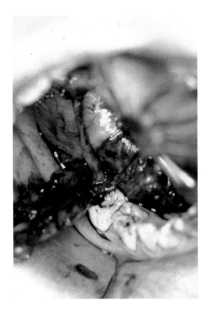

Figure 21.19 Submandibular duct repositioning with sublingual gland excision.

gland, which does not need to be removed. The intact ranula can then be dissected by a combination of scissors and swabs. The sublingual gland is identified as it envelopes the submandibular duct and is excised. The remnants of gland closest to the submandibular gland are often difficult to identify and separate completely, and it may be necessary to leave small remnants of glandular tissue in this area. Obvious residual glandular tissue should be cauterized to minimize leakage of saliva. Adequate haemostasis should be ensured at this point because postoperative bleeding can be a real problem.

Surgery for drooling

The most effective operation for drooling is excision of the sublingual gland with redirection of the submandibular ducts into the hypopharynx. Exactly the same procedure is carried out as for excision of the sublingual gland with a ranula, except that the mobilized submandibular duct on its cuff of mucosa is repositioned underneath the lingual mucosa to exit at the back of the tongue into the hypopharynx. Intraglandular botulinum toxin can be effective.

Submandibular gland excision

The submandibular gland is approached by transcervical approach; the incision is two fingerbreadths below the lower border of the mandible. A 3- to 4-cm incision is made, which is deepened through fat that bleeds; bleeding should be controlled using bipolar haemostasis to expose the platysma muscle (Figure 21.20). The platysma is divided, and the lower border of the submandibular gland is identified enveloped in the submandibular fascia. The fascia is incised, and an upper flap that includes submandibular fascia, platysma, fat and skin is developed. This approach and adherence to the gland will preserve the function of the marginal mandibular branch of the facial nerve. The superficial pole of the gland is mobilized posteriorly (Figure 21.21), if need be, by ligating the facial vessels (but this is not always needed), anteriorly by counter traction and inferiorly by finger dissection. The mylohyoid muscle is then retracted, and the gland is placed on traction. Finger dissection usually frees the gland up, and the lingual nerve is pulled down by countertraction exposing the submandibular ganglion and the associated thin-walled veins. The ganglion should undergo bipolar haemostasis and is dissected free. This allows the lingual nerve to spring free, and the gland will be adherent by a few fascial attachments and the submandibular duct. The submandibular duct should be traced as far forward on the floor of the mouth as possible, ligated and divided. Bipolar haemosta-

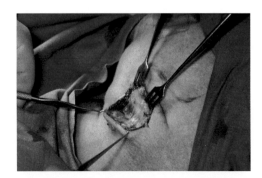

Figure 21.20 Submandibular gland excision. The skin incision is approximately two fingerwidths below the lower border of the mandible. After skin incision, control of bleeding and sweeping aside fat, platysma is seen.

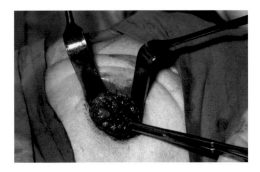

Figure 21.21 The submandibular gland lies immediately underneath platysma enveloped in fascia. Sticking to the glandular surface (in glands without tumour) is a safe way to protect the marginal mandibular branch of the facial nerve.

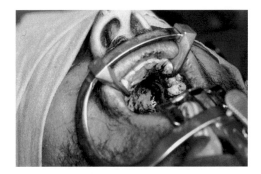

Figure 21.23 Excision of palatal pleomorphic adenoma by using a cleft palate gag to aid access. Subperiosteal stripping provides an adequate margin and heals well by allowing simple granulation to occur.

sis is carried out, and the defect has a drain placed and is closed in two layers.

Excision of palatal tumours

Most palatal salivary gland tumours are pleomorphic adenomas, and most of these arise at the junction of the hard and soft palates (Figure 21.22). For all tumours that overlie the hard palate, simple subperiosteal excision with a mucosal margin is adequate (Figure 21.23). Healing by secondary intention of the palate is excellent and can be achieved by using a dressing plate with a sedative and anodyne dressing such as Coe-Pak. If the tumour extends into the soft palate, the capsule of the tumour can be elevated from the underlying levator aponeurosis (which will granulate), leaving an acceptable margin of normal tissue and a

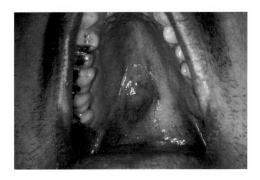

Figure 21.22 Palatal pleomorphic adenoma arising at a typical site.

good functional result. If the levator aponeurosis is breached, however, this has to be repaired and should be reconstituted with vascularized tissue, such as a buccal fat pad flap or a temporoparietal fascial flap.

Parotidectomy

Parotidectomy is divided into extracapsular dissection, (so-called) superficial parotidectomy, deep lobe parotidectomy, total facial nerve–preserving parotidectomy and radical parotidectomy in which the facial nerve is sacrificed. Any facial nerve–preserving parotidectomy is basically a dissection of the facial nerve. Most parotidectomies are approached via a cervical mastoid facial incision starting in the preauricular sulcus, looping underneath the earlobe around the mastoid and down into a neck skin crease. A skin flap is raised over the parotid fascia and the skin overlying the sternomastoid; this is elevated forward on a plane very similar to that used in a cutaneous face lift. The parotid fascia is identified, the great auricular nerve is identified and the posterior branch is preserved where at all possible (Figure 21.24). The groove between the parotid gland and the sternomastoid muscle is developed to identify the posterior belly of digastric muscle (Figure 21.25). This is the depth at which the facial nerve will be found. The preauricular incision is deepened in a relatively avascular plane between the auricular cartilage and the parotid gland, and this will

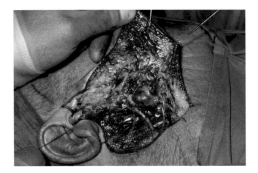

Figure 21.24 Parotidectomy – raising the skin flap. The greater auricular nerve and sometimes the external jugular vein are anatomical guides to the correct thickness of the skin flap.

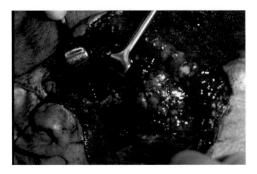

Figure 21.26 The cartilaginous 'pointer' indicates the location of the facial nerve trunk at the depth of the posterior belly of digastric.

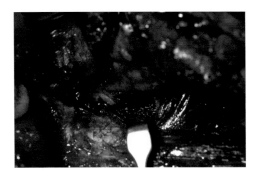

Figure 21.25 The posterior belly of digastric is the anatomical marker for the depth of the facial nerve trunk in parotidectomy.

take you down to the inferior portion of the cartilaginous canal of the external auditory meatus that points in the general direction of the facial nerve 1 cm deep and inferior to its tip The facial nerve will lie in the area indicated by the so-called cartilaginous pointer at the depth of the posterior belly of the digastric muscle (Figure 21.26). The remaining attached parotid gland can therefore be proceeded through quite quickly. A further method to localize the facial nerve is to identify the groove between the cartilaginous and bony external auditory meatus because its sharp lateral edge of bone will be felt. It lies immediately superficial and superior to the nerve at its point of exit from the skull, and it is a good fallback position if the nerve has not already been identified. Once the nerve is identified, the dissection should take place along the plane of the nerve lying just superficial to it (Figure 21.27). The procedure will vary

depending on whether tumour or sialadenitis is the indication:

- Sialadenitis – morselization of the gland lateral to the nerve is the quickest and the most effective way to remove it.
- Tumour – the nerve branch is identified above and below the tumour so adequate excision can be carried out.

When the tumour is confined to the deep lobe (i.e. medial to the facial nerve and usually behind the posterior border of the ramus of the mandible), it may be necessary to osteotomize the ramus and mobilize the segments to allow adequate three-dimensional access for safe excision of the tumour (Figure 21.28). It is the capacity to deal with the unexpected in salivary gland surgery that distinguishes the safe surgeon. Pure deep

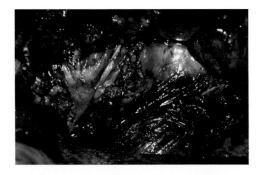

Figure 21.27 The superficial lobe is stripped of the underlying facial nerve, which has divided into its upper and lower divisions.

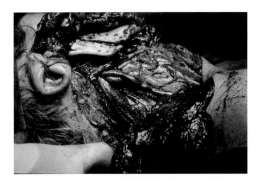

Figure 21.28 A vertical subsigmoid osteotomy has been used to mobilize the mandible for access to the 'deep lobe' of the parotid gland.

lobe tumours identified on imaging may be best approached using a labiomandibulotomy and the Attia approach along the floor of the mouth. The swinging out of the mandible provides excellent three-dimensional access to the lateral pharynx.

Some surgeons carry out parotid gland surgery only with a facial nerve monitor in constant use. Other surgeons find this an unwelcome distraction. Many confirm the facial nerve trunk at the beginning and end of the operation by using a facial nerve stimulator. The wound is closed with a drain and two-layered closure.

FURTHER READING

Albergotti WG, Nguyen SA, Zenk J, Gillespie MB. Extracapsular dissection for benign parotid tumors: a meta-analysis. *Laryngoscope* 2012;122:1954–60.

Cawson RA, Gleeson MJ, Eveson JW *Pathology and surgery of the salivary glands.* Oxford: Isis Medical Media, 1997.

Ciuman RR, Oels W, Jaussi R, Dost P. Outcome, general, and symptom-specific quality of life after various types of parotid resection. *Laryngoscope* 2012;122:1254–61.

Olsen KD, Lewis JE. Carcinoma ex pleomorphic adenoma: a clinicopathological review. *Head Neck* 2001;23:705–12.

Rinaldo A, Shaha AR, Pellitteri PK, Bradley PJ, Ferlito A. Management of malignant sublingual salivary gland tumours. *Oral Oncol* 2004;40:2–5.

22

Oral cancer

Contents

Aims and learning outcomes

For undergraduates:

- To be able to demonstrate the ability to recognize potential oral cancers.
- To describe how a patient with such a lesion should be referred.
- To discuss in general terms the aetiology, epidemiology and treatment of oral cancer.

For postgraduates:

- To be able to describe appropriate management for a range of stages of oral cancer.
- To be able to discuss premalignant lesions and their relevance.
- To be able to list a relevant range of investigations for patients with oral cancer.
- To be able to demonstrate the ability to take informed consent from a patient about to undergo surgical treatment of oral cancer.
- To be able to discuss the likely outcomes of treatment for a range of stages of oral cancer.

Epidemiology

Cancer of the oral cavity includes cancer of the lip, tongue, gingivae, floor of the mouth and palate. Of these, the most common sites are of the tongue and floor of the mouth.

Squamous cell carcinoma (SCC) comprises some 90% of oral cancer cases. Other types of oral cancer include those arising from salivary glands (see Chapter 21), bone and other connective tissues, melanoma and lymphoma.

There are about 6200 new cases each year in the United Kingdom. The incidence of oral cancer is increasing. Globally, cancer of the mouth and pharynx is the sixth most common type of cancer. Although less common in the United Kingdom (head and neck cancer is the 12th most common cancer for male patients), it is the most common in the Indian subcontinent (India, Pakistan and Bangladesh). There is a north-south divide in the United Kingdom, with higher incidence recorded in the northern parts of England, Scotland and Northern Ireland compared with the more affluent south.

Oral cancer is more common in men. Most patients with oral cancer are middle aged or older (98% >40 years old). The disease is, however, increasing in younger patients, in particular, in nonsmokers. Possible reasons given for this rise are the increased consumption of alcohol and involvement of high-risk strains of human papillomavirus (HPV-16 and HPV-18). HPV is an established cause of a rapid increase in oropharyngeal cancer (which is considered a separate cancer from oral cancer in some epidemiological data), particularly that of the tonsil and base of tongue, which are more frequently treated primarily nonsurgically, although this has led to a different series of post-treatment problems.

In Germany, there are 9500 new cases of oral cancer in men and 3500 new cases in women each year. In men in Germany, oral cancer therefore is the fifth most common type of cancer. On average, men are 66 years old and women are 70 years old when the disease is detected. Given that the United Kingdom and Germany have two very similar Northern European populations with similar interpretations of data, this difference in incidence is unlikely to be explained by the 20 million difference in population.

Aetiology

Most oral cancer (as in most of upper aerodigestive tract cancer) is the result of tobacco and alcohol consumption to 'excess' (>75% of cases). Our knowledge of risk factors associated with oral cancer is principally that of SCC. There is relatively little known about the aetiology of salivary cancer, sarcoma or mucosal melanoma.

Tobacco

There is overwhelming evidence that tobacco use in the form of cigarette, cigar and pipe smoking is associated with a more than 10-fold increased risk of developing oral cancer in comparison with nonusers. All forms of tobacco smoking are associated with increased risk. There is also evidence that heavier and prolonged use of tobacco is associated with a greater risk of having oral cancer as well as a second malignant disease. Smoking cessation is worthwhile

because the risk after abstention for more than 10 years becomes similar to that of nonsmokers.

The mechanism of tobacco carcinogenesis has been well researched. There are several hundred carcinogens identified in tobacco smoke (e.g. aromatic hydrocarbons and tobacco-specific nitrogen compounds). These agents act both locally and systemically. They interfere with DNA replication and lead to mutations, and they contribute to the molecular chain of events in malignant transformation.

Chewing tobacco, with or without areca (betel) nut, and snuff dipping (placing it buccally) are both associated with oral cancer. The areca nut is itself an oral carcinogen. It is associated with submucous fibrosis and epithelial dysplasia, leading to malignant transformation, particularly if it is used in conjunction with tobacco. The areca nut is chewed as a quid of betel leaves and slaked lime, with or without tobacco. It is popular in the Indian subcontinent, South East Asia and New Guinea.

Alcohol consumption

Because of the tendency for those who smoke also to consume alcohol, often in significant quantities, care is needed in interpreting the association of alcohol with oral cancer. There is good evidence that heavy alcohol consumption is associated with a significant risk of oral and pharyngeal cancer. For example, consuming 100 g of alcohol or more per day increases the risk of developing oral cancer by at least sixfold. Although certain alcoholic beverages may have significant contributory impurities, it is thought that the quantity of alcohol consumed is the main significant risk factor.

Alcohol is thought to contribute to cancer of the head and neck by local and systemic mechanisms. These include ethanol-induced increased permeability of oral mucosa (to carcinogens), carcinogenicity of active metabolites of ethanol, liver disease in heavy drinkers that results in reduced detoxification of carcinogens and poor diet associated with alcoholism.

Synergistic effect of smoking and alcohol

Smoking and high alcohol consumption are associated with a synergistic or multiplicative effect in terms of risk of oral cancer. Heavy drinkers who also smoke heavily have a more than 35 times greater oral cancer risk in comparison with those who do not smoke or drink.

Given that some 75% of patients with oral cancer smoke and/or drink alcohol, these factors should be targeted in preventing oral cancer.

Other factors

Consumption of fruit and vegetables has a protective beneficial effect. Certain diets such as salted fish (in Chinese food) have been associated with an increased risk of pharyngeal cancer.

Certain viruses are known to be closely related to human cancer (e.g. human immunodeficiency virus [HIV] and Kaposi's sarcoma, Epstein Barr virus and nasopharyngeal carcinoma, hepatitis B virus and hepatocellular carcinoma and HPV and cervical and anogenital cancer). The link between HPV and oral cancer is currently being investigated. The HPV-16 and HPV-18 strains are particularly implicated, and they are associated with base of tongue and tonsillar cancers, which have seen a marked increase in recent years (up to 15% per annum). People affected tend to be younger, are less likely to be smokers and (if nonsmokers) have much better outcomes in terms of survival. These findings have led to a number of studies involving treatment intensity reduction in patients treated by radiotherapy in a bid to reduce the very severe morbidity associated with many of the more recent nonsurgical oncological techniques (particularly chemoradiotherapy).

Irradiated tissue has a long-term risk of forming new malignant tumours. This is one of the many reasons to look at options other than radiation for treating cancers in younger patients.

Poor dental status had often been quoted as a cause of oral cancer. However, these patients often have confounding factors such as poor socioeconomic status, heavy alcohol and tobacco use and poor dietary habits.

Premalignant conditions and lesions

Oral leukoplakia (according to the World Health Organization definition) is a white patch or plaque that cannot be characterized, clinically or histopathologically, as any other disease. Erythroplakia can be similarly described but for bright red patches or plaques. Erythroleukoplakia (speckled leukoplakia) forms the third lesion commonly associated with a risk of malignant transformation. This risk has been reported to be 2% to 6% for leukoplakia (varies with sites [e.g. highest in the floor of the mouth]); 40% to 50% of erythroplakias have high-grade dysplasia or carcinoma present. Speckled leukoplakia is an intermediate risk (Figure 22.1).

Other lesions associated with malignant transformation include chronic hyperplastic candidiasis, submucous fibrosis (Figure 22.2) and sideropenic dysphagia. Less commonly, certain conditions such as dyskeratosis congenita (tongue leukoplakia), discoid lupus erythematosus (lip cancer) and lichen planus (1% to 3% incidence, lichenoid dysplasia being the main reason; Figure 22.3) have a risk of malignant change.

The management of these premalignant lesions, in particular leukoplakia, can be controversial. Cessation of smoking is beneficial, with spontaneous resolution seen in some 50% of lesions in some studies. Some clinicians prefer to observe these lesions closely with selective biopsies where there are worrying changes such as induration, contact bleeding, ulceration or conversion to erythroplakia. Surgeons, in particular, may advocate laser excision with the aim of achieving thorough histological analysis and reducing the incidence of malignant transformation (Figure 22.4).

Decision making depends on several issues, such as whether the lesions are localized (easy to remove) or widespread, the patient's compliance and preference and the clinician's resources. Biopsies are often carried out to assess the degree of dysplasia, in particular where there is speckled leukoplakia or erythroplakia. Many of these lesions have high-grade dysplasia, if not malignant transformation.

Vitamin A and related compounds (retinoids) have been used as chemopreventive agents. Some studies have demonstrated the resolution of leukoplakia with regular use of retinoids. However, the side effects associated with retinoid use can be considerable. Poor compliance and recurrence

(a)
(b)

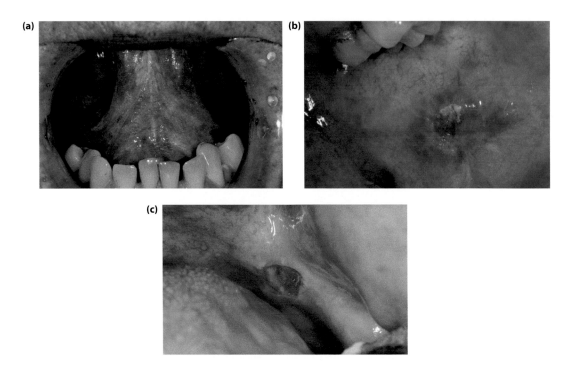

(c)

Figure 22.1 Examples of premalignant lesions: (a) leukoplakia, (b) speckled leukoplakia, (c) erythroplakia.

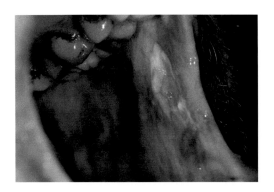

Figure 22.2 Submucous fibrosis is progressive, forming bands beneath the mucosa, and is associated with epithelial dysplasia. The fibrosed bands can cause severe trismus.

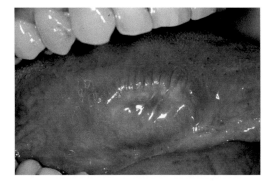

Figure 22.3 Biopsy of this tongue lesion showed features of lichen planus with epithelial dysplasia.

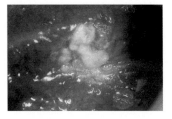

of lesions on cessation of these chemopreventive agents have limited the usefulness of this treatment modality.

The use of nonsteroidal anti-inflammatory drugs in chemoprevention of oral cancer is unsupported by evidence (and is a good example of research fraud [see Chapter 25]).

Figure 22.4 An area of leukoplakia that changed (it became indurated). This was early squamous cell carcinoma on histological examination after excision.

Diagnosis

Presentation

Oral cancer can be asymptomatic for some time, resulting in late presentation. In addition, significant numbers of oral cancer sufferers are alcohol-dependent recluses.

Early symptoms and signs of oral cancer include persistent mouth ulceration (often painless), lumps and white, red or speckled lesions. Later features may include recent onset of difficulty with speech or swallowing, numbness, neck swelling (lymphadenopathy) and unexplained loosening of a tooth or teeth. Any of these persistent lesions (>3 weeks) should be referred urgently for specialist opinion and possible biopsy. Although most oral cancer is clinically apparent (Figures 22.5 and 22.6), both patients and general practitioners may miss a small proportion. Some patients can present late with enlarging neck nodes (Figure 22.7). Fine needle aspiration cytology (FNAC) examination (using a needle and syringe to aspirate cells from a lump in an outpatient clinic setting) can be useful diagnostically.

The oral mucosa has a renowned ability to heal (Figure 22.8). It is therefore important for the specialist to see the suspected lesion intact (i.e. leave the biopsy procedure to the specialist). This will enable better recording and more accurate treatment planning.

Techniques to reveal high-risk lesions are available (e.g. toluidine blue rinse, optical techniques). It is generally accepted that these methods are not suitable for general use because of the significant proportion of false-positive and false-negative results.

Data collection, referral pattern, fast track system and delays

There is a drive from both professionals and governments to improve outcome in head and neck cancer. In the state-controlled systems of the United Kingdom, this has produced a top-down dogmatic administrative approach, with mixed benefits. These efforts included setting standards in quality and quantitative parameters in the form of guidelines and recommendations,

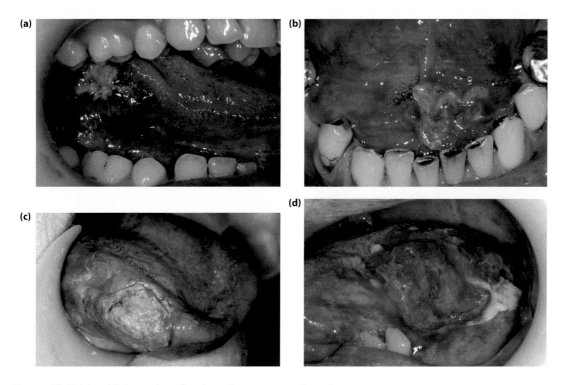

Figure 22.5 (a) to (d) Examples of early oral squamous cell carcinoma.

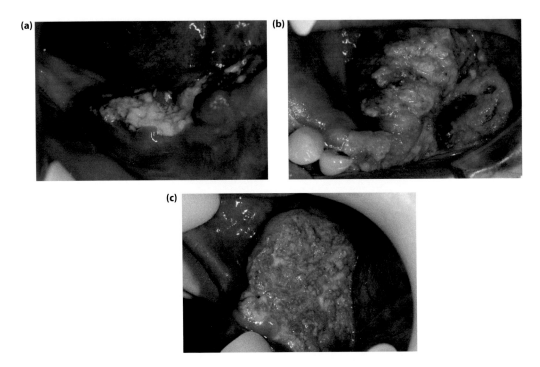

Figure 22.6 (a) to (c) Examples of advanced oral squamous cell carcinoma.

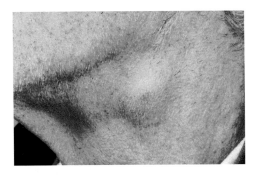

Figure 22.7 Enlarged cervical lymph nodes in adults mandates exclusion of head and neck cancer. Typical sites for this presentation are the tongue base, nasopharynx and posterior oropharynx.

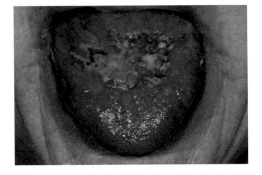

Figure 22.8 This woman has two lesions. Three weeks earlier she had a biopsy 2 cm from the tongue tip that showed squamous cell carcinoma.

political cancer strategies by various governments and expert group consensus views (in the United Kingdom, the National Institute for Health and Care Excellence [NICE] produced a document on head and neck cancer).

Data collection for cancer statistics is vital for improving outcome. In the United Kingdom, the Data Accumulation for Head and Neck Oncology (DAHNO) project aims to standardize this aspect and enable auditing and research on a national basis. The UK government's Cancer Strategy target for urgent referrals is aimed at reducing delays in urgent referral to appropriate cancer specialists. There is, however, the real risk of delays for cancer cases that had not been referred urgently. Part of these political initiatives in the United Kingdom are driven by unfavourable comparisons in cancer survival (in general) between the United Kingdom and other developed European countries. There is a degree of frustration with nationwide broad-brushstroke approaches to 'national cancer statistics' because at least one pan-European survey showed Scotland to have one of the best 5-year survival rates for oral cancer when rates were analyzed specifically. 'Lies, damned lies and statistics' is not a cliché for no good reason.

Breaking bad news, support and counselling

The diagnosis of mouth cancer is a major life event for the patient. It is important to ensure that a histological diagnosis is obtained because even experienced specialists can make a wrong diagnosis based on clinical grounds alone.

Breaking bad news and providing support and counselling should be carried out in a sympathetic, unhurried manner within a quiet and private environment (see Chapter 5). On receiving the news, patients can become significantly stressed psychologically and may not be able to take in or retain much information. It is important that support is available such as a trained nurse counselor, a contact number to ring and written information with or without an information leaflet on oral cancer (that the patient can read). The general medical practitioner, family physician or other referral source should be informed promptly.

Diagnostic workup

In addition to history and clinical examination, further investigations are necessary to evaluate the extent of the disease and the fitness of the patient to undergo treatment both medically and psychosocially.

The extent of disease is evaluated radiographically and by examination under anaesthesia.

Radiography

An orthopantomogram (OPG) will provide some information on bone invasion as well as the patient's dental status (Figure 22.9). Information on the patient's dental status will help identify existing or potential sources of dental infection. If radiotherapy is anticipated, these teeth should be dealt with by restoration or extractions to prevent osteoradionecrosis (ORN) from developing subsequent to extractions performed after radiotherapy.

Magnetic resonance imaging (MRI) of the primary tumour and principal draining lymph nodes and computed tomography (CT) scans of the chest and abdomen are routine staging scans (except for the larynx, for which CT of the primary tumour is preferred).

Either imaging technique (depends on local resources) can be used to assess the size of tumour, the structures involved or in close proximity to the tumour, the presence of cervical lymphadenopathy or any previously undetected pathology.

MRI provides good soft tissue details with minimal risk of artefacts around the jaw (from amalgams) (Figures 22.10 and 22.11). There is no radiation involved, but MRI is contraindicated for patients with metallic objects affected by the strong magnetic field (e.g. pacemaker or metal fragment in the eye) and in patients who are claustrophobic, unless open MRI is available.

CT scan is good for bony imaging, takes less time to complete and can stage the chest simultaneously. Its use is limited around the jaw because of amalgam artefacts.

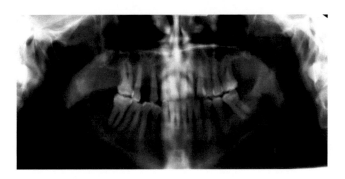

Figure 22.9 A large tumour invading the body of the mandible.

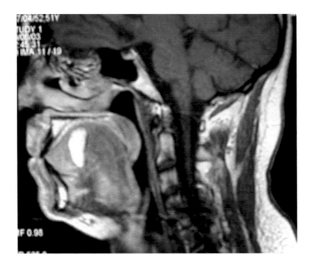

Figure 22.10 Magnetic resonance imaging can provide various viewing windows. This sagittal view of a tongue liposarcoma is seen as a high signal on the T2-weighted sequence.

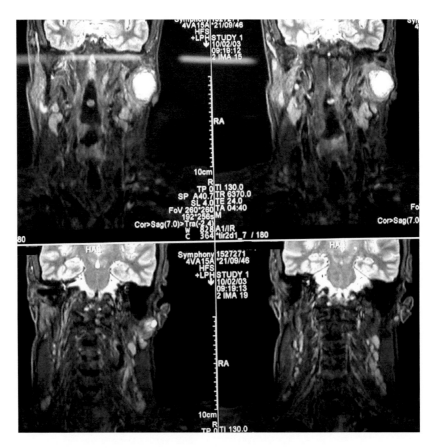

Figure 22.11 This four-frame magnetic resonance imaging view shows a carcinoma ex pleomorphic adenoma of the left parotid gland with involved lymph nodes.

Ultrasound scan with FNAC is an alternative method to assess the neck. However, it depends on the availability of specialized expertise.

Chest radiography and CT scans of the thorax are performed because most patients with mouth cancer are at risk of coexisting lung diseases, including lung cancer and distant metastases.

Positron emission tomography combined with CT scan (PET/CT) is a particularly useful method to detect distant metastases and tumour recurrences in previously treated patients. It relies on tumour cells preferentially picking up injected radiolabelled glucose. Radioactive signals produced from metabolism of this labelled agent are detected by a gamma camera and are shown as concentrated areas on the films (known as fluorodeoxyglucose [FDG] avid). The poor anatomical definition can be overcome by coregistration with MRI or CT scans. However, the limited availability of PET/CT precludes its widespread use.

Examination under anesthesia

Examination under anaesthesia is necessary when a thorough assessment of the tumour is not possible otherwise (e.g. extensive tumour, retching or pain). Patients with mouth cancer are also at risk of a second tumour. This is most likely to occur in the upper aerodigestive tract. An alternative method is to use a flexible nasoendoscope to augment the imaging findings described earlier.

Medical assessment (fitness for surgery, radiotherapy or chemotherapy)

This assessment includes history, examination, haematological and biochemical tests and cardiovascular (e.g. electrocardiogram, echocardiogram) and respiratory (e.g. pulmonary function tests, arterial blood gases) investigations (see Chapter 5). In addition, an anaesthetic assessment for these often high-risk patients is invaluable.

Assessment in practice

The key questions to answer are tumour resectability (and proximity to vital structures), the likelihood of neck (both sides) involvement and the presence or absence of distant metastases.

Primary tumour

Clinical assessment often yields substantial information on its own within the oral cavity. However, occasionally, other methods are required (e.g. in patients with extension of tumour into the pharynx, close to the mandible, retching or pain excluding a thorough examination). MRI is better than CT because CT images are often degraded by associated amalgam artifacts. More information on bone invasion can be gained using plain radiographs, MRI or CT scan and, very rarely, radioisotope scintigraphic bone scan.

Neck metastases

Clinical palpation tends to miss some 30% to 40% of neck metastases. Imaging techniques such as ultrasound, MRI or CT scanning and ultrasound-guided fine needle aspiration provide better accuracy (in ascending order). If a thorough histological analysis of neck specimens in necks that have clinically and radiologically negative findings is carried out, some 30% of patients with oral cancer will be found to have occult disease in the neck.

Distant metastases

Most distant metastases arising from oral SCC occur in the thorax. CT of the thorax is more detailed and accurate than plain chest radiography.

Staging and treatment planning

Staging of the disease

It is important that the staging nomenclature adopted is widely accepted and therefore must be simple and clearly defined. The staging process allows the clinician to have a uniform, communicable description of that patient's disease (i.e. the extent of the cancer). It helps in the treatment plan process, predicts prognosis and enables better audit (within and among different centres), as well as meaningful multicentre studies.

Tables 22.1 and 22.2 show the current staging nomenclature in use for oral SCC. There are other staging methods. However, to be effective, a staging method needs to be widely known (and therefore adopted universally), easy to use, reliable to score and ideally able to fulfill the roles stated earlier. Despite its several inadequacies, the TNM system remains the most universally used.

Table 22.1 Union for International Cancer Control and American Joint Committee on Cancer TNM classification

T – Primary tumour

- TX – Primary tumour cannot be assessed.
- T0 – No evidence of primary tumour.
- TCIS – Carcinoma in situ.
- T1 – Tumour 2 cm or less in maximum dimension.
- T2 – Tumour more than 2 cm but no more than 4 cm in maximum dimension.
- T3 – Tumour more than 4 cm in maximum dimension.
- T4 – Tumour invading adjacent structures (e.g. bone, deep extrinsic muscles, maxillary sinus or skin).
- T4a – Resectable.
- T4b – Unresectable.

N – Regional lymph nodes

- NX – Regional lymph nodes cannot be assessed.
- N0 – No regional lymph node metastasis.
- N1 – Metastasis in a single ipsilateral lymph node 3 cm or less in maximum dimension.
- N2a – Metastasis in a single ipsilateral lymph node more than 3 cm but not more than 6 cm maximum dimension.
- N2b – Metastasis in multiple ipsilateral lymph nodes, none more than 6 cm maximum dimension.
- N2c – Metastasis in contralateral or bilateral lymph nodes, none more than 6 cm maximum dimension.
- N3 – Metastasis in a lymph node more than 6 cm maximum dimension.

M – Distant metastases

- MX – Presence of distant metastasis cannot be assessed.
- M0 – No distant metastasis.
- M1 – Presence of distant metastasis.

Table 22.2 Stage grouping of TNM classification

Stage	T status	N status	M status
Stage 0	TCIS	N0	M0
Stage I	T1	N0	M0
Stage II	T2	N0	M0
Stage III	T3	N0	M0
	T1, T2, T3	N1	M0
Stage IVA	T4	N0	M0
	T4	N1	M0
	T1, T2, T3, T4	N1, N2	M0
Stage IVB	T1, T2, T3, T4	N3	M0
Stage IVC	T1, T2, T3, T4	N0, N1, N2, N3	M1

Sobin L, Gospodarowicz M, Wittekind C. *The TNM Classification of malignant tumours*, 7th ed. UICC, 2009.

Treatment plan

Once the staging process is completed, the definitive treatment plan can be formed. Treatment planning is generally carried out in a multidisciplinary team setting. The team usually consists of head and neck cancer specialists, surgeon(s), clinical oncologist(s) with radiotherapy expertise, a pathologist and a radiologist, as well as allied medical professionals such as a speech and language therapist, a dietician and a head and neck cancer nurse specialist. There are also other specialists associated with the service such as a dental hygienist, a maxillofacial technician, an occupational therapist, a psychologist and a physiotherapist. The team approach is aimed at removing bias in treatment planning and outcome assessment and at combining experience as well as expertise to ensure the best possible treatment that can be provided for the patient.

Treatment intention

It is important to be clear about the treatment intention for that individual patient. In the majority of cases, this is curative, although in some cases it is entirely palliative, which may be defined as 'active' (usually using low-dose and low-toxicity radiotherapy or chemotherapy) or best supportive care. Rarely, 'curative treatment with palliative intent' (i.e. the same intensity of treatment, often surgery and radiotherapy, as in treatment with curative intent) is offered in the belief that even if the cancer is not curable on the grounds of metastases, the best chance of effective symptom control lies with curative-intensity treatment.

The overall decision on accepting treatment must lie with the patient (when a competent adult). This decision is made by balancing the information on acute and chronic morbidity of treatment, relative chances of cure, morbidity associated with not having optimal treatment and individual quality of life decisions. All patients are different, and each patient has differing priorities. Patients should be enabled to make the most appropriate decisions for them, ideally with an adequate length of time, support and environment to come to a balanced decision.

Choosing a treatment modality

More than 90% of mouth cancers are SCCs. The natural progression of the disease involves invasion of local structures and spread to the regional cervical nodes and distant sites, principally the lungs. The invasive process is such that the microscopic front tends to be farther than macroscopically apparent. The more advanced the disease, the poorer the prognosis will be.

Standard curative treatment modalities for oral SCC are:

- Surgery.
- Radiotherapy.
- Combined modalities (surgery and radiotherapy).

Chemotherapy is generally accepted to not be curative for oral SCC. It is mainly used as a palliative tool or in combination with radiotherapy to enhance the effectiveness of radiotherapy (chemoradiotherapy). Chemotherapy can sometimes be used as a test of tumour responsiveness in which if the tumour regresses after a cycle or two of chemotherapy, radical radiotherapy is added (induction chemotherapy).

Surgery

Surgical tools are principally cutting implements – scalpel, cutting diathermy, laser or Coblator. These are simply different tools with different ways of cutting tissue; they are not anticancer tools, although some surprising properties have been ascribed to lasers of different types. It is important to respect the key principle of adequate excision margins whichever tool is used. For oral cancer, this macroscopic margin is 1 to 1.5 cm. The aim of surgery is to have a histopathological clearance of 5 mm. This would appear straightforward if such a large macroscopic clearance is being taken, but mucosal shrinkage and formalin-induced shrinkage often narrow these margins. There is some evidence to suggest that a clear margin of 2 mm after shrinkage produces the same statistically significant survival as a 5-mm margin. A positive margin equates to a poor prognosis.

Radiotherapy

This is a technique that uses radiation, principally photons or electrons. Previously, fast neutrons went through a subsequently disastrous period of popularity, and protons are currently being advocated as more dose-efficient targeted treatments.

The mainstays of treatment and those of proven effectiveness for most head and neck cancer are photons, where possible targeted using intensity-modulated radiotherapy (IMRT). The dose required to cure head and neck cancer (usually between 55 and 65 gray) is sometimes augmented (in a fashion that does not allow accurate dose estimation) by chemotherapy. This dose is extremely close to the point where necrosis of tissue occurs, and both soft tissue necrosis and hard tissue necrosis are complications of radiation treatment. This disorder is covered in more detail later.

Nonstandard treatments

These are treatments that have been demonstrated to be effective anticancer strategies but are not universally available or applicable. They should not be confused with 'alternative therapy', which consist of treatments that may or may not be useful adjuncts to overall patient management but have no anticancer effect (aromatherapy, homeopathy).

Photodynamic therapy

Photodynamic therapy (PDT) is quite frequently used for superficial skin cancers. It is often provided as a service by dermatologists and uses a topical photoactive substance (aminolevulinic acid [ALA]). For use in mucosal cancer of the head and neck in the United Kingdom, PDT is licensed only for palliative use or when other standard strategies have failed or are not possible. This therapy involves an intravenous injection of a photosensitizer (temoporfin) about 4 days before illuminating the tumour either with superficial or interstitial red light laser. During the entire process, the patient is light sensitive, and the drug is slowly leached out of the system by gradual exposure to artificial light and daylight, the major drawback of the technique. This process causes destruction of the tumour. Problems include calculation of light dose to all aspects of the tumour and the safety margin of normal tissue around the tumour. There are dramatic examples of effectiveness, but as many examples of spectacular failure. The evidence base is not sufficient for PDT to be internationally recognized as a standard treatment alternative in head and neck cancer, although in some other sites this has been achieved.

Electroporation

This treatment involves electrical stimulation of the tumour to increase its sensitivity to a chemotherapeutic agent, usually bleomycin. Similar to PDT, electroporation is currently a single-company process (and, similar to PDT, a second company is attempting to launch the technique after disappointing results for the initiating companies). The indications for electroporation are similar to those for PDT, but electroporation avoids the dangers of light sensitivity inherent in PDT.

Issues to consider in choice of treatment modality

Patient-related factors

The general health of the patient can have a major bearing on the choice of treatment modality to adopt. Many of these patients tend to smoke tobacco, drink alcohol and have significant related comorbidities. Preexisting medical problems such as heart and chest disease are common in patients with mouth cancer. In addition to fitness to survive anaesthesia and surgery, complications are more likely to arise following surgery. Radiotherapy should not be considered an easy option in medically compromised patients because it causes substantial associated morbidity, including a mortality rate in the literature for radical chemoradiation higher than that of surgery. This is discussed later.

The patient should clearly be involved in the decision. The patient should be competent to make decisions. Some patients rely on their carers, friends and family, and it would be helpful to include them in the process. It has also been shown that patients with good family and social support tend to do better. It should always be remembered that no other person can give consent for an adult, and for those patients deemed incompetent to consent to treatment, a formal legal process must be followed appropriate to that country and situation.

Tumour-related factors

In some instances (e.g. small tumours [stage I or II]), both surgery and radiotherapy are equally effective in terms of locoregional control and survival. Then, other issues such as functional outcome, quality of life and morbidity, as well as the patient's preference, will help the patient to decide on the treatment modality most appropriate to him or her. It is always worth remembering that although the other modalities can be repeated, radical radiotherapy can be given only once.

The proximity of certain structures influences the treatment modality. For example, where there is bone involvement, surgery is preferred to radiotherapy (better control and fewer side effects) Tumour involvement of the carotid arterial tree or the base of the skull can mean not being able to achieve a clear margin (not resectable – categorized in the TNM system as T4b). What may be nonresectable (or not reconstructible) in one surgeon's mind is entirely treatable in another's. This variation is universal. The use of multidisciplinary teams (in the United Kingdom), tumour boards (in the United States) and other forms of multidisciplinary expert working groups aims to reduce it, but the variation will never reduce to zero. In practice, a few tumour margins are positive. Adjuvant radiotherapy (given after surgery) is indicated to improve control but is never as good as achieving histologically clear margins (variously defined as a 2- to 5-mm tumour-free margin histologically).

The presence or high risk of neck disease is usually addressed by surgery. Certain tumour features (e.g. large tumours, thicker lesions, tongue site and histological features such as poor differentiation or perineural spread) may sway the decision toward neck dissection. There have been attempts at predicting the likelihood of nodal metastases accurately, but to date it remains an inexact science (~30% of tongue cancers staged clinically and by imaging as T2N0 will have at least micrometastases).

More advanced tumours are better controlled with surgery followed by adjuvant radiotherapy. As outlined earlier, chemoradiation may have a role to play in poorly differentiated tumours, in patients with extracapsular spread of tumour from lymph nodes or with positive margins after surgery – all signs of a 'high-risk' squamous cancer.

Clinician-related factors

Local expertise, resources and better outcome associated with a preferred modality within each team are practical considerations that often influence the treatment choice and can render national guidelines ineffective, even when apparent international 'gold standards' of care exist.

Treatment

Surgery

Surgery can be confined to tumour ablation alone, with or without reconstruction (see Chapter 23). Where there is regional node involvement, neck dissection is carried out at the same time. In many instances, reconstruction is simultaneous. If so, the surgery will be more extensive, in the form of a series of procedures (e.g. tracheostomy, neck dissection, access surgery, dental clearance, tumour ablation followed by immediate reconstruction and closure of the donor site). In such instances, a two-team approach is preferred because the workload is shared, and the total anaesthetic time is reduced, with the flap harvested while ablative surgery is performed.

Airway

There are several issues to consider as part of tumour resection. The airway must be secured during and after the surgery. If there is a significant risk to the airway (e.g. likely oral or neck swelling), a temporary tracheostomy should be performed (Figure 22.12).

Access for tumour resection

Adequate access is important because the presence of a positive margin adversely affects the outcome. Small anterior oral tumours can be approached through the mouth (peroral or transoral). Where better access is needed, surgical approaches such as lip split and access osteotomy (labiomandibulotomy) or a visor approach can be adopted (Figure 22.13).

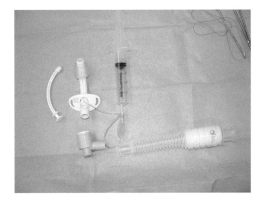

Figure 22.12 The individual components for a tracheostomy. Top left introducer, tracheostomy tube (check that cuff **before** you put it in), syringe to inflate cuff, bottom left to right, connector and flexible connecting tube – don't even think about starting before you have all of these immediately on hand.

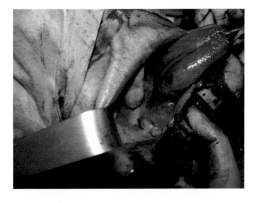

Figure 22.13 Labiomandibulotomy (splitting the lip and mandible) allows three-dimensional access to posterior tumours.

Tumour resection

The principal aim of ablative surgery with curative intent is the eradication of local disease by taking a margin of clinically normal tissue from all around the palpable edge of the tumour three dimensionally. This is usually possible for most tumours. There needs to be a balance between achieving cure with extensive radical surgery at the price of significant mutilation and an overly conservative approach resulting in insufficient tumour clearance to achieve better function. Most surgeons take a 1-cm normal tissue margin all around the tumour. On completion of the tumour resection, some surgeons take small specimens at selective margins for frozen sections analysis. This process takes about 20 to 30 minutes. It is, however, dependent on the site(s) sampled. Moreover, frozen section interpretation is never as accurate as definitive haematoxylin and eosin examination, so the risk of false reassurance while using this technique is ever present (Figure 22.14).

Some 70% of oral SCCs occur in a U-shaped area around the mandible, floor of mouth and tongue. In some instances, lesions close to the mandible can be difficult to assess in terms of bone involvement. If frank invasion has taken place (clinically or on periosteal stripping), then the tumour is likely to have involved the medullary space. If the mandible is involved (by the cancer), it will need to be included in the resection. The functional sequelae arising from a segmental mandibular resection with discontinuity of mandible are considerable even if the mandible is reconstructed immediately. Where the tumour is close but not involving the bone, a rim of the mandible can be taken, leaving a preserved lower border. The reconstruction is usually simpler and has a better functional outcome.

Certain vital structures need preserving (e.g. common and internal carotid arteries, which have a ~20% risk of stroke if they are ligated, although this possibility can be assessed preoperatively or even perioperatively, and cavernous sinus, which is not resectable). Cancers close to or involving such vital structures usually represent advanced disease with a poor prognosis. This situation helps illustrate the need for careful preoperative assessment.

Laser

This method of thermal surgery has a useful role in the treatment of premalignant lesions and early SCC. A laser beam is used instead of a scalpel for the surgery. The laser beam can be projected in a noncontact manner through a handpiece with a focusing guide length (e.g. carbon dioxide laser) or transmitted through a cable and cut on contact (e.g. diode laser).

The laser wound is left unreconstructed (i.e. 'raw'). Its advantages include a haemostatic effect (seals vessels smaller than 0.5 mm), less scarring and oedema and possibly less pain. The wound will epithelialize to leave a virtually normal-looking mucosa.

A similar result can be achieved using fine tip (Colorado needle) cutting diathermy at significantly lower capital cost. Both share a risk in that the surgical margin suffers from thermal artifact.

Transoral robotic surgery

There are a small number of surgical robots in the world market. These are inevitably concentrated in the developed world, most obviously in North America. Because these robots were developed to gain better three-dimensional access to areas of the body that are difficult to approach, there has been, unsurprisingly, interest in their use in oropharyngeal cancers. Currently at the phase of use and reporting by enthusiasts, it will be interesting to see whether these expensive and complex machines demonstrate benefits to patients in terms of survival and quality of life assessments to balance the obvious costs.

The status of the surgical margin is an important prognostic outcome. The presence of a close or positive (tumour present) margin considerably worsens the prognosis (Figure 22.15).

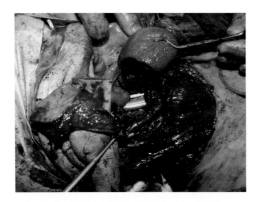

Figure 22.14 The defect left after resection of oral squamous cell carcinoma.

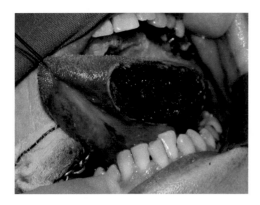

Figure 22.15 Tongue bed defect after laser excision.

Metastatic disease in the neck

The lymphatic drainage of the oral cavity is generally an orderly and sequential flow into the submental, submandibular and upper jugular chain. Malignant disease usually spreads in a similar orderly fashion, with the exception of previous treatment areas (either surgical or nonsurgical because both change the pattern of lymphatic drainage) and the skip metastasis phenomenon for tongue lesions to the lower jugular chain.

The presence of metastatic disease in the neck worsens the prognosis by about 50%. Unfortunately, it is not always possible to predict the presence of disease in the neck accurately. We know that overall, about 30% of oral cancers are likely to have spread to the neck on presentation, even though disease is not palpable clinically.

The decision to treat the neck depends on several factors:

- The presence of any enlarged node(s) is presumed to be metastatic disease until proven otherwise.
- There is a high risk of clinically undetected disease in the neck (occult metastases).
- If the patient is unlikely to comply with close follow-up, an initial more radical (i.e. do the neck dissection) approach is logical.
- Microvascular access for reconstructive free flap transfer is required.

To achieve regional control of the disease, lymph nodes in the neck can be treated surgically with neck dissection or irradiated. Surgery is usually the preferred option.

Neck dissection

The gold standard technique to achieve regional control of the neck surgically is radical neck dissection, which means removal of lymphatics and fat in all five levels in the neck (Figure 22.16). However, there are significant side effects associated with the procedure (Figure 22.17). The nomenclature for types of neck dissection can be confusing, but it has been classified to standardize the terminology (Table 22.3). The surgical treatment of the neck can be divided into elective and therapeutic neck dissections.

The most commonly chosen approach for the neck with clinically negative findings among patients with head and neck SCC is selective neck dissection as a staging or therapeutic surgical procedure. The reason comes from the early work of Lindberg, who demonstrated in 1972 that in patients with carcinoma of the oral cavity (tongue, floor of mouth), the lymph nodes most frequently involved included the following:

- Submandibular (level I).
- Jugulodigastric (level II).
- Midjugular (level III).

The low jugular (level IV) and posterior triangle (level V) lymph nodes were rarely involved. The same study demonstrated that the lymph nodes

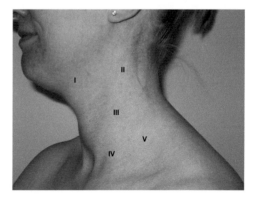

Figure 22.16 The basic description of cervical node distribution within the neck – level I, submandibular and submental nodes; level II, upper jugular chain from skull base to level of hyoid; level III, midjugular chain from level of hyoid to lower border of cricoid; level IV, lower jugular chain from cricoid to clavicle; and level V, posterior sternomastoid edge to anterior edge of trapezius from skull base to clavicle.

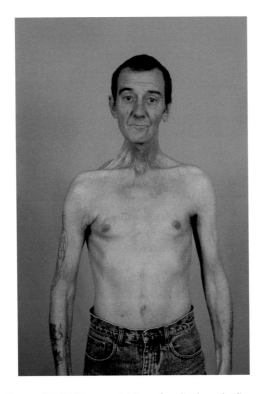

Figure 22.17 The morbidity of radical neck dissection. This patient has had bilateral neck dissections. The morbidity caused by the radical neck dissection is evident in the drooping shoulder, loss of neck volume and symptoms of shoulder pain, stiffness and anaesthesia. The side that underwent selective neck dissection is much less morbid.

most frequently involved in patients with carcinoma of the oropharynx were the jugulodigastric in all sites, including potential bilateral involvement. The lymph nodes of the submandibular or submental (level I) triangles were seldom involved in patients with oropharyngeal carcinomas. Lindberg also noted that SCCs arising from the base of the tongue frequently metastasized to both sides of the neck.

Shah, in a retrospective analysis in 1990 of 1119 radical neck dissection specimens, reported the following:

- The submental (IA), submandibular (IB), jugulodigastric (II) and midjugular lymph nodes were at highest risk for metastases from SCCs of the oral cavity.
- The jugulodigastric, midjugular and lower jugular lymph nodes were at highest risk for metastases from SCCs of the oropharynx, hypopharynx and larynx.

Davidson in 1993 reported a 3% incidence of histologically positive posterior triangle (level V) lymph nodes in a retrospective study of 1277 neck dissections in patients with SCCs of the head and neck.

Elective neck dissection is performed when there is no clinical evidence of involved lymph nodes in the neck. It is a useful staging procedure. To minimize

Table 22.3 Classification of neck dissections*

A. Comprehensive (removes all five levels of neck lymph nodes)

1. Radical neck dissection (removes XI, IJV and SCM).

2. Modified radical neck dissections.

   a. Type I (preserves XI).

   b. Type II (preserves XI and IJV).

   c. Type III (preserves XI, IJV and SCM).

B. Selective (removes only some of the levels of neck lymph nodes; preserves many structures)

1. Supraomohyoid neck dissection (removes levels I, II and III).

2. Anterolateral neck dissection (removes levels I, II, III and IV).

3. Lateral neck dissection (removes levels II, III and IV).

4. Posterolateral neck dissection (removes levels II, III, IV and V).

IJV, internal jugular vein; SCM, sternocleidomastoid muscle; XI, accessory nerve.

*Lateral and posterolateral neck dissections are used in laryngeal and hypopharyngeal cancers, not oral cancers (high-risk levels are I, II, III and IV).

the side effects, these procedures tend to be selective (only take the high-risk groups of lymph nodes to minimize side effects and therefore improve function). As many structures in the neck that are not involved in the spread of malignant disease as possible are retained. Although originally introduced as a staging procedure, the selective (elective) neck dissection removing levels I to IV has become the therapeutic standard in patients with N0 and low-volume node-positive neck findings when treating oral and oropharyngeal cancer surgically.

Interestingly, this approach is not universally applied and may reflect the particularly UK influence on the role of level IV – its anatomical versus radiological definition, relationship with skip lesions and consistency in technique and training in selective neck dissection.

German practice for SCCs consists of neck dissection of levels I to III as standard procedure. If the tumour is strictly on one side close to the body of the mandible or the lateral border of the tongue, neck dissection is performed only unilaterally and is expanded to the other side and to level V on the ipsilateral side only in cases of positive lymph nodes, as proven by frozen sections. If the tumour is located anteriorly in the mouth or behind the molars, neck dissection of levels I to III is conducted on both sides and is expanded to level V if the results of frozen section in level II or III are positive. This is clearly a different oncological strategy from that used in the United Kingdom and is based on a different premise and available resource (e.g. ready availability and reliance on perioperative frozen section). In the United States variation is even greater.

Therapeutic neck dissection is performed when we strongly suspect or know there is disease in the neck (e.g. enlarged lymph nodes by clinical or radiological criteria or positive FNAC results). To achieve good control, some surgeons may perform comprehensive neck dissection (taking all five levels of lymph nodes in the neck, usually including at least some of the noninvolved anatomical structures). This is technically described as modified radical neck dissection types I to III. However, in small-volume neck disease, it is reasonable to perform selective neck dissection as described earlier because if postoperative radiotherapy is indicated, the survival and recurrence figures are no different and the morbidity of selective neck dissection is less than that associated with radical neck dissection.

In many maxillofacial surgical oncological practices, it is now more common to perform an extended modified radical neck dissection (hyperradical, including skin or other structures in one area but preserving a viable structure, perhaps the accessory nerve, in another) than the classical radical (block) neck dissection.

A 'positive neck' is the one with clinical or radiological evidence of disease in neck lymph nodes. There is no randomized controlled evidence that would clearly define the best treatment for patients with a clinically node-positive neck. Patients with clinical N1 disease should be treated by appropriate neck dissection or radical radiotherapy with or without chemotherapy. Patients with clinical N2 or N3 disease should undergo the following:

- Comprehensive neck dissection and external beam radiotherapy.
- Radical radiotherapy and comprehensive neck dissection.

The reason is that in N2 or N3 disease, there is poor correlation between clinical and pathological responses following chemoradiotherapy.

Elective neck dissection is a controversial area, in particular for early-stage oral cancer. A possible disadvantage of leaving a neck alone and operating only when it becomes involved clinically is that positive neck findings carry a poorer prognosis because the disease is more advanced, a consequence of the detection of disease in the neck often coming when it has reached the N2 stage.

The disadvantages of neck dissection include unnecessary surgical morbidity (if results are found to be negative pathologically), a claimed 1% risk of mortality (this may well be a significant overestimate) and inefficient use of resources.

Complications commonly associated with neck dissections include those associated with general anaesthesia, bleeding, haematoma, infection, wound healing and scarring, as well as specific problems.

Specific problems arising from neck dissection include shoulder problems (pain, stiffness and deformity), neck problems (stiffness and pain), altered sensation and cosmetic deformities including the consequences of damage to the marginal mandibular branch of the facial nerve, deformed scarred neck and shoulder droop. Chyle leak is a complication that can be difficult to manage. It results from damage to the thoracic duct on the left or the lymphatic duct on the right. It occurs in up to 3% of neck dissections, with most occurring on the left side. Chyle is a mixture of lymph from interstitial fluid and emulsified fat from intestinal lacteals. It is estimated that 3 to 5 litres of lymph fluid will pass through the thoracic duct daily. In extreme cases damage to the thoracic duct with chyle extravasation can result in hypovolaemic shock, hyponatraemia and oedema, as well as serious nutritional consequences. It is recommended that high-output leaks more than 1 to 2 litres a day for more than 5 to 7 days should be actively treated. The management of a chyle leak may be classified into the following:

1. Intraoperative recognition of injury with repair.
2. Conservative postoperative management.
3. Management using interventional radiology or minimally invasive endoscopic surgery.
4. Reexploration and repair.

Alternatives to elective neck dissection (when no disease is demonstrable clinically or radiologically) include a watch and wait policy, close monitoring with regular ultrasound-guided FNAC (problem with follow-up compliance) and, currently on trial, sentinel lymph node biopsy, although this has been shown to have poor sensitivity in occult disease.

Types of neck dissection

It is inevitable that more advanced neck disease has a poorer prognosis. Important prognostic factors include extracapsular spread, multiple nodal disease or bilateral neck involvement and level IV or V involvement.

Radical neck dissection is effective in controlling bulky disease in the neck in less than 40% of cases when it is used alone (Figure 22.18), but when it is used with adjuvant radiotherapy, the control rate rises to around 80%. In patients with negative neck findings, radical neck dissection provides control in excess of 90% of cases. In smaller-volume disease, modified radical neck dissection is as effective as radical neck dissection but is associated with less morbidity.

Selective neck dissection has been shown to be effective in managing patients with clinically negative neck findings. It provides good control (<10% recurrence). This is similar to radical neck dissection for neck findings staged as N0 but with less morbidity. Where occult disease is present on histological analysis, regional control drops (up to 24% recurrence). The addition of adjuvant radiotherapy improves control to recurrence rates of 15%, an acceptable control rate in comparison with radical neck dissection. The key advantages of selective neck dissection are less morbidity and better quality of life outcomes.

Adjuvant radiotherapy is given to the primary tumour site where there is tumour present at the

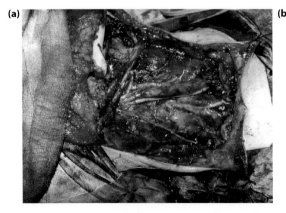
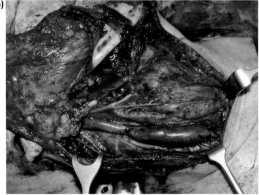

Figure 22.18 (a) Radical neck dissection; note the absence of internal jugular vein, sternomastoid muscle and accessory nerve. (b) Selective neck dissection; the structures missing in the radical neck dissection are preserved, and in some cases the cervical plexus can also be preserved.

margins, close to the margins, high-grade dysplasia or carcinoma *in situ* at the margins on histological analysis, bone invasion (T4 by definition) or large tumours.

Adjuvant radiotherapy is given to the neck following neck dissection where there is extracapsular spread, multiple intracapsular disease (more than two lymph nodes positive) or soft tissue disease or positive margins.

Radiotherapy

The use of ionizing radiation for therapeutic purposes in oncology dates from the end of the nineteenth century, after the discovery of radium by Marie and Pierre Curie. It is an effective and important treatment modality in head and neck cancer.

Radiotherapy works on the principle that rapidly dividing cells (e.g. cancer cells) are selectively destroyed by exposure to irradiation. Cells exposed to ionizing radiation form free radicals intracellularly, thus causing denaturation of large molecules including DNA. Although most of the changes are not apparent immediately, any attempt at division (to form new cells or repair injury) results in mitotic cell death. Rapidly dividing cells are most vulnerable, especially most cancer cells and normal fast-proliferating tissues such as mucosa and skin.

The unwanted effects can be divided into acute reactions and delayed effects with long-term late damage (Table 22.4). Such effects are dose dependent.

The efficacy of irradiation on tumour cells depends on their radiosensitivity (e.g. sarcoma is less sensitive than carcinoma), the oxygenation of the tissue (the better to create free radicals) and the tumour volume (small-volume tumours are better controlled than large tumours).

Radiation delivery has evolved from conventional external beam two-dimensional therapy to three-dimensional conformal radiotherapy. In a further advance, IMRT has been a significant technological advance because it allows sparing of formal tissue while delivering radical radiation doses to the target volumes. The potential of IMRT for sparing organs at risk has been demonstrated in patients with mixed head and neck cancers,

oropharyngeal and nasopharyngeal. The multicentre study PARSPORT (**Par**otid-**Sp**aring Intensity Modulated versus Conventional **R**adio**T**herapy in Head and Neck Cancer), which compared parotid-sparing IMRT with standard radiotherapy in patients with oropharyngeal and hypopharyngeal cancer, showed a significant reduction in xerostomia in the IMRT arm of the trial at 1 year after radiotherapy. IMRT has not yet been shown to improve tumour control or patient survival significantly compared with two-dimensional or three-dimensional radiotherapy. The only randomized controlled trial comparing IMRT versus three-dimensional radiotherapy reported to date, PARSPORT, had too small a sample size and too short a follow-up to investigate any differences in clinical outcome. IMRT also has disadvantages resulting from the complexity of IMRT planning and delivery process and the possibility of errors in planning or delivery.

There are three ways radiotherapy can be administered – by teletherapy (external beam), by brachytherapy (radiation source placed within or close to tumour) and with radioactive isotopes injected systemically and taken up by cancer cells (e.g. used in thyroid cancer). In oral cancer, only the first two are used.

Teletherapy (external beam radiotherapy)

This is the most widely used method. The machines used are megavoltage external beam radiotherapy linear accelerators (photons). The beam produced is precise in definition, direction and depth, thus allowing careful planning in terms of delivery (scan aided with computerized planning). The patient is immobilized in a clear custom made plastic shell (Figure 22.19), and multiple beams are used to maximize delivery to the tumour target volume planned yet minimizing adjacent tissue such as salivary glands, spinal cord and lens of the eye. The accuracy of this process is improved by CT planning and intensity modulation.

There are several regimens with variable dosage and fractions (a fraction is a single dose delivered) used. The optimal treatment time and number of doses remain controversial and dependent on the volume irradiated. A common regimen for head and neck cancer is around a total dose of 55 to 60 Gray (a gray is energy absorption of 1 joule/kg)

Table 22.4 Side effects of radiotherapy

	Features	Comments
Acute		
General	Tiredness, lethargy, fatigue.	Systemic effects of treatment.
Mucositis	Erythema, exudate formation, ulceration.	One of earliest to show because of rapid (12 days) mucosa epithelial turnover.
		Takes several weeks to heal after completion of radiation.
Skin reactions	Erythema, desquamation.	Slightly later (21 days).
		Healing similar to mucosa.
Hair loss	In line of radiation beam.	Usually temporary but can be permanent.
Loss of taste	Some change noticed.	Temporary because taste buds are fairly radioresistant.
		Mechanism related to salivary changes?
Xerostomia	Reduce saliva production, sticky saliva, dental caries.	Salivary glands sensitive to radiation.
		A common complaint despite attempts to reduce this side effect (e.g. shielding, avoiding beams).
		Saliva substitutes, vigilant dental care (including topical fluoride) important.
Infection	Acute bacterial and candidal infections.	Antifungal agents.
		Chlorhexidine mouthwash painful to use, best avoided.
Late		
Ischaemia and fibrosis	White atrophied scarred tissue with telangiectasia, dry skin and mucosa.	Hypocellularity, hypovascularity. Hypoxaemia.
Soft tissue necrosis	Chronic ulcers, with slow or poor healing.	For the foregoing reasons.
Radiation caries	Classically cervical caries, widespread.	Resulting from brittle enamel, poor saliva protection, sticky sugary diet, poor hygiene secondary to treatment.
Osteoradionecrosis	Exposed bone, which can be painful and progress to pathological fractures, dehiscence, halitosis	Prevention better than cure – eliminate dental sepsis sources before irradiation, avoid trauma (ill-fitting denture), perform atraumatic extractions in high-risk teeth and possibly administer HBO.
		Treatment possibly difficult – sequestrectomy, HBO and radical surgery used.
Malignancy	New malignancy developing in irradiated area years later.	Small but real risk.

HBO, hyperbaric oxygen.

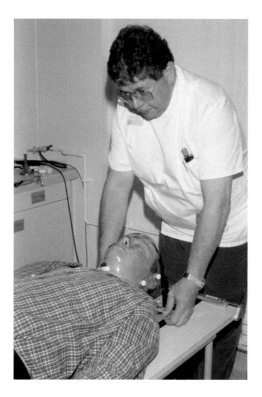

Figure 22.19 Positioning a patient using a customized mask for external beam radiotherapy.

delivered as 20 fractions over 28 days. The optimal radiotherapy treatment is balanced between achieving control of disease and too much irradiation causing necrosis or significant late effects.

The therapeutic effect of radiotherapy can be reduced by delays between fractions (allow tumour cells to repair and repopulate), by a patient who continues to smoke and in whom radiotherapy is delivered after surgery (adjuvant radiotherapy), by relative hypoxia and by a long delay between surgery and the start of radiotherapy (6 weeks is regarded as optimal).

Other radiotherapy beams used include electrons for superficial tumours; the penetration of electrons is very limited, causing less collateral damage but rendering it ineffective for deeper tumours. Fast neutron particles went through a vogue but were seen to create much more morbidity for no greater benefit than photons. Proton beam therapy is another modality. It is relatively new, and setting up the equipment is very expensive. The proton beam has less scatter than conventional photon-based radiotherapy because of the large size of the particle and is believed to be particularly effective for tumours that are difficult to access (skull base and paediatric cancers). Its use is restricted to highly specified cases in the United Kingdom. However, the technique is widely used, and some would say inappropriately used, in the United States and in parts of Europe. Maslow's analogy of the hammer and the nail should always be borne in mind.

Brachytherapy (interstitial radiotherapy)

The principle of this method is to deliver ionizing radiation by inserting radioactive source(s), usually removable iridium-192 implant wires, into tumour by using slotted guide needles or plastic tubing. This method delivers a high intensity of radiation into its immediate vicinity, with a rapid fall in dosage in the surrounding tissue. The number of needles inserted is calculated according to volume and dosage required. The needles are inserted manually or using a remote computerized loading system (to avoid staff irradiation) while the patient is under general anaesthesia, with radiological checks. Because the patient is radioactive, he or she is kept in a protected and isolated environment. A common regimen involves delivery of a total dose of around 65 to 70 grays over 6 to 7 days.

This technique is not suitable for patients with poor compliance or claustrophobia. Tumours very close to or involving bone are also unsuitable for treatment using this approach. It is mainly used for small tumours with the key advantage of good functional outcome. It is an effective treatment modality but does not address the neck. The posttreatment area is often necrotic and very painful. This creates real difficulty in the first few months in terms of distinguishing between persisting disease and radionecrosis (Figure 22.20).

Adjuvant and neoadjuvant therapy

The rationale for postoperative radiotherapy is that a small volume (microscopic) of malignant cells may be left within the surgical bed through spillage or incompletely excised in the margins. Where frank tumour is present, radiotherapy is less effective, and in such instances, further resection is advocated. However, this may not always be possible (vital structure proximity, inability or unwillingness of the patient to have further surgery or flap reconstruction *in situ*). It has been

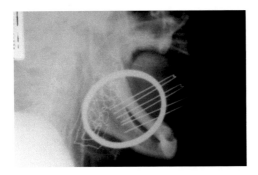

Figure 22.20 Radiograph of iridium wires *in situ* for brachytherapy.

shown that irradiating the operated tumour bed or neck helps reduce the chance of recurrence by some 50%. Ideally, this is carried out within 6 weeks of surgery.

Side effects of radiotherapy

Unlike surgery, in which many of the side effects are manifested quickly, the side effects of radiotherapy build up gradually. These can be divided into general, acute and delayed (see Table 22.4).

Of cases of ORN, 95% will occur in the mandible. ORN is often associated with dental extractions of teeth in an irradiated mandible. The general dental practitioner has an important role in preventing this unpleasant complication (Figure 22.21).

ORN is defined as irradiated bone that becomes devitalized and exposed through the overlying skin or mucosa without healing for 3 months, without recurrence of tumour.

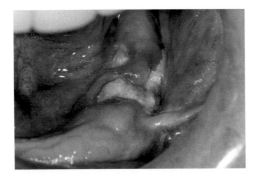

Figure 22.21 An example of osteoradionecrosis. Treatment of this condition can be more demanding than that of the original cancer. Do not lightly remove teeth from patients who have had radiotherapy to the mouth and jaws.

The Notani classification is quickly applicable to all cases of mandibular ORN after clinical examination and dental panoramic tomography and is as follows:

I. ORN confined to dentoalveolar bone.
II. ORN limited to dentoalveolar bone or mandible above the inferior dental canal or both.
III. ORN involving the mandible below the inferior dental canal or pathological fracture, or skin fistula.

There are several theories attempting to explain the pathophysiology of ORN. Marx in 1983 presented the triad of:

- Hypoxia.
- Hypovascularity.
- Hypocellularity.

More recently, the radiation-induced fibrosis theory was presented by Lyons and Ghazali. The key event in the development and progression of the condition is the dysregulation of fibroblastic activity in the irradiated area, which produces atrophic tissue with damage to microvessels and allows increased leakage of inflammatory mediators. The presence of tumor necrosis factor-alpha, platelet-derived growth factor, fibroblast growth factors and reactive oxygen species in the irradiated tissue then triggers a further inflammatory response with increasing damage to local tissue.

Approaches in the management include pentoxifylline (acts against TNF-alpha) and vitamin E (scavenger of reactive oxygen species) as part of the PENTOCLO protocol, as follows:

- 800 mg pentoxifylline
- 1000 IU vitamin E   5 days/week
- 1600 mg clodronate (non–nitrogen-containing bisphosphonate)
- 20 mg prednisolone
- 1 g ciprofloxacin   2 days/week

This regimen is continued (if tolerated) for 16 ± 9 months. Interestingly, the evidence base for this lies in nothing more than a case report and series from the same French authors. Personal experience shows a high incidence of intolerance related to unwanted effects of these drugs. It is ironic that this study also includes a bisphosphonate, one of the drugs known to cause bone necrosis, albeit a different type.

Other options are the hyperbaric oxygen (HBO) protocol that includes 20 dives; if improvement is noted, then they are followed by 10 dives at an atmospheric pressure of 2.4 atm. This protocol, originally described by Marx, has never benefitted from published work replicating his extremely good results. Despite this, it is used by many centres treating this condition and is subject in the United Kingdom to the HOPON (Hyperbaric Oxygen to Prevent Osteoradionecrosis) trial, which is attempting to create some form of evidence base in the treatment of this devastating disease affecting cancer survivors.

HBO remains used in the United States both for the treatment of ORN and in the form of prophylactic use before dentoalveolar procedures (e.g. extractions, implants) in irradiated jaws.

Personal experience over a 20-year period managing an escalating number of cases of ORN favours localized débridement and fresh vascularized coverage of viable bone ranging from minor local procedures to vascularized free tissue transfer (usually fibula) combined with antibiotics and HBO. No doubt the debate will rage on for many years while cancer survivors continue to endure this terrible consequence of effective nonsurgical oncological treatment.

Chemotherapy

The role of chemotherapy in oral cancer is at present small but will continue to evolve even if only because drug companies will continue to seek new markets for existing products. To date, the impact of a range of drugs on oral cancer treatment has been very disappointing. Surgery and radiotherapy remain the two key treatment modalities on a curative basis. Chemotherapy agents commonly used in head and neck cancer are 5-fluorouracil, cisplatin or carboplatin and methotrexate. Epidermal growth factor receptor (EGFR)–targeting drugs, tyrosine kinase inhibitors and taxanes have all been used in trials. A limited role for cetuximab and taxanes has been identified.

Chemoradiation (combining chemotherapy with radiotherapy) in head and neck cancer demonstrated improved outcome for nasopharyngeal

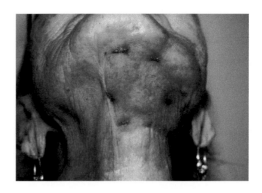

Figure 22.22 This woman developed skin metastases despite therapeutic surgery and radiotherapy for her large buccal carcinoma. Chemotherapy provided good palliative control with short-term resolution of her skin deposits.

cancer and certain poorly differentiated SCCs with the additional benefit of organ preservation. A meta-analysis of studies showed improved locoregional control with survival improved by some 8% to 15%, depending on the study (both the European Organization for Research and Treatment of Cancer [EORTC] and the Radiation Therapy Oncology Group [RTOG] groups have produced convincing data). However, the combination of chemotherapy and radiotherapy is associated with increased morbidity and mortality. All the studies failed to contain a surgical control arm, and none identified or excluded patients who were nonsmokers with HPV-driven cancers. Currently we are seeing the consequences of the widespread application of these hyperradical regimens and, in some cases, quite devastating long-term morbidity in the survivors. The continued use of chemoradiation will need appropriate cases and almost certainly not those cases that are relatively low risk (HPV driven) or equally treatable using surgery as a single modality.

Chemotherapy by itself has a useful role in palliation in some instances (Figure 22.22).

Preferred treatment modalities in practice

Small oral malignant tumors can be treated effectively (with similar cure rates) using either radiotherapy or surgery. The aim is to keep to a single treatment modality, thereby reducing the side effects. In such instances, a better functional outcome (e.g. tongue base better with radiotherapy) or the prospect of fewer side effects (surgery is better when tumour is close to bone) will influence the decision. The patient's preference after full information on the risks and benefits has been given must also be taken into account.

Large tumours usually require both modalities. The neck is treated surgically if the lymph nodes are enlarged, involved or at high risk of being involved or where microvascular access is required.

Outcome of treatment modalities, prognosis and quality of life issues

The prognosis of oral cancer depends on the stage of the disease. Early-stage tumours have around 70% to 90% 5-year survival rates, and tumours in more advanced stages drop to 20% to 50%.

The development of distant metastases means that the disease is incurable using current modalities. The incidence of lung metastases has been reported to be up to 20% clinically and close to 50% when assessed by means of postmortem examination. It is more likely with more advanced disease and with locoregional recurrence. Patients with lung metastases usually die within a year.

These patients are also at risk of developing second primary tumours, especially patients who had smoked (and consumed alcohol) heavily for a prolonged period and who continued to smoke following their cancer treatment. Inevitably, a second cancer, although most likely to develop in the same area, may not be easily diagnosed or treated, and some patients will die of this new cancer.

Patients with oral cancer tend to have significant medical problems associated with smoking and excess alcohol consumption (e.g. cardiovascular and respiratory disease [comorbidity]). A significant proportion of these patients will die of these and other associated diseases. It is not unusual for patients with head and neck cancer to have lung cancer either at diagnosis or later on.

It is often claimed there has been very little progress in terms of survival outcome in oral cancer over the last few decades. Nevertheless, oral cancer survival figures in the United Kingdom actually compare favourably with survival figures in other countries in Europe, unlike with many other cancers. Survival outcome data of specific units appear to be much better than the often quoted crude overall 56%; this finding implies that specific treatment systems and standards of care can improve survival figures. The major advancement since the 1990s has been in reconstructive techniques and, with it, improved quality of life outcomes. Quality of life is clearly an important issue as our understanding of oral cancer as a chronic disease improves.

Rehabilitation and follow-up

It is clear that patients with oral cancer pay a significant price to be rid of their malignant disease. They may have physical problems (e.g. speech, eating, swallowing, shoulder dysfunction, neck stiffness, cosmetic deformities including scars, numbness, donor site problems from reconstructive surgery, xerostomia, loss of teeth), social problems (e.g. work-related issues, financial hardship, difficult interactions with family and friends) and psychological problems (e.g. coping with illness, loss of previous lifestyle, fears of recurrence).

Some of these problems can be lessened with rehabilitative measures such as physiotherapy and occupational therapy, support groups and counselling, as well as dental rehabilitation, including extensive restorative dental treatment

Follow-up surveillance is generally undertaken on an outpatient basis. The aims include monitoring, diagnosis and management of complications or side effects of treatment, diagnosis of recurrence at an early stage to improve salvage rates and finding second malignant tumours. Recurrences are likely in the first 2 years, and follow-up appointments tend to be tailored accordingly. There is about a 3% to 5% chance of developing a second primary tumour (cancerization theory of field changes related to exposure to smoking and alcohol, with most new malignancies arising in the same upper aerodigestive tract region).

Recurrence

Recurrence of the primary tumour is most likely to occur in the first 2 years following treatment.

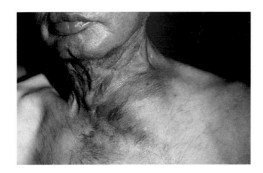

Figure 22.23 This patient had aggressive tongue cancer. He was lost to follow-up and returned with a large metastatic mass low in the neck. He also had lung metastases.

Patients at high risk include those with more advanced stages of disease at diagnosis, aggressive tumour features, positive margins and nodal disease including extracapsular spread. Recurrence can be local, regional or in distant sites (Figure 22.23).

Salvage treatment can be carried out using radiotherapy including brachytherapy (not possible if patients have had radiotherapy to that area), surgery or both. Unfortunately, patients are frequently at an advanced stage of disease, and curative treatment options are limited.

Palliation

Palliative treatment is an important treatment modality because not all cancer will be curable (e.g. tumour is not resectable, distant metastases are present, patient is not fit for active treatment or has an untreatable recurrence).

The aim of palliative treatment is to maintain the patient's quality of life. This is achieved by alleviating any suffering (e.g. pain control), as well as providing emotional, social and spiritual support to the patient and relatives. Palliation can be viewed as 'active' when an intervention, usually chemotherapy (in some cases up to six lines of chemotherapy are tried) or very limited radiotherapy, is used, and as 'best supportive care' when no active intervention is used.

The approach is similar to other treatment in being multidisciplinary team based, with good communication among the general medical practitioner, charitable support (in the United Kingdom, Macmillan and, to a lesser extent, Marie Curie nurses) and district nurses and social services. In addition, hospital or hospice-based expertise from palliative care teams, pain management teams and the caring environment of hospices can make an invaluable contribution to the quality of the end of a patient's life.

FURTHER READING

Ad VB, Chalian A. Management of clinically negative neck for the patients with head and neck squamous cell carcinomas in the modern era. *Oral Oncol* 2008;44:817–22.

Bhide SA, Nutting CM. Advances in radiotherapy for head and neck cancer. *Oral Oncol* 2010;46:439–41.

Brennan PA, Blythe JN, Herd MK, Habib A, Anand R. The contemporary management of chyle-leak following cervical thoracicduct damage. *Br J Oral Maxillofac Surg* 2012;50:197–201.

Davidson BJ, Kulkarny V, Delacure MD and Shah JP. Posterior triangle metastases of squamous cell carcinoma of the upper aerodigestive tract. *Am J Surgery* 1993;166:395–8.

Delanian S, Chatel C, Porcher R, Depondt J, Lefaix JL. Complete restoration of refractory mandibular osteoradionecrosis by prolonged treatment with a pentoxifylline-tocopherol-clodronate combination (PENTOCLO): a phase II trial. *Int J Radiat Oncol Biol Phys* 2011;80:832–9.

Elsheikh MN, Rinaldo A, Ferlito A, Fagan JJ, Suárez C, Lowry J, Paleri V, Khafif A, Olofsson J. Elective supraomohyoid neck dissection for oral cavity squamous cell carcinoma: is dissection of sublevel IIB necessary? *Oral Oncol* 2008;44:216–9.

Ferlito A, Rinaldo A, Robbins TK, Leemans RC, Shah JP, Shaha AR, Andersen PE, Kowalski LP, Pellitteri PK, Clayman, GL, Rogers SN, Medina PK, Byers RM. Changing concepts in the surgical management of the cervical node metastasis. *Oral Oncol* 2003;39:429–35.

Kerawala CJ, Heliotos M: Prevention of complications in neck dissection. *Head Neck Oncol* 2009;1:35.

Lindberg R. Distribution of cervical lymph node metastases from squamous cell carcinoma of the upper respiratory and digestive tracts. *Cancer* 1972;29:1446–9.

Lyons A, Ghazali N. Osteoradionecrosis of the jaws: current understanding of its pathophysiology and treatment. *Br J Oral Maxillofac Surg* 2008;46:653–60.

Mazeron R, Tao Y, Lusinchi A, Bourhis J. Current concepts of management in radiotherapy for head and neck squamous-cell cancer. *Oral Oncol* 2009;45:402–8.

McLeod NMH, Pratt CA, Mellor TK, Brennan PA. Pentoxifylline and tocopherol in the management of patients with osteoradione-crosis: the Portsmouth experience. *Br J Oral Maxillofac Surg* 2012;50:41–4.

National Cancer Institute (United States). www.cancer.gov. In the UK: www.ncri.org.uk.

Shah JP, Johnson NW, Batsakis JG. *Oral cancer.* London: Martin Dunitz, 2003.

Shah JP. Patterns of cervical lymph node metastasis from squamous carcinomas of the upper aero-digestive tract. *Am J Surg* 1990;160: 405–9.

Watkinson JC, Gaze MN, Wilson JA. *Head and neck surgery,* 4th ed. Oxford: Butterworth Helnemann, 2000.

Woolgar JA. Histopathological prognosticators in oral and oropharyngeal squamous cell carcinoma. *Oral Oncol* 2006;42:229–39.

23

Reconstruction of the mouth, jaws and face

Contents

Aims and learning outcomes

For undergraduates:

- To be able to describe the differences between a flap and a graft.
- To be able to describe the nature of oral and facial wound healing.
- To be able to discuss some common flaps and grafts.

For postgraduates:

- To be able to describe the role of various modalities of wound healing.
- To be able to outline a range of flaps and grafts.
- To be able to describe the steps in harvesting some common flaps and grafts.

Introduction

One of the most common reasons for reconstruction of the mouth, jaws and face is repair of deformity following resection of tumours. This resection often involves destruction of complex normal anatomy with significant functional sequelae. Historically, these patients were left disease-free but mutilated and severely impaired functionally. Such deformity can have a major impact on the patient's quality of life. The disfigurement is often easily seen and associated with psychological sequelae. Other needs for reconstruction include traumatic and congenital defects.

Immediate flap reconstruction following ablation is the optimal approach because the operation is single stage with minimal distortion from scarring, thus allowing functional and psychological rehabilitation to proceed. There is some evidence that simultaneous reconstruction improves disease-free survival.

The advocates of delayed reconstruction justify this approach on the basis that recurrence is possible and may be masked by the reconstruction, with a consequent delay in retreatment. They also believe that the time and effort of immediate reconstruction is 'wasted'. The main problem with this approach is that patients with a greater risk of recurrence tend to be those with larger defects and a greater functional need for reconstruction, and they benefit from adjuvant radiotherapy. Delayed reconstruction is seldom as successful, and so these patients are left functionally more compromised, with a poorer quality of life and potentially with a lower long-term survival benefit.

Surgical advances in head and neck reconstruction have resulted in a progressive trend from unreconstructed deformities or grafted wounds to locoregional flaps, two-staged repairs and currently immediate microvascular reconstructive surgery.

Reconstructive philosophy

The reconstructive surgeon operating in such a complex area needs to consider the following issues:

1. Defect size, site and tissue character.
2. Flap characteristics (e.g. tissue quality and quantity available, pedicle length, vascular reliability including vascular caliber), success rate, donor site morbidity and complications.
3. The functional outcome of options available (e.g. appearance, chewing, quality of life, sensation, shoulder function, speech and swallowing).
4. Rehabilitation (e.g. implants).
5. Cost factors and resource requirements.
6. Patient's general health (i.e. comorbidity can influence reconstructive options).
7. Patient's preference.
8. Surgeon's preference (and expertise).
9. Alternative options (e.g. obturator or no reconstruction).

Tumour ablation should never be compromised for the sake of reconstruction.

Classification of defects

In addition to the size, location and anatomical complexity, the defect can be divided into type of tissue that needs to be reconstructed:

1. Soft tissue.
2. Bone.
3. Composite.
4. Special tissue (e.g. nerve).

In practice, bone defects usually have some soft tissue component involved as well. It is often easier to think of the dominant tissue that is missing in the defect.

Reconstructive techniques

Many different reconstructive techniques are available. These range from minor, technically simple procedures such as grafting to state of the art complex composite microvascular free flap transfers. Table 23.1 shows the reconstructive options available and their advantages, disadvantages and indications.

A classification frequently quoted is the reconstructive ladder. This ladder starts at the bottom rung with the simplest technique (e.g. open wound healing by granulation) and progresses to prefabricated free flaps at the top. It is a useful concept, reflects the expertise involved and, when linked with consequences of failure, as in 'snakes and ladders', aptly reflects the 'fall' should that technique not work. Failure can result from haematoma, infection or thrombosis. These mechanisms result in ischaemia, necrosis and flap loss.

It is important to realize that although the more sophisticated technique often has greater benefits, it is likely that a higher price will be associated with its failure (e.g. a free flap is usually an all or none phenomenon, and every graft or flap harvested has accompanying donor site morbidity). This field may be the most in need of recalling Boyes' law – 'The ability to do an operation is not an indication'. Even more graphically – Keep it simple, stupid.

Open wound healing

In certain circumstances, leaving a superficial open wound to heal can be the best option. This includes laser wounds (Figure 23.1), as well as some defects in young children.

There is clearly a limit to this option because deep or extensive wounds usually heal slowly with scarring and resulting deformity.

Healing by primary intention

This is the most common reconstructive method used when the defect is small and the surrounding

Table 23.1 Options for reconstruction of the mouth, jaws and face

Options	Advantages	Disadvantages	Indications
Leave to heal (open wound)	Simple. No donor site.	Contracture, scarring. Wound dressings needed.	Superficial wounds. Laser wounds (good healing).
Primary closure	Simple. No donor site. Linear scar. Heal fastest.	Dehiscence risk. Adjacent tissue distortion.	Small defects with lax adjacent tissue. Should be used whenever possible.
Graft	Relatively simple. Skills possessed by most surgeons.	Reliance on healthy bed to take. Limited character and bulk (cosmesis).	Superficial wounds where primary closure is not feasible.
Local flap	Matching tissue characteristics. Ease of harvest.	Can further distort local function if large defect.	A popular option for small to medium defects.
Distant pedicled flap	Large tissue transfer from healthy region.	Poorer tissue match. Donor site morbidity. Additional larger procedure.	Medium to large defects.
Distant free transfers	Can tailor best tissue available to suit defect. Healthy tissue with good vascular supply allowing better healing.	Complex procedure requiring specialized expertise. All or none phenomenon – failure will result in defect remaining. Anastomoses (and flap) at risk if patient is unstable medically.	Reconstruction of choice for most significant defects in most patients fit for major surgery.
Prefabricated flaps	Better flap quality with modification or prefabrication.	Extra surgical procedure with prefabrication. Can risk flap outcome with previous surgery.	Ideal for traumatic or congenital defects (less suitable for patients with cancer who have disease progression).
Prosthesis	No surgical reconstruction needed. Allows inspection of defect for recurrence.	Needs expertise of prosthetist. Limited by patient's compliance and dexterity.	Low-level maxillary defects.

tissue is slack enough to allow advancement for closure of the wound. It provides the best outcome because the adjacent area provides similar quality tissue without the need for a separate donor site wound. The wound should also heal faster and, apart from suture removal, requires relatively simple aftercare.

Healing by primary intention is not a viable option when there is inadequate adjacent tissue because closure under tension will simply break down.

Grafts

A graft is the transfer of tissue by complete separation from the donor site to the recipient site. This potentially dead piece of tissue then gains a new blood supply by ingrowth of new vessels from the donor bed. This process works on the principle that the tissue's nutritional requirement is initially met by fibrin attachment with diffusion of oxygen from the plasma of the tissue bed (coined 'plasmatic

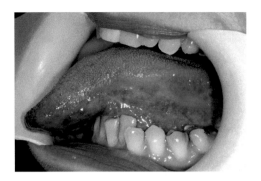

Figure 23.1 The result after granulation following laser excision of a small squamous cell carcinoma of the lateral tongue.

imbition'). Capillary ingrowth with establishment of a new vascular supply follows shortly.

The graft can be from the same individual (autograft), from another individual of the same species (allograft) or from different species (xenograft). Autografts are better for several reasons, including immunocompatibility, lower rates of infection and ultimately better outcomes.

Skin grafts

Skin grafts can be harvested as follows (see Chapter 18):

1. Split-thickness grafts (all of the epidermis and part of the dermis) – the donor site will resurface by epidermal cell migration.
2. Full-thickness grafts (the epidermis and dermis layers) – the donor site needs to be closed because no epidermal structure remains to resurface, and if left, the site will heal slowly with a contracted scar.

Skin grafting is a simple and popular soft tissue reconstructive technique. It requires a healthy bed to take. The donor site is dictated by factors such as size of graft required, appearance of donor site scar and harvested tissue, presence or absence of hair, access during surgery and mobility of the patient after surgery. Split-thickness skin grafts can provide viable reconstruction for the tongue in some cases (Figure 23.2 (a) and (b)).

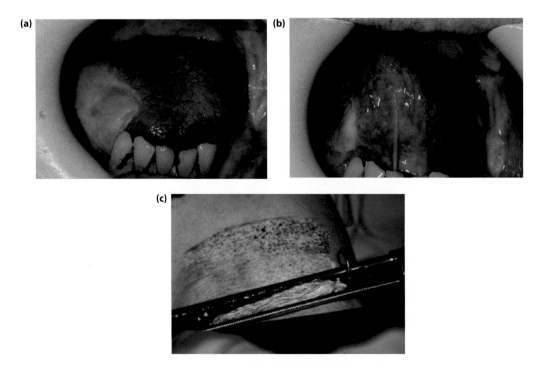

Figure 23.2 (a) A split-thickness skin graft repairing a postexcisional defect on the left lateral border of the tongue. (b) The mobility of the tongue is maintained. (c) Harvesting a split-thickness skin graft with a Watson knife.

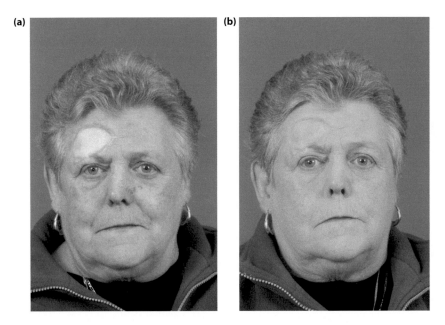

Figure 23.3 (a) The aesthetic result is often unfavourable, and (b) the patient may need cosmetic camouflage when a split-thickness skin graft is used on the face.

Split-thickness donor sites include the upper and lower limbs as well as the abdomen. Grafts can be harvested manually with a specialized knife or an electric dermatome (Figure 23.2 (c)). The donor site requires dressing changes over a period of weeks, and patients can experience more pain at the donor site than at the recipient site. The donor site can also be paler in appearance (Figure 23.3 (a) and (b)).

Full-thickness skin grafts for the face are usually harvested from the face (preauricular, post-auricular, upper eyelid or nasolabial fold), neck or abdomen. The choice of donor site depends on the colour match, the size required and the patient's and surgeon's preferences. The donor site is primarily closed, leaving a linear scar preferably in an inconspicuous site.

Both split-thickness and full-thickness skin grafts are useful in repairing superficial oral and facial defects. The full-thickness skin graft is particularly effective in nasal, eyelid and forehead defects. Split-thickness skin grafts can be meshed (make holes to increase graft size) to cover large defects. In some instances (e.g. surplus skin graft or an infected recipient site), placement of the skin graft can be delayed for up to 3 weeks provided the harvested skin graft is stored at 4° C and moistened with saline on paraffin gauze.

Split-thickness skin graft takes more readily (thinner tissue requires less vascular ingrowth) but has a poorer outcome (tendency to contract, with a thinner, characterless look) than full-thickness skin graft (Figure 23.4). The success rate is generally high. Failure is usually the result of mobility of the graft, haematoma or infection.

Mucosal grafts

These grafts can be harvested from the buccal mucosa (primary closure) or the palatal mucosa (will reepithelialize). The advantages of using a mucosal graft to reconstruct oral defects are a good tissue match and the ease of harvesting in the same operative field. However, it introduces a scar in the same area and may further impair function. This graft is useful for gingival or alveolar repairs and as inner lining in eyelid repair.

Fascial grafts

The fascia is a strong band of tissue, and it can be harvested from the temporalis fascia or from the fascia lata in the thigh (Figure 23.5). Uses in the head and neck include dural repair in craniofacial procedures and facial slings (as part of static facial reanimation in the treatment of a paralyzed face).

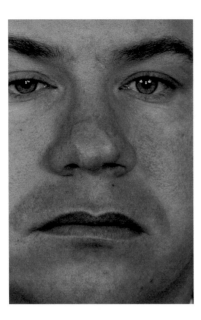

Figure 23.4 The good aesthetic result from full-thickness skin grafting.

The graft will contract and scar considerably if it is used in the mouth or on the skin surface.

Bone grafts

Bone grafts can be:

1. Cancellous (medullary component, which is mushy but rich in bone-formative components).
2. Cortical (hard structure useful for supporting role).
3. Corticocancellous block (Figure 23.6 (a)).

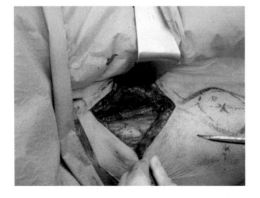

Figure 23.5 Fascia, in this case fascia lata from the thigh, can be taken as a robust graft for internal support.

Bone grafting is an established and relatively simple hard tissue reconstructive technique. A bone graft is used to provide a rigid structure (form, contour and mechanical support) and osteogenic potential (Figure 23.6 (b)). Osteogenic potential occurs by providing a scaffolding structure (osteoconduction role), which is later replaced by ingrowth of new bone. This active process is thought to take place using the grafted bone's osteogenic (osteoinductive) potential, in particular, the bone morphogeneic proteins. Research in the field of bone engineering, synthesis, prelamination and application is currently quite active (see Chapter 25).

Bone grafts can be used to fill bone cavities, augment bone deficient areas or replace and reconstruct bony loss (Figure 23.6 (c)). Cancellous bone grafts are commonly used in secondary cleft repair (see Chapter 20), and they provide osteogenic potential in treating nonunion of fractures (with rigid fixation). Rigid bone grafts are often used to provide continuity and support in jaw defects and to replace orbital volume in trauma.

Common donor sites for nonvascularized bone graft harvesting are the iliac crest (cancellous and cortical), tibia (cancellous), rib, calvaria and mandible. Vascularized bone grafts are covered in the section on free tissue transfer (free flaps).

There are various commercially available synthetic bone substitutes (e.g. demineralized bone matrix, calcium carbonate, hydroxyapatite) which can add bulk and some scaffolding to native bone but are seldom useful entirely on their own (although an exception to this is in the calvarial bone graft site, where synthetic graft heals well). Cadaveric bone has not found favour in mainstream maxillofacial reconstructive surgery. A short, low-morbidity, operation to acquire the patient's own bone from a regenerable source is usually best.

Bone grafting is generally successful. The requirements for successful bone grafting include a healthy bed (to enable vascularization), relative immobility (for bony union) and freedom from infection. The autogenous bone graft is initially devoid of blood supply and is revascularized by ingrowth of capillaries from the adjacent bed. The existing bone 'scaffold' is eventually replaced by its resorption and the deposition of new bone. Cortical bone tends to take longer (but can provide

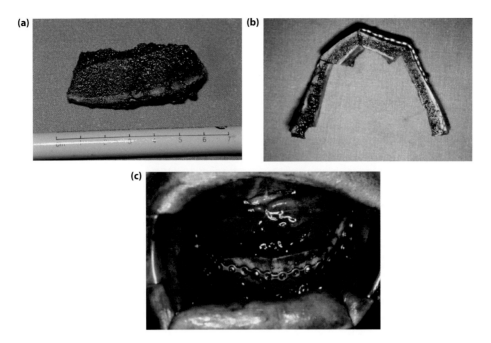

Figure 23.6 (a) Bone can be harvested for cancellous or corticocancellous grafts. (b) Mandibular reconstruction with shaped corticocancellous bone; the graft will survive if it is immobilized in a well-vascularized environment. (c) Inset free corticocancellous bone graft with plate.

useful mechanical support during this time) than cancellous bone. Cancellous bone can be incorporated into the host skeleton within 3 months.

Other than donor site morbidity (e.g. with iliac crest harvest, scarring, numbness on side of leg and groin, aching and deformity), the main adverse event is bone graft loss. The presence of infection is a contraindication to free bone grafting because the success rate is dramatically reduced. In patients with cancer, an irradiated tissue bed or adjuvant radiotherapy is commonly associated with bone graft loss. In these instances, vascularized bone transfers have a substantially higher success rate.

Cartilage grafts

Cartilage grafts are useful in specific areas of reconstruction, particularly for the nose. The best source is from the patient (autogenous grafts). Three donor sites are commonly used – the nasal septum, the ear and the rib. Cartilage has a low rate of rejection and can provide good support for overlying soft tissue. It has little or no antigenicity and can be harvested as a composite graft incorporating thin skin or mucosa.

Nerve grafts

Nerve reconstructions are usually carried out as free cable grafts, although nerve transfers can be incorporated as part of a vascularized free tissue transfer. The cable nerve graft gains its blood supply from the tissue bed and provides the scaffolding for reinnervation. Common applications for nerve grafts in the head and neck region are facial nerve reconstruction following radical parotid surgery and reinnervation of the mental nerve following mandibular resection with loss of the inferior alveolar nerve. Nerve grafting requires microsurgical reanastomosis under magnification.

Common donor sites for head and neck reconstruction include the great auricular nerve and the sural nerve. The superficial branches of the radial nerve have been used as part of a vascularized technique. Although often deemed technically successful, the reinnervation generally comprises some 30% of a complete recovery. It is worthwhile in facial nerve reconstruction because there will often be better facial tone even if complete reanimation is not achieved. Success using cadaveric reconstituted nerve grafting has been reported, and this may obviate the donor site arguments against nerve grafting.

Flaps

A flap is transferred tissue that has its own blood supply. Reconstruction using grafts is limited by the need for a well-vascularized recipient site because a graft depends on initial plasmatic imbibition followed by vascular ingrowth resulting in 'take'. A flap is much less dependent on the recipient site for take because it brings its own, new, blood supply. The use of flaps with their own blood supply allows more tissue bulk and predictable healing and viability (Figure 23.7). The greater tissue bulk in flaps can provide better form, structure and character in comparison with grafts. The better the blood supply, the larger and more complex the amount of tissue will be transferable.

There are two main patterns of blood supply for flaps – random and axial. A random pattern flap relies on general subcutaneous blood flow. Because there is no specific vascular supply (e.g. a named blood vessel), there is a limit to the amount of tissue transferable before distal flap necrosis occurs. In random pattern flaps, this is usually a ratio of 1:2 for base to length of flap. In the head and neck, because of its rich vascular network, a ratio of 1:3 and sometimes more is safe. Examples of random

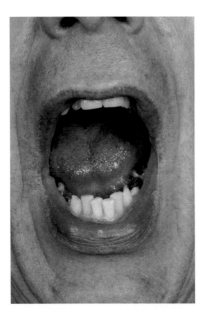

Figure 23.7 A local buccal mucosal advancement flap has preserved function in this patient who had a small buccal mucosal cancer excised.

pattern flaps used in head and neck reconstruction include local mucosal and skin flaps, as well as the nasolabial flap (see Chapter 18).

An axial flap is based on a specific vascular pedicle running in the subcutaneous plane. It supplies an area of overlying skin (the vascular territory is termed the angiosome). The vascular supply of an axial pattern flap is more reliable than that of a random pattern flap; provided the vascular pedicle is safely included, much larger and longer flaps can be raised. Examples of axial flaps include the forehead flap and the deltopectoral flap.

Myocutaneous flaps such as the pectoralis major flap or the latissimus dorsi flap are usually a combination of the two patterns of blood supply – an axial muscular supply with a random patterned supply to the overlying skin by small 'perforating' vessels. The skin paddle depends on small musculocutaneous vessels arising from the vascular pedicles deep to the muscle. The axial blood supply means that muscle only flaps can also be raised. Myocutaneous flaps tend to be bulky, although the denervated muscle atrophies with time.

Classification of flaps

See Table 23.2.

Pedicled flaps

Local flaps

This is a popular reconstructive method for small defects, particularly when the wound bed is not suitable for grafting (e.g. through-and-through defect or cortical bone surface) or the wound is too big for primary closure. It uses adjacent tissue, which has the ideal characteristics required for the defect. The blood supply depends on random

Table 23.2 Classification of flaps

A. Pedicled.
- Local flaps (e.g. tongue flap, buccal fat pad, nasolabial or submental flaps).
- Distant flaps (e.g. deltopectoral [axial pattern], pectoralis major flap [myocutaneous]).

B. Free (microvascular tissue transfer).
- Radial forearm.
- Fibula.
- Deep circumflex iliac artery (DCIA).
- Anterolateral thigh.
- Rectus abdominis.

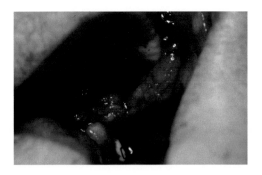

Figure 23.8 The buccal fat pad flap is a useful local piece of well-vascularized tissue.

patterned subdermal plexus of vessels. The rich vascular supply of the face and oral cavity is well suited to this technique.

Factors to take into consideration when raising such local flaps include likely cosmetic results and ensuring that the blood supply entering the flap at its base is not compromised by tension or kinking. Examples of local flaps in the oral cavity include buccal mucosa advancement flaps and the buccal fat pad flap (Figures 23.8 and 23.9). Local flaps to reconstruct facial defects are dealt with in Chapter 18. A common example is the nasolabial flap.

Nasolabial flap   This is a random pattern flap and relies on the rich vascular network of the face. It is a safe, reliable two-staged technique (inset to allow vascularization from the adjacent tissue bed before division of the pedicle 2 to 3 weeks later).

A finger of skin is raised (inferiorly based for oral defect) and tunneled through the cheek and buccal mucosa to repair the adjacent floor of mouth, tongue or alveolar defects. Occasionally,

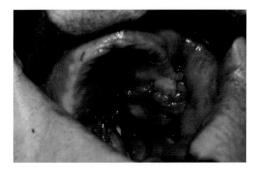

Figure 23.9 The flap mucosalizes by epithelial cell seeding but tends to scar and fibrose.

the tip of the flap may necrose. Bilateral flaps are often used for small to moderately sized anterior floor of mouth defects. The donor sites are closed primarily and heal well with minimal cosmetic defect within the nasolabial folds (Figure 23.10 (a), (b), (c) and (d)).

Regional (distant) flaps

A regional flap is usually defined as any flap raised outside the local area (below the mandible) and transferred to reconstruct head and neck defects. Examples of large pedicled distant flaps used in head and neck reconstruction are the deltopectoral flap and the pectoralis major flap.

Deltopectoral flap   This axial patterned skin flap is based on the first four perforating branches of the internal mammary artery (Figure 23.11). The flap is medially based and is transversely orientated on the upper chest. It is a two-staged technique, initially rotated to repair large wounds in the neck and lower part of the face. The donor site and pedicle are temporarily dressed and at the second stage 2 to 3 weeks later, the pedicle is divided and the proximal component is reinset to the chest. The distal defect of the donor site is skin grafted. This flap has been superseded by other flaps but remains a good fallback option.

Pectoralis major flap   This reconstructive technique was the 'workhorse' for oral cavity defects in the 1980s. It remains an important reconstructive option (e.g. if a patient is not fit or suitable for free flaps, if no microvascular facilities or expertise are available or if an initial free flap had failed).

The vascular pedicle is based on the pectoral branch of the thoracoacromial artery. It can be raised as a skin paddle (myocutaneous) or a muscle only flap. The pectoralis major muscle is associated with a large skin territory (allowing a good-sized skin paddle and usually primary closure of donor site), good muscle bulk (useful to protect neck vessels when tunneled into position), and a good arc of rotation enabling variable positioning for reconstruction of any head and neck defects up to the zygomatic arch. It is relatively easy to raise without the need to reposition the patient and is generally very reliable. However, it is bulky and can be too rigid for certain oral defects that require a more pliable reconstruction.

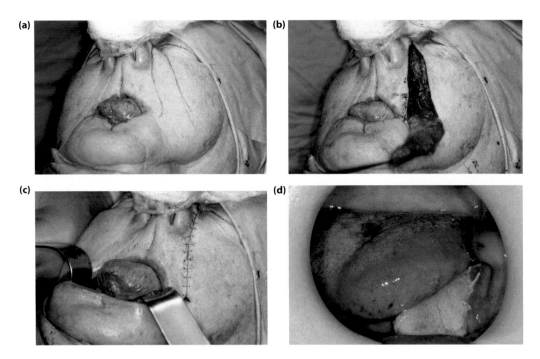

Figure 23.10 (a) Outline of a nasolabial flap. (b) The nasolabial flap is raised in the fat plane above the muscles of facial expression and is a random pattern skin flap. (c) The flap is passed through the cheek, and the majority of the donor site defect is closed primarily. Division of the flap base, inset and final closure take place at 3 weeks following initial operation. (d) Final result.

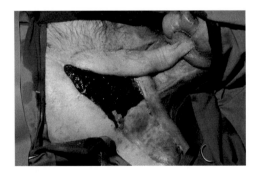

Figure 23.11 A deltopectoral flap before division and inset.

Figure 23.12 (a) to (d) shows an example of a pectoralis major myocutaneous flap, and Figure 23.13 (a) to (g) shows a muscle only flap.

Free flaps

Microvascular or free tissue transfer has been the major advancement in reconstructive surgery since the 1980s. It involves the harvesting and detachment of tissue with its blood (and sometimes nerve) supply and transferring it to repair a complex defect. The blood (and nerve) supply of the transplanted tissue is then reestablished by reanastomosis of its vascular pedicle to suitable vessels (and nerve) at the recipient site by using microvascular techniques (Figure 23.14 (a) and (b)).

Microvascular surgery

The ability to anastomose blood vessels by using operative magnification has revolutionized reconstructive surgery. The surgery is complex and demands certain specific processes.

- Preoperative assessment – this includes clinical examination and usually imaging. The aim is to ensure that there is no abnormal pathology or aberrant vascular anatomy that will threaten the success of flap transfer or the safety of the donor site (e.g. viability of the foot following harvest of a fibula flap).
- Perioperative issues – a two-team approach is commonly adopted, with one team carrying out the ablation and the other raising the flap simultaneously. The diameter of vessels involved commonly ranges from 1 to 3 mm.

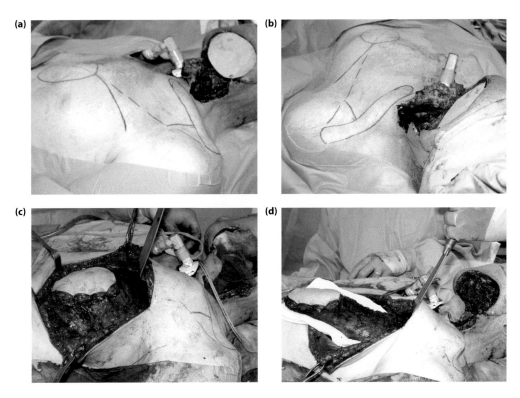

Figure 23.12 (a) A template is marked to match the defect. (b) The skin markings for a pectoralis major myocutaneous flap. (c) The skin island is incised and the muscle is exposed; a subcutaneous island is created to pass the flap into the neck. (d) The isolated pectoralis major flap before rotation.

The vessels are joined from end to end or from end to side using 9-0 to 11-0 sutures and microsurgical instruments used under an operating microscope or loupes.

Postoperative monitoring – the flap's viability is most at risk within the first 48 hours of surgery. Although various monitoring tools are available, including implantable Doppler, microdialysis and laser flow Doppler, regular clinical monitoring by visual inspection remains a mainstay. Venous occlusion results in a blue, engorged flap (Figure 23.15), whereas arterial blockage (more difficult to detect) results in a white, flaccid flap. Flap salvage relies on prompt detection, reexploration, identification and correction of kinking, haematoma or vascular occlusion.

Benefits of free flaps

There are several advantages to the use of free flaps. Complex defects are better reconstructed with a completely new blood supply (healthy fresh tissue promotes healing). Distant tissue can now be used (no longer limited by an attached pedicle), and the type (and amount) of tissue harvested can be better tailored to the defect. This complex technique is now considered so reliable that it is often the first choice for reconstruction. Table 23.3 compares pedicled flaps with free tissue transfers.

Common free flaps used for oral defects

The radial forearm free flap is generally considered to be the workhorse for head and neck reconstruction, in particular oral soft tissue defects. It can be used for bony defects as a composite flap, although other, better options exist such as the fibula, deep circumflex iliac artery (DCIA) and scapula flaps. The scapula flap is particularly suited for complex defects because multiple tissue types at different orientations are possible based on the same vascular pedicle. The major disadvantage is the need to turn the patient midoperation. For this reason

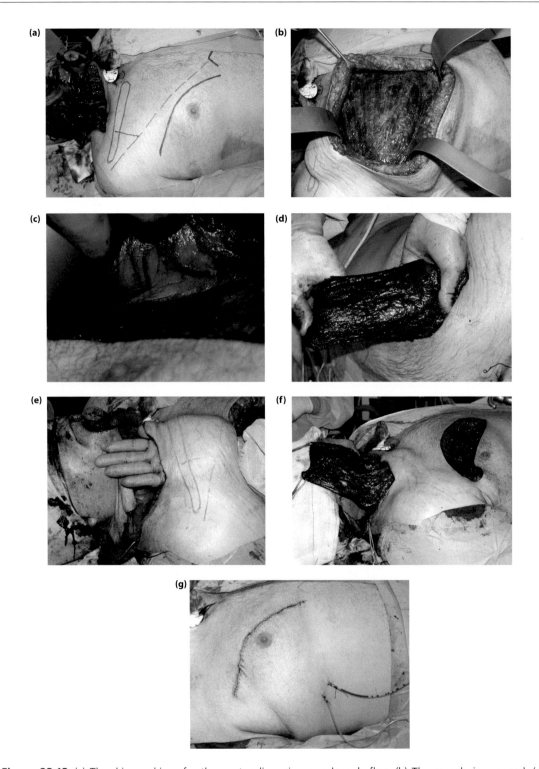

Figure 23.13 (a) The skin markings for the pectoralis major muscle-only flap. (b) The muscle is exposed. (c) The acromiothoracic vessels that supply this flap. (d) The muscle flap fully elevated based on its pedicle. (e) The subcutaneous tunnel has been developed. (f) The muscle flap is passed into the head and neck via the subcutaneous tunnel. (g) The chest is closed primarily (this is usually possible when a skin paddle is raised as well).

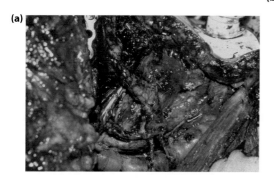
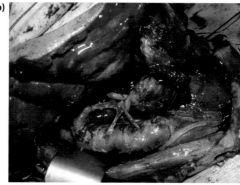

Figure 23.14 (a) An example of arterial and venous microanastomosis. (b) Controversy exists on whether more, as shown here, or fewer venous anastomoses are advantageous.

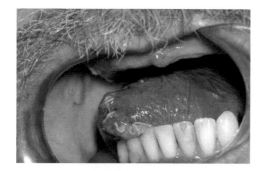

Figure 23.15 A congested flap. This is the usual mechanism of failure of free flaps – compromise of venous drainage, usually caused by compression of the venous pedicle or venous thrombosis.

some teams use a combination of flaps that can be harvested with the patient supine.

Common flaps with their blood supply may include:

1. Radial – radial artery.
2. Pectoralis major:
   - Thoracoacromial artery.
   - Lateral thoracic.
   - Internal mammary.
3. Scapula – circumflex scapular branch of the subscapular artery.
4. Latissimus dorsi– thoracodorsal artery.
5. Anterolateral thigh – lateral circumflex femoral artery.
6. Fibula –peroneal artery.
7. DCIA – deep circumflex iliac artery.
8. Trapezius.

- Superiorly based – occipital artery, paraspinal perforators.
- Lateral island – transverse cervical artery.
- Inferiorly based: transverse cervical and dorsal scapular arteries.

9. Deltopectoral – perforator arteries from the internal mammary. The blood supply to the extension of this flap beyond the thoracoacromial artery and deltopectoral groove is nonaxial.
10. Rectus – dual supply: superior and inferior epigastric – most flaps are raised on inferior epigastric vessels.
11. Paramedian – axial flap based on the supratrochlear artery.
12. Nasolabial – technically random; the small vessels of the subdermal plexus are generally orientated along its long axis.
13. Submental neck skin and platysma muscle based on the terminal branches of the facial and submental artery – useful when neck dissection is not needed (i.e. nonmalignant cases).

Radial forearm free flap The skin paddle for this well-established flap is based on the radial artery, its venae comitantes and optional cephalic vein (Figure 23.16 (a)). It provides soft, thin and pliable skin and fascia with, if required, bone, nerve or tendon. The quality of the skin is well suited for reconstructing intraoral defects, where the aim is to provide coverage and at the same time allow residual oral tissue such as tongue and floor of mouth the flexibility to continue to function (Figure 23.16 (b)). It has a reliable long pedicle

Table 23.3 Comparison between pedicled and free flaps

Variable	Pedicled flap	Free flap	Overcome problem
Technique	Less complex.	Microvascular expertise and equipment needed.	Usually local expertise is available.
Duration of surgery	Shorter.	Longer.	Two-team approach shortens operating time.
Reliability	Generally more reliable but can still fail, especially partial skin necrosis.	Total flap failure rate ~5%.	In specialized unit, both are now reliable.
Character of flap	Bulkier and restrictive. Tissue available limited by pedicle length.	Type of tissue required can be tailored better. Wide tissue options available because distant sites can be transferred.	
Donor site morbidity	Yes.	Yes.	See Table 23.5.
Duration of hospital stay	Perceived to be associated with less morbidity but shown to have longer hospital stays.	Shorter stay unless complications develop.	

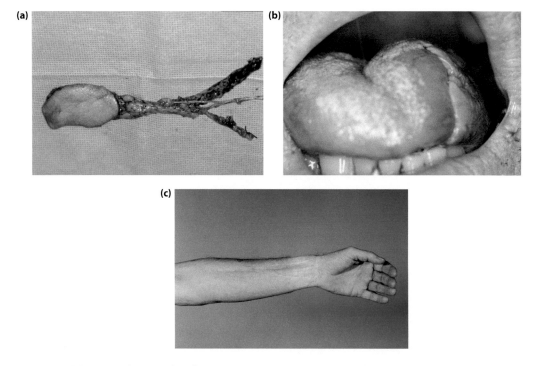

Figure 23.16 (a) A radial forearm free flap harvested with the radial artery, vena comitans, cephalic vein and lateral antebrachial cutaneous nerve of the forearm. (b) A forearm flap *in situ* showing tongue mobility by providing a stretchable layer of tissue in the ventral tongue and floor of the mouth. (c) The radial forearm donor site defect after closure using the ipsilateral full-thickness forearm skin graft technique.

and good vessel caliber, and it allows simultaneous harvesting during head and neck ablation, thus reducing operating time. The donor site can be repaired with a local flap or, more commonly, with a full-thickness or split-thickness skin graft (Figure 23.16 (c)).

The radial bone component is limited with regard to length and height (Figure 23.17 (a)), and it is therefore less suitable for implants. The donor site radius has a significant risk of fracturing (Figure 23.17 (b)), although this can be overcome by prophylactic plating (Figure 23.17 (c)). Interestingly, the thin bone strut and the potential donor site defect have led to a real international polarization of views on the use of the composite radial forearm free flap. In the United Kingdom, techniques to overcome the donor site defect, including prophylactic plating and full-thickness skin grafting, possibly coupled with patients with very atrophic mandibles who require composite resection, have meant that the radial forearm free flap has been retained as part of a range of flaps for composite reconstruction. In Germany and parts of North America, the technique is virtually never used and sometimes is heavily criticized. Whether this is because donor site management techniques have not been adopted or whether the atrophic mandible or maxilla with malignant disease is much less of an issue is unclear.

Fibula free flap This flap provides a long (up to 25 cm), vascularized, tubular (although really more triangular), thick cortical bone capable of reconstructing an angle-to-angle mandibular defect (Figure 23.18 (a)). The flap can be raised either without skin (Figure 23.18 (b)) or with a skin paddle. The bone is suitable for implants and, when harvested carefully, provides a reasonable skin paddle. The vascular pedicle can be lengthened significantly by trimming the proximal bone and is based on the peroneal artery and associated venae comitantes. The donor site can be primarily closed for very small skin paddles; this leaves a reasonable donor site scar. Most skin flaps have to be split skin grafted, which delays donor site healing. Full-thickness skin grafting of this defect does not work anything like as well as it does on the forearm, and we have abandoned it.

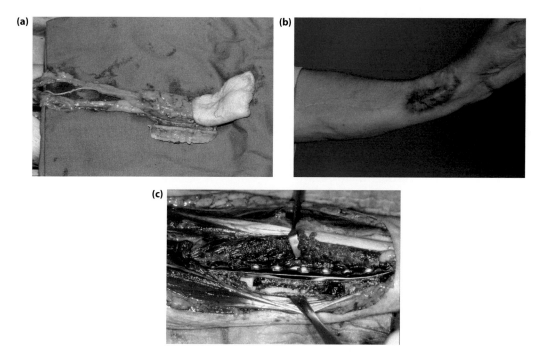

Figure 23.17 (a) The composite radial forearm free flap uses up to 40% of the thickness of the radius but still only provides a thin strut of bone. (b) As many as 25% of composite forearm defects fracture. (c) Prophylactic plating prevents this complication.

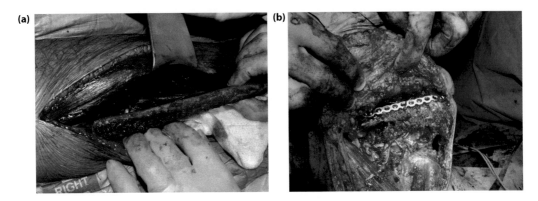

Figure 23.18 (a) The free fibula is a long bone and skin flap based on the peroneal vessels. (b) It provides dense implantable bone, although not the bone height of the iliac crest flap. The pedicle length is a great advantage.

It is important to assess the vascular supply of the donor leg. Magnetic resonance angiography is recognized internationally as the technique of choice. Duplex Doppler ultrasound assessment combined with a plain radiograph has been shown to be reliable in detecting any abnormal anatomy or pathology that may threaten the success of the flap and viability of the foot. Simple assessment of pulses as the only preoperative assessment, although still advocated by some surgeons, has been abandoned by most. Joint stability is not a problem if the surgeon preserves at least 6 cm of fibula bone at the knee and ankle. Patients will have numbness on the dorsum of the foot and may have some weakness in dorsiflexing the big toe.

Complex defects In some instances, a single flap reconstruction is not adequate or optimal. The scapular flap, with its numerous options, is an excellent choice for such complex defects. However, this technique involves turning the patient perioperatively and increases shoulder morbidity. An alternative is to use combination flaps (Figure 23.19 (a), (b), (c) and (d)).

Innervated flaps Certain flaps can be harvested with either their nerve supply (sensory, motor) or a vascularized nerve incorporated.

A sensate flap (e.g. radial forearm flap) can be useful if there is a recipient nerve in the head and neck (e.g. a divided lingual nerve). Reinnervation of a sensate flap can be an advantage when reconstructing the soft palate, pharynx and lip to aid functional rehabilitation, especially with swallowing and speech. Facial reanimation is a common

reason for motor reinnervation. It can also be useful to maintain muscle bulk or tone in patients who have undergone total glossectomy.

As a working principle, it is now believed that limited sensory recovery usually occurs in thin flaps without direct nerve anastomosis and that recovery in thick flaps even with neural anastomosis is very limited. There is no good justification for damaging a recipient site nerve to attempt sensate recovery of a flap, although if such a nerve is resected in tumour ablation or trauma, then reanastomosis of an unavoidably sensate flap is rational. Motor nerve harvest and anastomosis follow similar principles when reconstruction of solid tissue is the primary aim of the procedure. Facial nerve reconstruction in isolation is quite a different consideration.

Prefabricated flaps In a bid to improve the character of some free flaps further, the donor site tissue planned for transfer can be modified. For example, a cartilage structure harvested from the costal margin carved to resemble a pinna can be set into the soft tissue of a forearm distally. Once established, this modified tissue (prefabricated structure) can be transferred as a free flap to replace a missing ear. Similar procedures have been described for mucosa and bone. Inevitably, these flaps are part of a delayed reconstructive process.

'Perforator' flaps There remains debate about what exactly is meant by the term perforator flap. Some surgeons claim that almost all flaps are perforator flaps, whereas others list a few named flaps in which visualization of the perforating vessels from the named flap vessel to the supplied tissue

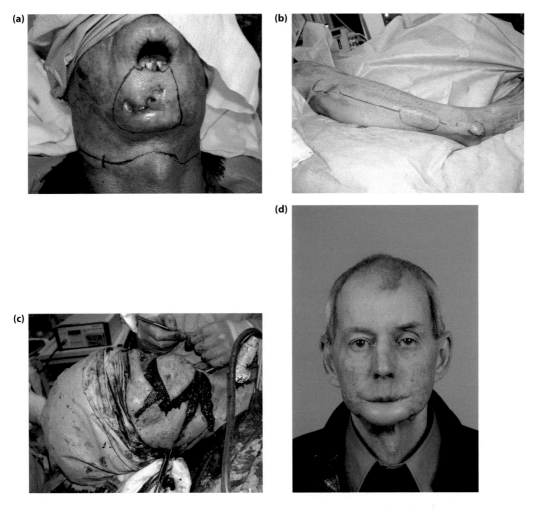

Figure 23.19 (a) Complex multitissue defects may require multiple flaps, (b) in this case an osseocutaneous fibula and a chimeric (c) anterolateral thigh flap. (d) Postoperative appearance.

(usually skin) is the defining parameter. Probably the most accurate and useful approach is to define these flaps as those in which a defined area of tissue is supplied by an unnamed vessel that perforates fascia to supply skin and is identified, dissected from surrounding tissue and anastomosed when reconstructing an area with that flap. The advantages of the flap – that no significant blood supply is impeded and that only the required reconstructive tissue is harvested – would be clearly shown while easily demonstrating the disadvantages, which are that the pedicle is actually very short and the diameter is small.

Although the anterolateral thigh free flap is the most widely described perforator flap,

most surgeons actually dissect the length of the descending branch of the lateral circumflex femoral vessels (thereby removing a named but relatively unimportant vascular tree), to give a long pedicle and large-diameter vessels. The actual perforating component (going through fascia to supply skin) is a relatively short length of vessels requiring i.m. dissection in 80% of patients. The skin paddle of the fibula often has visible perforating vessels to the skin, but these are seldom dissected through muscle and fascia to isolate them. The lateral sural artery perforator flap is variably dissected as a soleal branch of the peroneal vessels – all short expendable vessels but they are anatomically named. The relative significance of retaining the tissue (usually muscle) at the donor site is very debatable, with the possible exception of the transverse deep inferior epigastric perforator flap used for breast reconstruction in younger women or for soft tissue trauma coverage where there is an arguable advantage in retaining a semifunctioning rectus abdominis muscle.

Outcomes

Free flap success rates are usually reported to be in excess of 95%. Inevitably, there are local variations with types of flap and expertise available. The presence of coexisting medical conditions (usually cardiorespiratory diseases, as expected in smokers) can have an important bearing on likelihood of complications, which in turn can affect viability of free flaps during the immediate postoperative stage. A free flap technique offers many advantages, but it is an all or none phenomenon. Total flap loss results in a persisting defect and a weakened patient. A second reconstructive procedure can put that patient at significant risk. Table 23.4 lists the factors affecting free flap success.

Donor site morbidity should always be considered during treatment planning. Table 23.5 shows some specific drawbacks, including morbidity associated with various flaps.

Defects and reconstructive options

Ventral tongue and floor of the mouth

The main aim in reconstructing these defects is to allow maximal movements of the residual tongue so that the best possible speech, eating and swallowing can be achieved. Small lesions can be lasered (and left to heal; see Figure 23.1), excised and skin grafted (see Figure 23.2) or primarily closed with sutures (longitudinal better than transverse to reduce tethering). Larger defects can be repaired with a local flap (e.g. nasolabial flap; see Figure 23.10) or a radial forearm free flap (see Figure 23.16).

Where the majority of the tongue has been removed, there will be little or no residual function. This defect is best reconstructed with bulk (e.g. pedicled pectoralis major flap; see Figure 23.12) or large free flaps such as latissimus dorsi (Figure 23.20 (a), (b) and (c)) or rectus abdominis flaps (see later).

Buccal mucosa

The main requirement for this defect is to obtain closure by covering the area with a pliable lining while allowing for normal mouth opening. Superficial lesions can be excised with a laser and left to heal or skin grafted. Small deeper defects can be closed with a local flap. A large and deep defect is better repaired with a radial forearm free flap (Figure 23.21 (a) and (b)). Through-and-through defects require bipaddled repair.

Mandible

Where a segmental resection is required for bone invasion by cancer (Figure 23.22 (a)), it is likely that the area will be irradiated as an adjuvant measure for local control. A free nonvascularized bone graft is unlikely to survive such hostile treatment. Ideally, a vascularized bone flap followed by implant insertion should be considered for optimal rehabilitation. Suitable flaps include the fibula (good length; Figure 23.22 (b)), which can be combined with other flaps because of its long pedicle (Figure 23.22 (c) and (d)), and DCIA (large bone stock but much shorter pedicle; Figure 23.23 (a), (b) and (c)) free flaps.

Anterior segments if left unreconstructed will leave severe deformity and collapse of the chin with drooling. There are few reasonable alternatives to composite free flap reconstruction. Lateral

Table 23.4 Factors affecting free flap success

Local factors:
- Surgical mishaps (e.g. microsurgical suturing, pedicle tension or compression).
- Wound complications (e.g. haematoma, bleeding or wound infection).

General factors:
- Systemic hypotension with inadequate arterial flow.
- Increased coagulability (excessive transfusion, donor site bleeding).
- Vascular spasm (cold environment, smoking).

Table 23.5 Strengths and weaknesses of common free flaps in head and neck reconstruction

Drawbacks and morbidity	Flap	Common usage	Strengths
Soft tissue flaps			
Scar visible on forearm (skin graft can be lost). Numbness in superficial radial nerve distribution.	Radial forearm.	Widely used for oral defects.	Good supple skin paddle. Reliable long vascular pedicle. Can be harvested same time as ablation (two-team approach).
Risk to radial nerve. Shorter pedicle. Difficult to harvest at same time as head and neck ablation.	Lateral arm.	Reasonable alternative to radial forearm free flap.	Scar can be closed primarily and is easier to hide.
Patient requires turning. Winging of scapula. Poor colour match to face.	Latissimus dorsi.	Large soft tissue paddle.	Large soft tissue flap. Reliable vessels. Can be used with scapular system. Primary closure, hidden scar.
Skin perforators can be tenuous. Poor colour match to face.	Anterolateral thigh.	Large skin paddle.	Large soft tissue paddle with optional adjacent fascia lata and muscle. Allows two-team approach. Primary closure, hidden scar.
Hernia, abdominal wall weakness. Poor colour match to face.	Rectus abdominis.	Very large soft tissue coverage.	Large soft tissue paddle with rectus sheath. Allows two-team approach. Hidden scar.
Bone flaps			
Poor bone stock. Radial fracture risk (prophylactic plating will overcome this).	Radial forearm composite.	Lateral edentulous defects with large soft tissue defect.	Good skin paddle. Long pedicle and reliable vessels. Allows two-team approach.
Skin paddle needing careful harvesting. Skin graft required to donor site for larger skin paddle. Risk of vascular compromise to foot. Risk of weak dorsiflexion of big toe, numbness on foot.	Fibula.	Long bony defects.	Long bone (up to 25 cm). Good vascular pedicle.
Wide dissection and difficulty in obese patients. Shorter pedicle, bulky skin paddle.	Deep circumflex iliac.	Large bone stock for implantation.	Bone easy to contour. Best bone stock for implants. Allows two-team approach.
Need to turn patient. Two-team approach difficult. Shoulder disability risk.	Scapula.	Complex defects with bone.	Allows separate skin paddles and bone (complex defects).

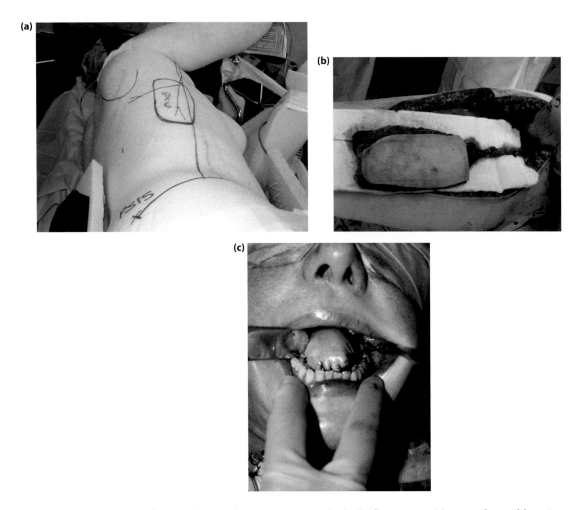

Figure 23.20 (a) Bulky defects such as total glossectomy require bulky flaps to provide some form of function such as the latissimus dorsi free flap; surface markings of the flap. (b) The flap and its neurovascular pedicle. (c) The flap in situ. This patient can communicate effectively and maintain her own weight without supplemental feeding.

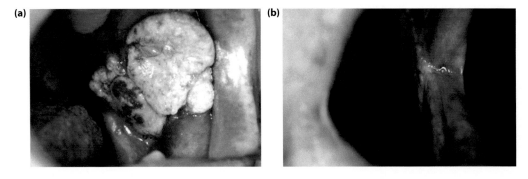

Figure 23.21 (a) A full-thickness buccal mucosa squamous cell carcinoma. (b) Reconstruction with a bipaddled radial forearm free flap.

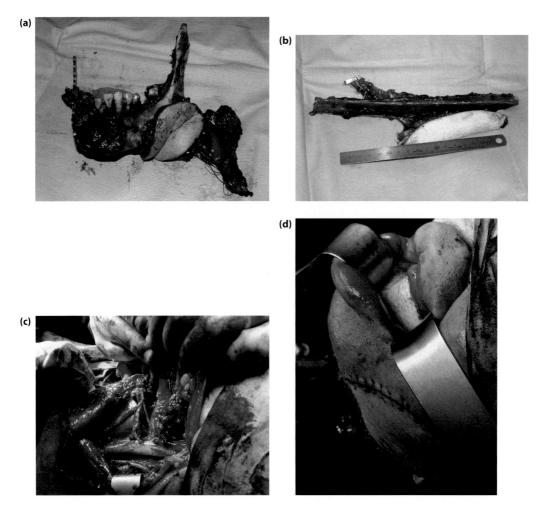

Figure 23.22 (a) A complex bony and soft tissue defect. (b) The fibula free flap provides bone, skin and a long vascular pedicle. (c) This allows combination with other flaps such as (d) the anterolateral thigh free flap.

defects, although best restored by composite flaps, can be simply treated with a reconstruction plate to maintain continuity with an enveloping bulky soft tissue flap such as the pectoralis major when the patient is not fit for a free flap procedure.

Available options include:

1. Free bone grafts – a corticocancellous block graft is taken from the anterior or posterior iliac crest. Free bone grafts are still a good option for defects that are not bigger than approximately 5 cm, provided the soft tissues are in good condition. Gaps larger than 5 cm are not really suitable for this means of bridging a defect, whereas in most cases of malignancy, when

a large part of the surrounding soft tissues is lacking, healing cannot be ensured. Previous or anticipated radiotherapy would also be a contraindication to the use of free bone grafts. Studies comparing the anterior and posterior iliac crest as donor sites reveal less morbidity when the posterior site is used.

2. Reconstruction plates – these are rigid plates that are applied along the lower border of the mandible. They were made with the intention of bridging a defect, thus stabilizing occlusion and facial contour. They are currently used to fix corticocancellous blocks or vascularized bone grafts to the remaining mandible. There are several types of these plates on the market,

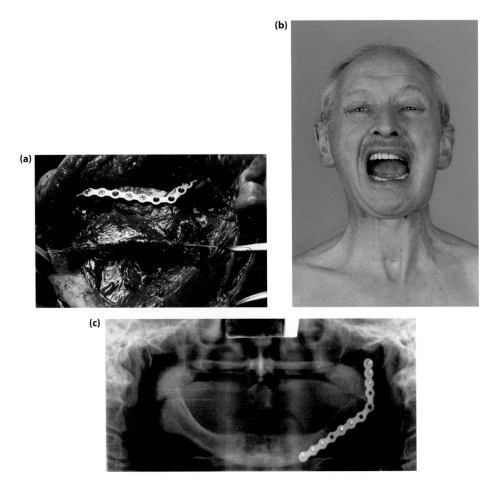

Figure 23.23 (a) The deep circumflex iliac artery (DCIA) with internal oblique free flap. (b) Postoperative function. (c) Postoperative radiograph.

but the overriding principle is to have one single plate of sufficient thickness and width to hold the fragments in place – approximately 3 mm thick and 5 mm wide. A special feature is the locking screw. This is supposed to minimize compression between the plate and the underlying bone and thereby optimize the vascularity surrounding the graft.

3. Free flaps – these include fibula, DCIA and scapula.
4. Particular bone cancellous marrow grafts – they must be placed in a frame.
5. Transport disc distraction osteogenesis – a segment of bone is cut adjacent to the defect (transport disc) and is moved gradually across the defect.

Maxilla

The main aims of rehabilitating this defect are to achieve coverage and to seal the oral cavity from the floor of nose and antrum. This has been traditionally managed with an obturator. Where facial skin and the orbit can be preserved, it remains a reasonable option, by allowing the patient to speak, eat and look normal while the obturator is worn.

There is a trend toward microvascular reconstruction with the aim of doing away with the prosthesis. This technique has a better outcome for larger defects than obturation and is much preferable if facial skin is involved in the defect. It is technically more challenging, and care is

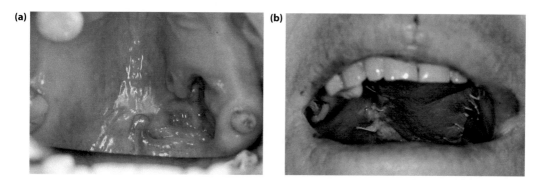

Figure 23.24 (a) A squamous cell carcinoma of the palate that resulted in a low-level maxillectomy. (b) Sealing the mouth from the nose and the antrum by using a radial forearm free flap.

required to ensure that adequate pedicle length and suitable vessels are available for anastomosing the flap. Flaps commonly used include DCIA, fibula, rectus abdominis, latissimus dorsi and radial forearm free flaps. Figures 23.24 (a) and (b) and 23.25 (a), (b), (c) and (d) show some reconstructive options.

Lip

The lip is an important area in terms of cosmesis and function (lip seal, speech and eating). Full-thickness defects of up to one third of the lip can be primarily closed. Intermediate full-thickness defects can be reconstructed with local flaps (see Chapter 18), or Abbe flaps. An Abbe flap involves rotating a wedge of lip from the opposite side of the lip by using a two-staged technique. Total full-thickness lip defects can be repaired using bilateral fan flaps or with a free tissue transfer with tendon slings.

Pharynx

An intact oropharynx is vital for swallowing and speech. Partial defects can be repaired using a rigid bulky flap such as the pectoralis major with the aim of allowing remaining tissue to have some function. If the defect requires the creation of a circumferential tube, alternatives include free soft tissue transfers such as a tubed radial forearm (largely historical now) or anterolateral thigh and jejunal free flaps.

Prosthetic rehabilitation

The use of nonbiological materials to reconstruct certain head and neck defects is an established and effective option. These defects include auricular (implant-retained ear prosthesis), maxillary and total rhinectomy defects (prosthesis retained with undercuts or implants). It is important to assess the patient's compliance and dexterity (to keep implants clean and to remove and reinsert prostheses) at the planning stage. This preoperative assessment and planning should be carried out with a prosthodontist and maxillofacial technician so optimal results can be achieved.

Maxillary prosthesis

This removable reconstructive option involves taking an impression before surgery to make a dressing plate. When the surgical defect is created, the dressing plate is used with a suitable obturator material (gutta percha or silicone) to provide support for the cheek, create an undercut to aid retention of the prosthesis and seal the oral cavity from the nasal and antral cavities to enable speech and swallowing. The plate can be secured with wires or screws. The inner wall of the defect is usually grafted with split-thickness skin to speed up healing, and coronoidectomy is performed to stop dislodgement of the obturator by mandibular lateral excursions.

The dressing plate and obturator are removed several weeks later for impressions to reconstruct an interim removable obturator. This is followed by a

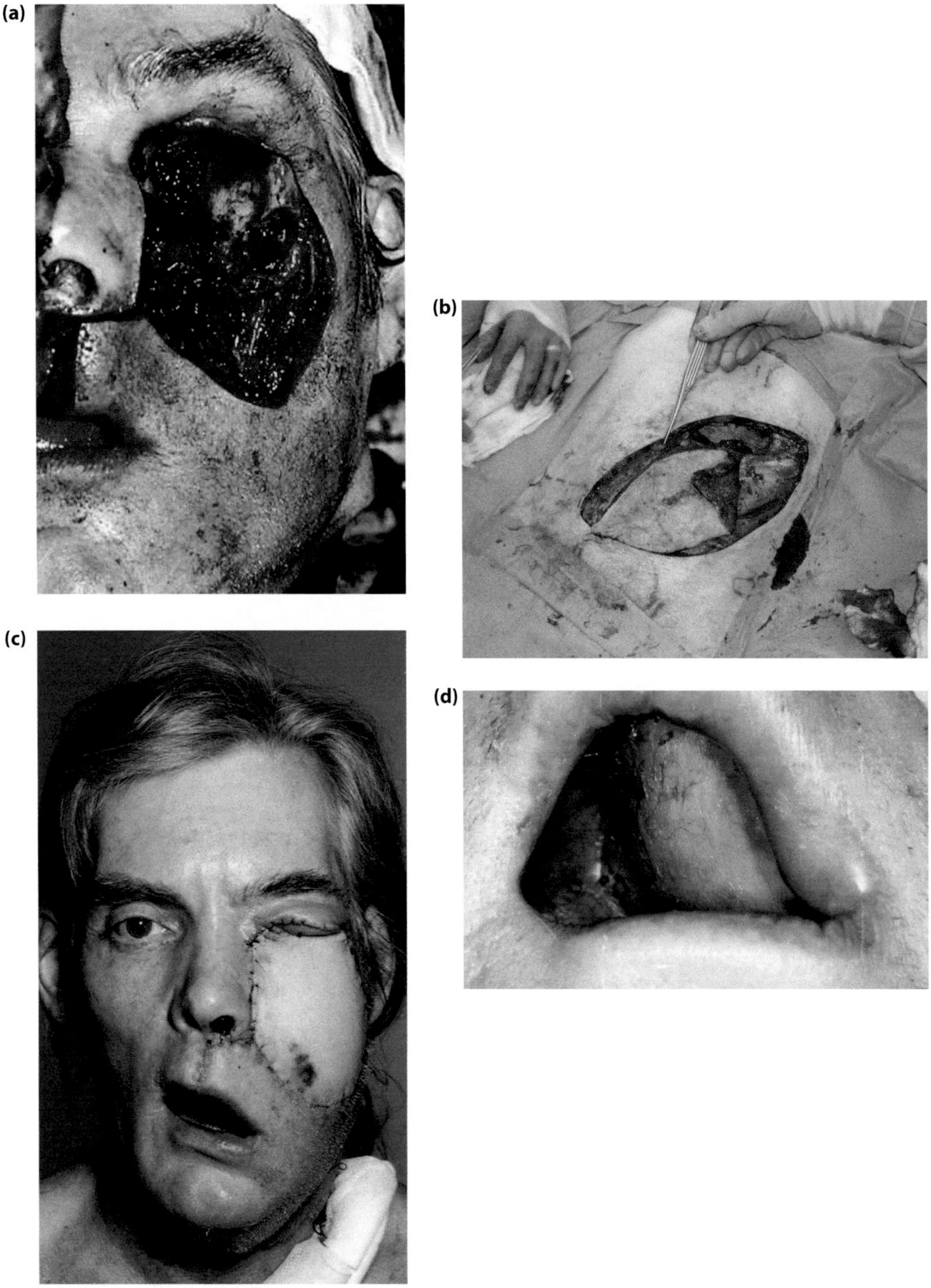

Figure 23.25 (a) A complex bone and soft tissue defect of the maxilla and orbit. (b) The rectus abdominis free flap can be segmentalized. (c) Early facial result. (d) Early oral result.

definitive prosthesis some months later. The prosthesis can be a single piece hollowed (to reduce weight and aid retention) or two-pieced (soft bung superiorly with rigid conventional oral plate) prosthesis.

Existing teeth within the same arch can be used to improve retention of the prosthesis with the aid of clasps. The maxillary obturator prosthesis for low-level defects is an excellent reconstructive option – so much so that these patients tend to refuse any secondary flap options if offered.

Solitary ear prosthesis was traditionally retained with glue (unsatisfactorily!). The advent of osseointegrated implants heralded a major improvement in this area (see Chapter 15). Larger complex defects involving the skin can be 'reconstructed' using multipieced obturators retained with implants, interconnecting joints or spectacles. However, the skin component coloration tends to fade with time and sun exposure. Facial components look good when they are still, but facial movements display gaps. However, they are better than patches.

Osseointegrated implants

It is inevitable that ablation surgery will alter the movements, pliability and anatomy of the oral and facial structures. Although clever use of undercuts and interconnecting multipieced prostheses are effective, retention of prostheses can remain a problem.

The introduction of osseointegrated implants has been a major advancement in overcoming this problem (see Chapter 15). Placement of implants requires adequate bone stock (reconstruction with DCIA or fibula free flaps preferred to radial composite free flaps) and good patient compliance and dexterity (to maintain a high standard of hygiene), as well as clinical resources (funding, expertise and further surgery). At some sites, however, these implants can give a prosthetic reconstruction unachievable by surgical treatment alone (Figure 23.26 (a), (b) and (c)).

Implants can be inserted at the same time as the flap, but accurate alignment for prosthetic use is much more difficult. When the implants are inserted following adjuvant radiotherapy (usual approach in practice), most clinicians advocate hyperbaric oxygen therapy to reduce the risk of osteoradionecrosis.

Summary

It is important to reiterate that ablation must not be compromised for the sake of reconstruction. In addition, the comorbidity of the patient has a significant bearing in predicting outcome and must be considered as part of the treatment plan.

The advantages of each reconstructive technique should be weighed, and the best possible option available (bearing in mind available expertise)

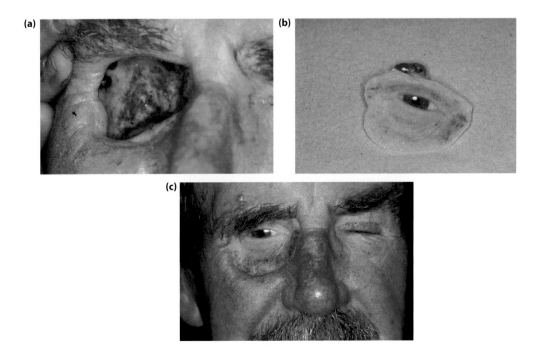

Figure 23.26 (a) Orbital osseointegrated implants. (b) Orbital prosthesis. (c) Implant-borne orbital prosthesis *in situ*.

to suit the patient and the defect should be used. Donor site morbidity should be taken into account.

Reconstructive techniques have advanced significantly. The larger and more complex the defect, the more impaired the patient will be functionally. Patients need to be counselled in a realistic manner with full input from a speech and language therapist, a dietician, a cancer nurse specialist and other allied head and neck specialists to enable the best possible outcome to be achieved.

Technical innovations include preoperative virtual planning of both the resection and the reconstruction, to allow precision positioning of the osteotomies and shaping of the retaining plate with preplanned jigs. Whether the time saved justifies the additional cost and the preoperative delay in most patients requiring osseous reconstruction (malignant disease) or whether this technology will be reserved for benign resections only (see Chapter 25) remains to be seen.

Ultimately, the reconstructive option chosen should be a joint decision between the surgeon and the patient based on a balance of risks (including comorbidity) versus benefits, as well as an honest assessment of the expertise available at that unit. The goal must be to use the simplest and most reliable technique possible to achieve the best possible rehabilitation.

FURTHER READING

Urken ML, Cheney ML, Blackwell KE, Harris JR, Hadlock TA, Futran N. *Atlas of regional and free flaps for head and neck reconstruction*, 2nd ed. Baltimore: Wolters Kluwer/Lippincott Williams & Wilkins, 2012.

Wolff KD, Hölzle F. *Raising of microvascular flaps: a systematic approach*, 2nd ed. Berlin: Springer, 2011.

Specific literature includes the following:

Chim H, Salgado CJ, Seselgyte R, Wei FC, Mardini S. Principles of head and neck reconstruction: an algorithm to guide flap selection. *Semin Plast Surg* 2010;24:148–54.

Erba P, Ogawa R, Vyas R, Orgill DP. The reconstructive matrix: a new paradigm in reconstructive plastic surgery. *Plast Reconstr Surg* 2010;126:492–8.

Goh BT, Lee S, Tideman H, Stoelinga PJW. Mandibular reconstruction in adults: a review. *Int J Oral Maxillofac Surg* 2008;37:597–605.

24

Facial aesthetic surgery

Contents

Aim

- To introduce the topic of aesthetic facial surgery.

Learning outcomes

- To be able to describe the range of common techniques available.
- To be able to discuss the relevance of those techniques to patients' aspirations.
- To be able to describe the basic steps in the more common procedures

Introduction and patient assessment

Aesthetic facial surgery entails the practice of a branch of surgery for which there is usually no medical requirement. It aims to change the appearance of the patient for aesthetic reasons alone and at the patient's request. It is the patient who has decided that he or she is not happy with his or her appearance. Although fraught with potential problems, aesthetic facial surgery can be an immensely satisfying branch of surgery.

As for any patient, a full medical and drug history should be sought. The patient's problem should then be explored using open questions initially (remember, the patient's perception of the problem may not be the same as yours). This will give some idea of the scale of the patient's perceived problem and where the patient thinks, anatomically, the problem lies.

Age is no barrier to aesthetic surgery, but it is worthwhile establishing why the patient wants surgery now, whether the patient is younger, older or at the more usual age for those requests.

Once the problem has been elucidated and the patient's wishes considered, what can and cannot be achieved, as well as potential complications, must be explicitly explained to the patient. If the patient's expectations are unrealistic, he or she will be more likely to be dissatisfied with the result and much less tolerant of any complications.

In assessing the patient, full consideration must be made of the sex, race and build of the patient. A patient whose complaint is that the nose is too large may, in fact, have mandibular retrognathism. In that case, orthognathic surgery rather than rhinoplasty would be the correct operation. The general racial characteristics of the patient should be maintained, although in some sectors, alteration of racial characteristics can be a principal request – 'westernization' of Asian faces has been a recognized practice.

Preoperative photography is mandatory (and simply sensible) in any aesthetic surgery.

Rhytidectomy

Rhytidectomy, or facelift, addresses the sagging skin and wrinkles of ageing. The elasticity of skin diminishes with age as collagen weakens. A stable successful rhytidectomy should be directed toward deeper connective tissue layers as well as skin.

The areas of the face addressed by rhytidectomy are essentially the lateral face and neck (jowl) bilaterally extending to the modiolus and cervical midline. The commonly used incisions are shown in Figure 24.1.

A skin-only facelift may relapse in as short a time as 6 months. The superficial musculoaponeurotic (SMAS) layer, which lies immediately above and

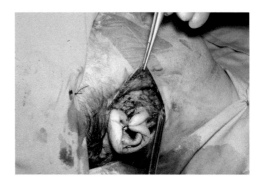

Figure 24.2 Facelift incision and undermining of the skin flap.

often intermingles with the parotid fascia and continues superiorly as the temporoparietal fascia and inferiorly as the platysma, can be lifted. This technique greatly reduces relapse by providing a robust component that can be fixed in a less temporary fashion.

The incision is made preauricularly, underneath the lobule of the ear, over the posterior aspect of the pinna and extended into the hairline at a right angle to it. A plane is formed in the subcutaneous fat (Figure 24.2), and extensive skin flaps are raised. They extend to the midline in the neck and to the modiolus in the cheek.

The SMAS layer may be dissected out as separate flaps, dissected with the skin flaps or not dissected out but rather hitched up and sutured to the temporal fascia with nonresorbable suture. The flaps are pulled upward and backward (separate SMAS flaps allow a differential pull), and excess skin is excised.

Potential complications are haematoma, infection, flap necrosis, relapse, greater auricular nerve injury and facial nerve injury. Because of the risk of flap necrosis, some surgeons recommend that the patient should be a nonsmoker or give up smoking before surgery.

A large area addressed by rhytidectomy is the neck, and platysmal plication may be performed at the same time. This procedure tightens the platysma muscle by suturing its two sides together in the midline via a small, horizontal submental incision.

There are probably more variations on the 'facelift' than on any other single procedure with a principal single outcome. The operation ranges from endoscopic through minimally invasive, mini to deep plane and subperiosteal lifts. The most

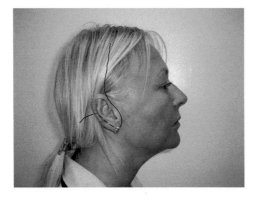

Figure 24.1 The incision line for rhytidectomy superimposed on a volunteer (the model is far too young to benefit from the discussed operations).

common tried and tested approaches are the classical skin only lift, the 'mini facelift', which does not address the temporal region or the platysma, and the SMAS lift as described.

Cervicofacial rhytidectomy is considered one operation, but it can be separated into its neck and its face component.

The facelift is often a two-part procedure:

- One for the lower face and jowls.
- One for the midface.

The upper face, less commonly discussed, also needs to be addressed.

Facelift procedures for the lower face and midface

Standard two-plane lift

The standard two-plane lift involves the elevation of a skin flap of variable length from preauricular and temporal incisions. After elevation of the skin flap, an SMAS flap is elevated, typically from below the zygomatic arch, then preauricularly, lateral to the anterior border of the parotid gland, usually extended past the earlobe and continued as a platysmal flap. The SMAS flap can be extended medially 3 to 5 cm, sometimes a little farther along the jowls, but more superiorly it ends before the level of the lateral border of zygomaticus major. SMASectomies and plication of the SMAS and platysma are common. The results of this approach are excellent for the jowls and lower face, but they do little to restore a more youthful appearance to the midface.

Extended superficial musculoaponeurotic system flap

The advocates of this method claim that by extending the SMAS flap medially well over the zygomaticus muscles, long-term improvement can be achieved for the nasolabial folds and consequently the midface (Mendelson 1992). Although injury to the facial nerve branches to the zygomaticus muscles is unlikely, branches to the upper lip orbicularis are vulnerable under the malar fat pad. The SMAS is often so thin medially that posterosuperior traction on it accomplishes little.

Two-plane lift with additional mobilization or suspension of the malar fat pad

A relatively extended skin flap is elevated to reach and mobilize the ptotic malar fat pad. It is repositioned and suspended with sutures to the temporal fascia. Problems are encountered with this method because of disruption of suborbicularis planes leading to prolonged oedema and possible distortion of the lateral canthus. This operation has good long-term results but is **not** without risks.

Extended supraplatysmal plane skin flap

In the extended supraplatysmal plane skin flap, a long, thick skin flap is elevated off the SMAS-platysma complex, thus leaving **all** the fat attached to the skin flap. In practice, this becomes difficult medially, where the SMAS thins out. All the facial retaining ligaments are released, and the skin flap is elevated. The SMAS and platysma are also generally plicated for additional support, or if thick enough, an SMAS flap or SMASectomy can be performed. The malar fat is in theory elevated, attached to the underside of the skin flap.

Deep plane or composite lift

The deep plane or composite lift is essentially an extended SMAS flap technique but leaving the skin attached to the SMAS. This long, thick skin muscle flap is closed under tension.

The neck flap and the face flaps do not connect over the mandible, unlike in most traditional two-plane lifts. There are real risks of complications and lengthy recovery.

Subperiosteal lift

The subperiosteal lift is primarily directed to the midface. In brief, the periosteum is elevated off the cheek bone. Once it is released inferiorly, the periosteal flap with all the overlying upper lip levator muscles, SMAS, malar fat pad and skin is repositioned more superiorly and posteriorly, thereby bringing the malar fat pad into its former position.

- Subciliary.
- Intraoral incision.
- Subperiosteal temporal lift (usually endoscopically).

Other simpler lifts

- Webster lift.
  - Shorter skin flap.
  - Simple plication.

- S-lift.
  - Short skin flap, smaller incision.
  - Simple plication.

- Suspension lift.
  - Gore-Tex sutures.

- Minimal access cranial suspension (MACS) lift.
  - Jowl correction.

- Minimal preauricular access.

Blepharoplasty and related procedures

Puffy or sagging eyelids are common complaints. Accurate diagnosis is essential. The complaint of sagging upper eyelids is often the result of sagging of the eyebrows, as opposed to excess tissue in the upper eyelid. In this situation the treatment is a brow lift first and then possibly an upper blepharoplasty. In assessing the eyelids, the appearance of bagginess may be caused by skin or fat or both. The word *blepharoplasty* was first used by Van Graefe in 1818 to describe a procedure for repairing defects in the eyelids secondary to tumour excision. The eyelids are one of the first structures of the face to develop structural changes related to ageing. Ageing results in changes in elasticity of the orbital septum, the tarsus and the orbicularis muscle. Clinically these changes lead to excess skin, wrinkles, pseudoherniation of orbital fat and baggy and tired-looking eyes. Ageing-induced changes in the skin are characterized by development of pigmentary anomalies. Because skin quality is not altered by blepharoplasty, adjunctive therapies such as dermabrasion, chemical peeling or laser skin resurfacing may need to be incorporated into rejuvenation strategies. Blepharoplasty will not on its own treat malar bags or the tear trough deformity.

Lower lid blepharoplasty

The formation of bags under the eyes has more to do with problems with periorbital fat than

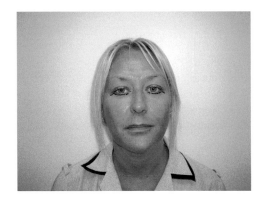

Figure 24.3 Schematic of a lower lid blepharoplasty incision on the same model.

with skin. The incision runs just under the lashes and then extends out laterally in a crow's foot (Figure 24.3). A musculocutaneous flap is raised, revealing the orbital septum and underlying fat. There are three fat pads – larger central and medial ones and a smaller lateral one. Where there is a prominent nasojugal groove, the fat is redraped to fill this groove and even out the bagginess of the lid. If this is not the case, the orbital septum may simply require tightening, which is achieved by bipolar diathermy burns that induce pinpoint areas of fibrosis and tightening. If fat requires removal, this should be minimal and is achieved as much by diathermy to make it shrink as by excision. Excessive fat removal can lead to a sunken appearance, which is difficult to correct. Skin removal should be minimal.

Potential complications are haemorrhage, infraorbital nerve injury and ectropion.

Upper lid blepharoplasty

In contrast to the lower eyelids, upper eyelid bagginess is largely the result of excess skin (although see the next section, on brow lift). An assessment of the amount to remove may be made by pinching the skin of the eyelid until the eye starts to open. This is the minimum that should be removed (Figure 24.4). The patient should be warned that the eyelids will not meet immediately postoperatively, but this will settle in about 2 weeks. In addition to skin removal, a small amount of muscle may need to be removed. As with the lower eyelids, there may be a small amount of fat herniation that

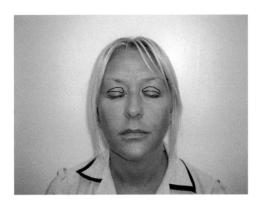

Figure 24.4 Schematic of an upper lid blepharoplasty excision.

may require reduction, but there is no lateral fat pad (this is the lacrimal gland, and it should be left well alone).

Brow lift

The eyebrows may become ptotic with age. The results are lateral crow's feet and hooding with concomitant overactivity of the forehead musculature with rhytid formation. The brow lift aims to address this issue. There are several techniques, the choice of which is determined largely by the height of the forehead. The distance between the upper edge of the eyebrows and the hairline should be approximately 5 cm. This distance may be lengthened or shortened by a particular brow lift, and this should be borne in mind when planning.

- **Coronal** – this incision is made well into the hairline (4 to 5 cm), and a strip of scalp is excised. This procedure tends to lengthen the forehead.
- **Pretrichial** – the incision is made at the hairline, and scalp is excised. This tends to shorten the forehead. It can result in an abrupt change from skin to hair, thus giving a slightly artificial appearance.
- **Midforehead** – the incision is within the forehead and is suitable for patients with deep rhytids. It shortens the forehead, and the patient should understand that there will be a visible scar that will be red for a year or so.
- **Direct brow pexy** – this simply excises tissue directly above the eyebrows. Again, there will

be a noticeable scar. This procedure is particularly indicated for patients with damage to the temporal branch of the facial nerve.
- **Endoscopic brow lift** – five small incisions are made within the scalp, and subperiosteal dissection is carried out endoscopically. The scalp is pulled posteriorly and is fixed to the skull with screws, which are removed after a few weeks. Although it can potentially lengthen the forehead, this approach is very popular.

Specific complications of brow lifts are scarring, alopecia and scalp paraesthesia.

Otoplasty (pinnaplasty)

The arterial supply of the ear arises from the superficial temporal and the posterior auricular arteries. The sensory supply of the ear is from the auriculotemporal, great auricular and vagus nerves. The auricle is fully formed at birth. It reaches 85% of its final size by the age of 3 years and is virtually adult size by 6 years.

Bat ears can be a source of misery for children as a result of teasing at school. They are caused by an excessive angle between the pinna and the skull, congenital absence of an antihelix or a combination of both. Again, proper evaluation of the exact problem is required because it may stem from the pinna with an absence of an antihelix or the conchal bowl creating an excessive concho-occipital angle (Figure 24.5 (a)).

There are various techniques. In the technique of anterior scoring, skin is excised in the posterior pinna after assessing the amount of reduction required. The skin excision is purely to remove the excess that will be left at the end of the procedure. The cartilage is incised and dissected off the anterior skin. The cartilage is then scored parallel to the long axis of the pinna, and further scores may be made at right angles to these. This procedure allows the intact posterior elastic cartilage to pull the pinna back, thus creating a rounded natural antihelix. The pinna will be lying at a more natural angle and can be sutured into position. An alternative is to thin the cartilage posteriorly with a burr and suture the cartilage to the mastoid process. This has the advantage of avoiding dissecting the skin over the anterior surface of the cartilage, but it

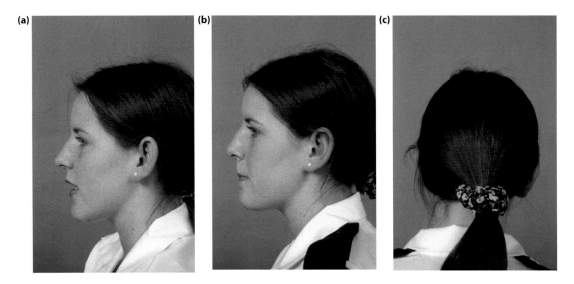

Figure 24.5 (a) Preoperative prominent ears. The increased conchal angle protrudes the ears, whereas the absence of an antihelix flattens them, increasing the apparent prominence. (b) After pinnaplasty using a combined Mustarde (suturing) Furness (conchal excision) technique. (c) Posterior view.

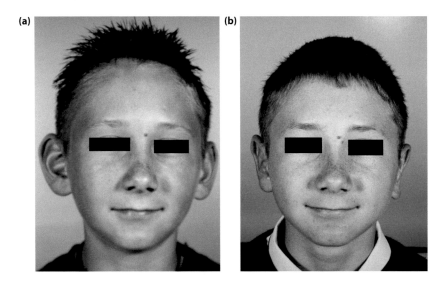

Figure 24.6 (a) Preoperative view of prominent ear correction. (b) Postoperative view of prominent ear correction.

works against the natural logic of using the elastic fibres. An alternative well-established technique is direct suturing using permanent mattress sutures (traditionally white silk) to recreate the antihelix as described by Mustarde. An excessive concho–occipital angle can be reduced by excision of the appropriate amount of cartilage from a posterior approach (Figure 24.5 (b) and (c) and Figure 24.6 (a) and (b)).

Potential complications are haematoma, dissatisfaction with the result, relapse and telephone deformity of the ear.

Rhinoplasty

Rhinoplasty is one of the most satisfying techniques in aesthetic surgery, but it is also one of the most demanding. As with all the previously discussed topics, evaluation of the problem is critical. The nose consists of skin, fibrofatty connective tissue, hyaline cartilage and bone. As a rule, rhinoplasty can address problems related to cartilage and bone, but it cannot alter the skin of the nose, which can vary from paper thin to thick and fleshy with many sebaceous glands.

The nose should be assessed with a view to maintaining the aesthetic balance of the patient's face as well as retaining racial characteristics. As already highlighted, mandibular retrognathism may make a perfectly acceptable nose appear large, but the nose will be in proportion following a mandibular advancement procedure.

The nose should be examined from all angles, including above and below. The various components to assess are tip projection, supratip break, dorsal hump, nostril symmetry, septal deviation and skin quality. Although there may be several components that deviate from the ideal, detailed discussion with the patient should highlight what the patient is dissatisfied with because it may not require as complex a procedure to deal with the specific complaint (Figure 24.7 (a)). It is vital that once the surgery has been planned, one does not change from this plan during the operation unless very detailed and specific consent has been given by the patient to allow this change. Remember that all aesthetic surgery is purely elective, and adherence to what the patient has agreed to accept is vital.

Vast arrays of incisions may be used in performing a rhinoplasty; however, there are essentially two approaches – open or closed. The closed approach, which remains the most popular, involves intranasal incisions either through the alar cartilages (intracartilaginous) or between the alar and upper quadrilateral cartilages with a connecting preseptal transfixion incision (Figure 24.7 (b)).

An open rhinoplasty leaves a small scar across the columella, whereas a closed rhinoplasty does not. The bony surgery usually involves removal of a dorsal hump (if present), thus leaving an 'open roof'. Lateral osteotomies from the piriform aperture along the junction of the nasal bones to the maxilla allow this to be closed to leave a narrower dorsum with a smooth, straight profile (Figure 24.7 (c)).

The alar cartilages may require attention if the nasal tip needs to be addressed. This usually involves either trimming the lower lateral cartilages or suturing the medial crura.

Increasing tip projection:

- Tip sutures – this procedure involves the removal of any intervening interdomal tissue and suturing the middle crura to one another with medial crural sutures.
- Columellar strut – this is when a cartilage strut is placed into a pocket between the medial crura of the lower lateral cartilages to provide a supporting structure.

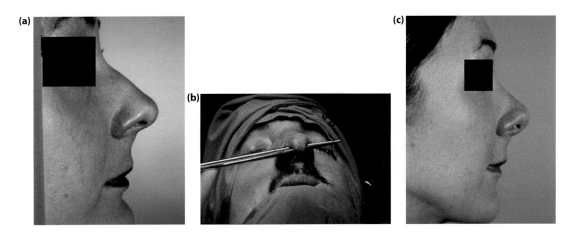

Figure 24.7 (a) This patient's main concern was the dorsal nasal hump. (b) A different patient's transfixion incision that connects the intranasal intracartilaginous or intercartilaginous incisions for access to the nasal skeleton. (c) The postoperative result of the patient in (a).

- Tip graft – when even further increased projection is needed, an onlay graft can be sutured over the tip.

Decreasing tip projection:
- Medial or middle crural release – in this procedure used for minimal deformity, release of ligaments and placement of sutures between the middle crura and caudal septum will set back the lower lateral cartilage complex to a certain degree.
- Cephalic trim – excision of a portion of the cephalic margin of the lower lateral cartilage will further disrupt support of the nasal tip. A medial crural-septal suture may be used to secure the tip in a more posterior position.

Increasing tip rotation – small increases in tip rotation may be achieved by simple excision of the cephalic border of the lower lateral cartilages.

Decreasing tip rotation – a septal extension graft of cartilage harvested from either the septum or the rib and fixed to both the dorsal septum and medial crura will serve to push the tip inferiorly and derotate the nose. The tip may be reduced, or a submucous resection of the cartilaginous septum may be carried out. Straightening a deviated cartilaginous septum is difficult.

Where tissue is required to be added rather than removed, a graft from the pinna or septum can be used (e.g. to augment the dorsum or project the nasal tip). Much time is spent discussing the best form of postoperative dressings and support, but the actual tissue manipulation is the crucial component of this operation (Figure 24.8).

Potential complications are epistaxis, septal haematoma or abscess, decreased nasal aperture with concomitant breathing difficulties and dissatisfaction with the result.

A common comment by surgeons experienced in rhinoplasty is to beware the young male patient requesting rhinoplasty. Dissatisfaction and complaints are frequent in this patient group.

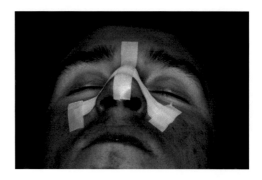

Figure 24.8 A light tape dressing after dorsal hump reduction and minimal tip work in a young male patient.

Genioplasty

Genioplasty is movement, or reshaping, of the chin. There are a number of approaches to this operation, usually depending on the training of the surgeon. Conventional genioplasty is an orthognathic procedure using similar principles (Figure 24.9 (a) and (b)). The chin is approached from an intraoral incision that exposes and protects the mental nerves. Bone cuts are made horizontally to retain the lingual muscle attachments. The chin is reduced by excising a middle portion of bone and inset to preserve the aesthetics of the cortical chin shape. It can be advanced by sliding forward. It is internally fixed using miniplates (Figure 24.10). Small asymmetries can be corrected in this fashion.

Variations on the advancement genioplasty have become popular in the treatment of obstructive sleep apnoea (see Chapter 19). Specific miniplates have been designed to make this operation more predictable. One technique twists the chin around 90°. The concept has an evidence base and is founded on advancement of the genial attachments of the tongue musculature.

Augmentation genioplasty by implant is used by some ear, nose and throat and plastic surgeons. This implant is often inserted by a skin incision under the chin (which is invisible from an anterior view). Silastic, coral and other synthetics are used. The main problems are implant infection and resorption of the underlying bone.

Almost inevitably, the aesthetic result using the patient's own bone is superior to that using synthetic materials.

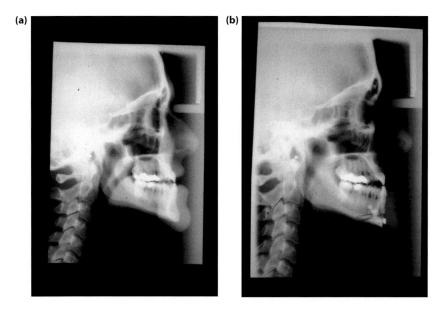

Figure 24.9 (a) Preoperative lateral cephalogram of a prominent chin. (b) Postoperative lateral cephalogram of the same case.

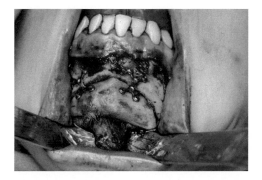

Figure 24.10 Internal fixation of a genioplasty.

Miscellaneous procedures

Facial rejuvenation – this procedure destroys the very superficial layer of the skin (different agents affect the skin to different depths). After healing, the finer rhytids will have disappeared. This procedure can be carried out using chemicals such as glycolic acid, trichloroacetic acid or phenol. A similar procedure can be carried out with carbon dioxide laser.

Botulinum-alpha toxin – botulinum toxin prevents acetylcholine release at the neuromuscular junction and paralyzes the muscle. Its use is widespread, particularly for the treatment of rhytids. Rhytids are formed at right angles to the direction of pull of the underlying musculature. Paralysis of these muscles with botulinum toxin decreases the wrinkling present and can prevent future rhytid formation. The solution is injected into the muscles in the affected area, most commonly the forehead, the glabella and the crow's feet. In the forehead the injection should be at least 1 cm above the eyebrow to prevent unwanted ptosis. The injection sites should not be massaged because this makes the solution dissipate unpredictably. The patients (or clients) should remain upright for 4 hours and should not undertake strenuous exercise that day. Otherwise, it is a remarkably safe procedure. The effect can be variable but will usually last 6 months to 1 year. Repeated injections over time may have a more permanent effect but antibody production is now recognized to make some patients "resistant" to treatment. Patients should be warned of paralysis of their facial muscles as a potential side effect. Botulinum toxin also is useful in treating blepharospasm, masseteric hypertrophy (Figure 24.11 (a) and (b)), temporalis hypertrophy (Figure 24.12) and Frey's syndrome. The doses of different brands of botulinum-alpha toxin (e.g. Botox, Xeomin, Dysport) are not interchangeable, and one should be familiar with the manufacturers' instructions.

Fillers – collagen and hyaluronidase solutions, sometimes combined with local analgesia, are used to fill out subcutaneous hollows, either deep (e.g. the nasolabial folds) or tiny (e.g. labial rhytids). Sometimes these fillers are used as a temporary solution to traumatic or acne scarring.

Dermabrasion – this works in much the same way as the rejuvenation procedures, but it uses a large burr to smooth rough areas of skin or scarring. It is particularly useful for severe skin damage (e.g. from severe acne). Laser resurfacing acts in a similar way.

Rhinophyma – this condition is caused by an overgrowth of sebaceous glands in the nasal skin (Figure 24.13). The lay perception that the condition is caused by excessive alcohol intake is erroneous. It can be quite dramatic in appearance but is relatively easily treated. The tissue can either be excised or dermabraded, and mechanical removal may be used in conjunction with a carbon dioxide laser. The tissue should be sent for histological examination because basal cell carcinoma may mimic benign rhinophyma.

Implants and bony resculpting – facial contours that appear excessive because of underlying bone may in part be corrected by osteotomies (Figure 24.14), particularly of those areas where reduction of the outer cortical shape may result in a distorted contour (Figure 24.15). It should be borne in mind, however, that the postoperative appearance is unpredictable because there is not a 1:1 relationship between bone removed and reduction in soft tissue contour. Similarly, where there appears to be a tissue deficit,

(a) (b)

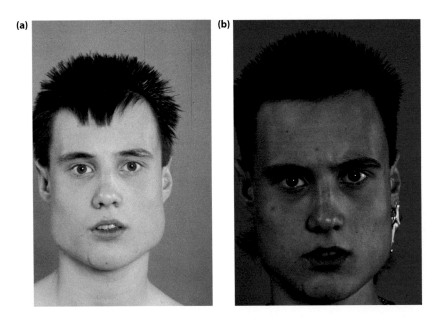

Figure 24.11 (a) Before treatment of bilateral masseteric hypertrophy. (b) After treatment of the same case.

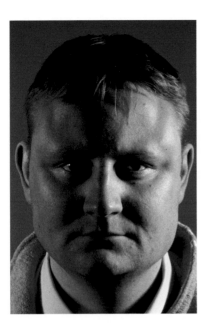

Figure 24.12 Masseter and temporalis hypertrophy.

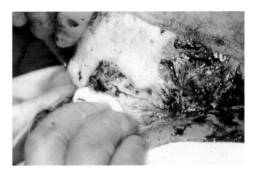

Figure 24.14 Supraorbital ridge reduction osteotomies in a gender reassignment case.

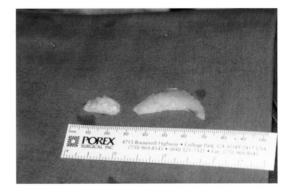

Figure 24.15 Bone resculpting.

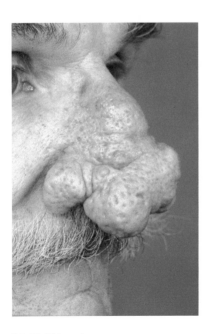

Figure 24.13 Rhinophyma.

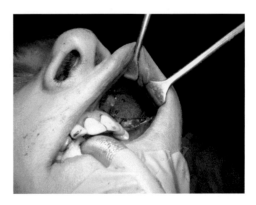

Figure 24.16 A synthetic implant (Medpor) placed transorally for malar augmentation.

then alloplastic onlays may be employed (Figure 24.16).

Minor soft tissue procedures – minor procedures that cross the demarcation between pure aesthetic surgery and trauma surgery include scar revision and correction of traumatic defects such as torn earlobes (Figure 24.17 (a) and (b)).

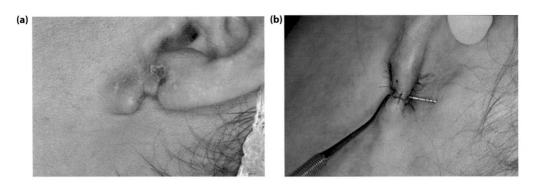

Figure 24.17 (a) Preoperative view of a torn pierced ear. (b) Immediate postoperative view.

FURTHER READING

Choucair RJ, Hamra ST. Extended superficial mus-culoaponeurotic system dissection and composite rhytidectomy. *Clin Plast Surg* 2008;35:607–22.

Eremia S, Willoughby MA. Rhytidectomy. *Dermatol Clin* 2005;23:415–30.

Hadlock TA, Cheney ML, McKenna MJ. Facial reanimation surgery. In Nadol JB, McKenna MJ. *Surgery of the ear and temporal bone.* 2005. Philadelphia. Lippincot Williams and Wilkins. 461–72.

Mendelson BC. Cosmetic surgery for the ageing face. *Aust Fam Physician* 1992;21:907–10, 913–5, 918–9.

Warren RJ, Aston SJ, Mendelson BC. Facelift. *Plast Reconstr Surg* 2011;128:747e–64e.

25

Cutting edge

Contents

Aim

- To gain information about scientific methods and the ability to investigate a scientific problem from the first steps to publication of the results.

Learning outcomes

- To be able to converse using research terminology.
- To be able to state the problem concisely.
- To find the appropriate methods to investigate solutions for the problem.
- To be able to describe the basic information, methodology and results from the investigation and objectively discuss and interpret the findings.
- To describe how these innovations could affect patient care.

Introduction

The past few years have seen remarkable developments in the practice of oral and maxillofacial surgery. Innovation can be from basic laboratory research – so-called translational research – which translates from the laboratory to the clinical arena. For example, Figure 25.1 shows an attempt to use bone marrow biopsies to predict outcomes of patients with oral squamous cell carcinoma to personalize appropriate treatment. An alternative is commercially sponsored technical innovations, most obvious in the drug world but seen in our field more frequently among the instrument manufacturers (Figures 25.2, 25.3, 25.4 and 25.5). These pictures demonstrate presurgical virtual planning that creates stereolithographic models and surgical positioning jigs for use in resection and reconstruction of benign osseous disease (in this case, an extensive ameloblastoma).

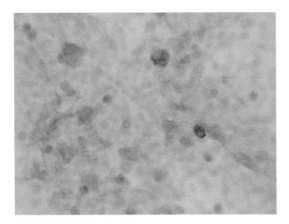

Figure 25.1 The trephining of small quantities of bone marrow from the iliac crest may enable detection of the high-risk patient with oral cancer as a simple outpatient test. This sample shows metastatic cytokeratin-positive squames in the bone marrow.

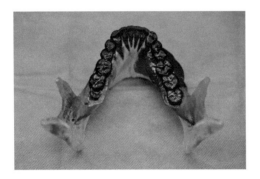

Figure 25.2 Modern stereolithographic modelling rendered in acrylic.

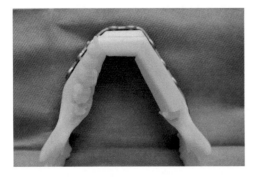

Figure 25.3 This modelling can allow prebending of titanium plates for fixation.

The routine use of free flaps in reconstructive surgery and new technology, especially in the field of imaging techniques, stereotactic navigation and preoperative surgical planning of reconstructive procedures, have advanced and continue to improve surgical practice, to the benefit of our patients.

Further development in technology such as robotic surgery may (or may not) prove important. Equally vital is research at the human end of patient care. As surgeons, we must resist the temptation to conform to stereotypes generated by either ourselves or others. Quality of life research in oral and maxillofacial surgery, particularly in the area of oral cancer, has contributed greatly to our understanding of what is important to our patients. This needs to be extended into hitherto underresearched areas, such as sexuality and intimacy in cancer and facial trauma survivors, and linked to tactics from the nonsurgical areas of medical practice to not only identify but also improve our patients' quality of life after treatment.

Predicting the future is always difficult. Many of the issues the research of the last decades seemed certain to resolve have not been, and totally unexpected advances have been made.

Research terms and procedures

Before you start thinking about research, you must have a methodology of how to read a paper. When you read a research paper, your aim is to understand the scientific contributions the authors are making to the literature. This may be a difficult task and may require going over the paper several times. Do not assume that the authors are always correct. Use the same approach for every paper you read. A useful framework may be to prepare a one-page review that should include the following:

1. The aim of the work.
2. A more extensive outline of the main points of the paper, including assumptions made, arguments presented, data analyzed and conclusions drawn.
3. An examination and notation of the limitations of the work.
4. A summary of your opinion of the paper and how it may be improved and further planning on how you are going to apply the findings in your practice.

The second aspect to consider is how to do a systematic review. You should familiarize yourself

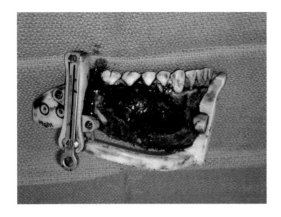

Figure 25.4 It can also enable design of a cutting jig for planned resection ....

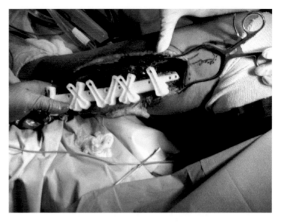

Figure 25.5 ... and reconstruction. The template allows accurate positioning of osteotomy cuts on the fibula while it is still vascularized at the donor site, thereby reducing ischaemic time.

with the PRISMA (Preferred Reporting Items for Systematic Reviews and Meta-Analyses) guidance on how to write a systematic review. Once you are familiar with how to evaluate a paper critically and understand the methodology of how to write a systematic review, the next logical step is to write your own paper or design your own research.

Literature

Before you start, find out what has already been done. One of the most important objectives before you start trying to answer a research question with either clinical or experimental content is to acquire knowledge of the current literature.

When you are confident that you understand the available literature, you should start to put your knowledge into action, and you should be able to develop your scientific question. The following two points may help:

1. Make a plan with aims that you can follow.
2. Given that you are able to write your aims down in a concise manner, you can start, because you are focussed.

These points sound very simple, but while working and writing them down you have the opportunity to reflect. Things will also become indistinct because they will become more complex with time. Then it is quite helpful to remember the aims you had in the first place.

Statistical methodology

Before you fully commit to the process of data collection, it is important to think about the analysis of the results. You should try to put any previous experience into planning. Ask yourself the following – What is the question? Why is it important? Where will the investigation be conducted? What will need to happen? Who will do it? How will the results be identified and disseminated?

In relatively easy projects such as a case series or a cohort study, the process of data collection and analyses may be straightforward.

For more complex studies such as a double-blind randomized controlled trial, a formal statistical plan should be in place well in advance of acquiring data. Having an expert statistician is very important because biomedical statistics have become increasingly complex. Knowing the number of patients or outcomes that will be needed for a study to reach statistical significance (the 'power' calculation) may demonstrate that the study is not feasible immediately.

You should know the basics of statistics to be able to analyze the work of other researchers and to have meaningful discussions with experts, although meaningful results require expert backing.

Basics include a t-test (e.g. comparison of normally distributed data in means), a Mann-Whitney U-test (e.g. comparison of scores), the Fisher exact test (comparison of the distributions), linear regression analysis (e.g. factors influencing treatment or survival) and the Kaplan–Meier method (e.g. survival analyses). Sometimes trying to understand statistics can be overwhelming. There are several available resources including introductory series in *BMJ* and the *British Journal of Oral and Maxillofacial Surgery*.

How to start writing a paper

There are several ways to write a paper. A basic understanding of the subject is essential. Many authors have embarrassed themselves by writing outside their area of knowledge and making simple obvious errors.

General information and its clinical relevance to the subject should also be explained. The introduction should be brief (a discussion later extends the relevant information), and references to the recent literature should be included.

Materials and methods should be detailed, usually in collaboration with the statistician with whom you worked out your strategy. This also helps the statistician to understand the problem and the relevance of the study completely. Afterward, it is very important to write down your results objectively, without any interpretation of data. In this part, it is not necessary to explain why what you have done is wonderful. It is just necessary to explain that it counts. Nothing more. In the discussion section, the interpretation of data should be given in comparison with data reported by other researchers who have already published their work. Here you can explain just what you have achieved and its importance. It may be important to demonstrate clearly why your results are unique. This may be the case in studies with very surprising results. You are able to interpret your data and show its relevance for the future, and you give further details on planned studies, changes of practice and so on. It is important to show the reader why your study may be relevant.

Where do you want to place your paper?

After you have carried out your research and written the draft manuscript, you should adapt it to the journal's guidelines. This is sometimes very difficult because every journal has its own style and requirements.

Please realize that it is every editor's pet hate to receive papers submitted from authors who have clearly not bothered to read the 'Instructions to Authors'. Failure to do so results in a very poor chance of successful dissemination of your results. To make it simple, do not bother sending a manuscript to a journal until you have read the instructions to authors. Do not even start writing the manuscript until you have some idea of your target audience and journal.

It is important to send your work to a journal that is relevant for you and your work. Although some journals do not have a high impact factor (IF – the rather simplistic but ubiquitous performance indicator for scientific journals and something many universities use as a surrogate for quality), this should not be the most important thing for you. Initially, it is more important to you that your article is published. Let the IF game come later in your career if it becomes relevant. This will maximize your chances of publication.

It is also important that the journal you try to publish in (at least after getting started) is indexed and accessible via PubMed, which creates peer visibility.

You will doubtless be exposed to the 'open access' option to make this article available for everybody in the world free of subscription or download charge. It may be helpful to understand that this concept started out as an altruistic notion that knowledge should be free to all. Nothing is for nothing, however, and in most cases this requires payment from the author. In most science fields, the work is funded by research grants, and in some instances the grant-awarding body will insist that part of the grant is used to fund 'open access'. Unfortunately, small, highly specialized surgical disciplines (among others) suffer in this approach because very few are able to gain access to substantial research funding. To most of us, 'open access' becomes 'pay to publish', which is worryingly close to vanity publishing and exactly the opposite of the intentions of the altruistic 'knowledge for all' movement.

Journals in this field are moving to a 'hybrid open access system' in which pure open access is available at a price (if the paper is grant funded), but more conventional publishing options that do not involve paying a fee are retained.

Always keep in mind – start simple, take early advice and know that good research will engender awareness irrespective of the journal in which it was published.

Your paper in the eye of a reviewer

One of the most difficult aspects for every researcher is to have his or her work rejected. This will happen more than once in the career of every researcher, and in most cases very simple reasons are the cause. Usually, the journal will provide a reason for the rejection and will make suggestions, but sometimes it depends on the scope of the research and the methodology of the work chosen.

If you have a good, objective method for your investigation and it can overcome the 'so what' criticism, it will be less difficult to publish your paper.

There are also political reasons for rejecting some papers. These can range from government edict to interspecialty rivalry.

Try not to let rejection discourage you. It is important to read the reviews given by the reviewers. Constructive comments will always improve the manuscript and should be taken into consideration without emotion, even if sometimes the comments do not make sense or illustrate that the reviewer did not understand the paper. It happens. That is life.

It may be better not to change everything, but clarify the methods and the results that generated the queries. Sometimes you will have the opportunity to resubmit your article, and this usually implies that if you make the requested changes, the paper will be accepted. You should always answer the questions of the reviewer precisely and give feasible reasons why you have done something in a particular manner if you do not want to change the content. It is not always necessary to change everything suggested, but more important, the reviewer's opinion should be respected and taken into consideration. At this stage of the review process, there should be no simple errors, and sometimes there is a need for additional assistance to understand clearly the perspective of the reviewer or the editor. Journals with a high IF have to filter out even quite good papers.

If not, and the rejection is outright, reassess the paper. Usually, taking the comments seriously and targeting another journal will improve your chances. Multiple attempts may be necessary until your work is accepted.

Summary

Whatever your own clinical interest, there is likely to be an area in which you can contribute to future developments. The place of clinicians in research is important. Your role as an 'end user' of research with unique insight into the needs of those for whom you care can determine the priorities for research and development. In addition, you will have several opportunities to find access to research methodology and science during training and clinical practice.

You should be aware of routine work and ask yourself why the practice you are doing is generally accepted or not. Personal or departmental audit, your own observations in daily routine and practice may not just enhance the outcome of your treatments, but they could also have more general applicability.

FURTHER READING

Greenhalgh T. How to read a paper: assessing the methodological quality of published papers. *BMJ* 1997;315:305.

Harris M, Taylor G. *Medical statistics made easy*, 2nd ed. Banbury, UK: Scion Publishing, 2008.

www.prisma-statement.org. PRISMA (Preferred Reporting Items for Systematic Reviews and Meta-Analyses) website.

26

Getting into oral and maxillofacial surgery

Contents

Useful sources of career information in oral and maxillofacial surgery

For those who are interested in or have made the first steps on embarking on a career in oral and maxillofacial surgery, the following information may act as a support.

The definition of the scope of oral and maxillofacial surgery is taken from the intercollegiate surgical curriculum project in the United Kingdom. This varies widely internationally, although a close parallel in terms of scope and hospital-based practice exists between the United Kingdom and Germany, some other parts of Europe and specific states/provinces in North America.

Scope of oral and maxillofacial surgery

Oral and maxillofacial surgery deals with the diagnosis, evaluation and treatment of conditions affecting the mouth, jaws, face and head and neck region. Internationally agreed guidelines define the current scope of the specialty as follows:

- Treatment of dentoalveolar and oral pathology.
- Preprosthetic surgery including implantology.
- Diseases and disorders of the temporomandibular joint.
- Craniomaxillofacial trauma – hard and soft tissue.
- Benign and malignant conditions of the salivary glands.
- Benign and malignant conditions of the head and neck.
- Congenital, developmental and acquired craniomaxillofacial deformity.
- Other nonsurgical conditions affecting the face, mouth and jaws (e.g. oral mucosal disease, cervicofacial infections, orofacial pain).
- Aesthetic facial surgery.

It is accepted that a full range of surgical techniques is required for each of the foregoing categories including, where relevant, reconstruction

USEFUL WEBSITES

Organization	Abbreviation	Website
American Association of Oral and Maxillofacial Surgeons	AAOMS	www.aaoms.org
British Association of Oral and Maxillofacial Surgeons	BAOMS	www.baoms.org.uk
British Dental Association	BDA	www.bda-dentistry.org.uk
British Medical Association	BMA	www.bma.org.uk
Organization	**Abbreviation**	**Website**
European Association for Cranio-Maxillo-Facial Surgery	EACMFS	www.eurofaces.com
Faculty of Dental Surgery, Royal College of Surgeons of England	FDSRCS Eng	fds@rcseng.ac.uk
General Dental Council	GDC	www.gdc-uk.org
General Medical Council	GMC	www.gmc-uk.org
International Journal of Oral and Maxillofacial Surgery	IJOMS	www.ijoms.com
Joint Committee on Intercollegiate Examinations	JCIE	www.intercollegiate.org.uk
Joint Committee on Surgical Training	JCST	www.jcst.org
Oral and maxillofacial courses, Royal College of Surgeons of England	OMF courses at RCS England	maxfac@rcseng.ac.uk
Royal College of Physicians and Surgeons of Glasgow	RCPS Glasg	www.rcpsglasg.ac.uk
Royal College of Surgeons of Edinburgh	RCS Ed	www.rcsed.ac.uk
Royal College of Surgeons of England	RCS England	www.rcseng.ac.uk
Royal College of Surgeons of Ireland	RCSI	www.rcsi.ie

using distant donor sites and microsurgical techniques.

As a specialty, oral and maxillofacial surgery varies greatly around the world. Even within Europe, substantial differences exist in the training and scope of practice between neighbouring countries. The old (and in some areas reemerging) dental specialty of 'oral surgery' overlaps with the dentoalveolar aspects of the discipline, and other surgical specialties (e.g. ear, nose and throat and plastic surgery) overlap with other aspects to a greater or lesser extent in varying degrees around the world. This book attempts to draw together a consensus in scope and approach, but it is heavily based in the UK scope, which has most in common with that in German-speaking countries. Despite that similarity, the differences in training are vast. For the sake of comparison, the training processes for completion of training in the United Kingdom, Germany and the United States are discussed here.

Specialist training in the United Kingdom

Entry to specialist training

Specialist training is the recognized pathway to achieving a Certificate of Completion of Training (CCT) in Oral and Maxillofacial Surgery. Under current guidelines, this certificate is mandatory for UK trainees who wish to apply for consultant positions in the United Kingdom. European trainees are eligible but must demonstrate 'equivalence' of training and assessment procedures.

The postgraduate deans working with the Specialist Advisory Committee (SAC) in Oral and Maxillofacial Surgery have the responsibility of ensuring that the training programmes are of a suitable standard to allow trainees to achieve a CCT. This responsibility is discharged on behalf of the Specialist Training Authority, the body that ultimately recommends the award of CCT and inclusion on the Specialist Register held by the General Medical Council (GMC).

Currently entry to specialist training follows a period of basic surgical training culminating in the attainment of the Membership of the Royal College of Surgeons (MRCS) diploma of one of the UK Royal Colleges of Surgeons. Appointment to a Specialist Registrar (StR) post is by centrally (nationally) organized competitive interview and is based on meeting certain prespecified criteria.

The emphasis in the early years of specialist training is on the acquisition of generic surgical competencies and basic specialist competencies. This normally includes experience in other surgical specialties, with the acquisition of relevant transferable knowledge and skills. This approach allows trainees to move laterally, should they wish it, into another related specialty in the early years of training. They will be able to take with them 'transferable credits' that will be accepted as counting toward accreditation in their new specialty.

Pathway to specialist training

Trainees in oral and maxillofacial surgery require formal (registrable) dental and medical qualifications. The route taken to the entry point for specialist training differs slightly depending on which qualification is taken first. (In many ways, the time taken for a second degree can actually be considered as part of specialist training for oral and maxillofacial surgeons.)

Starting from dental surgery

At present, most UK trainees start in dentistry and take medicine as their second degree. It is envisaged that a number of generic professional competencies will be achieved during the 2 years of General Professional Training that will follow dental qualification. This will allow transfer of 'credits' that should considerably shorten or obviate the need for a second foundation year after medical graduation. This concept is further supported by the realization that those dental surgeons who return to study medicine because they wish to train in oral and maxillofacial surgery have already made a definite career choice. Consequently, there is no need for any career orientation, which is a major reason for most medical graduates to be exposed to a variety of specialties in the second foundation year. A possible plan for the training pathway would therefore be as follows:

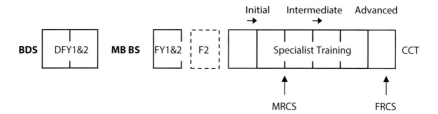

Initial ———————————→ Intermediate → Advanced

| MB BS | F1 | F2 | | BDS | | Specialist Training | | CCT |

MRCS   FRCS

Starting from medicine

Trainees who qualify first in medicine will probably opt to study dentistry following exposure to oral and maxillofacial surgery in the second foundation year or, more probably, in the early years of training in other related specialties. They will have achieved the relevant generic competencies during the 2 foundation years and can therefore reenter specialist training immediately following dental qualification.

Active support from the universities and the Department of Health for a shortened medical or dental course would help to reduce the training period further. This should be possible if the principle of 'transferable credits' is accepted for undergraduate education, as it will be in postgraduate training.

The mandatory requirements for progress from the initial to the intermediate stage of specialist training in oral and maxillofacial surgery are:

■ Medical and dental qualification.
■ GMC and General Dental Council (GDC) registration.
■ Satisfactory completion of the foundation year(s) (demonstrated by successful completion of an Annual Record of Competent Progress [ARCP] or equivalent – changes regularly).
■ Satisfactory progress through the early years of specialty training, including time spent in related disciplines, with the acquisition of defined competencies (ARCP or some similar semiobjective workplace assessment).
■ Success in the MRCS examination (specialty format yet to be agreed).
■ Success in competitive central recruitment into specialty training.

What do you actually do (operations) when training in oral and maxillofacial surgery?

To give the neophyte an idea of what he or she will be expected to do as a UK oral and maxillofacial surgical trainee progressing through training, the key indicative procedures in oral and maxillofacial surgery are given.

Specialist Advisory Committee core procedures in oral and maxillofacial surgery

These procedures were devised to create a 'marker' operation in each of the subspecialist areas of oral and maxillofacial surgery, the idea being if you mastered that operation, most of the related operations could be assumed to be safe in your hands.

These conditions and/or procedures are those that are considered core to the specialty. All trainees should have been routinely exposed to them, and have acquired the relevant clinical competencies, before the award of a CCT. Trainers should ensure that trainees are fully assessed in the management of these conditions and procedures in particular.

Important note – competence in these conditions and procedures will be taken to denote competence in the management of closely related pathology or less complex procedures in the same anatomical area.

Summary

The specialist training programme in oral and maxillofacial surgery aims to furnish trainees with the knowledge, skills and attitudes to acquire a CCT in the specialty. It is designed so that trainees will make progress through the stages from novice to competent practitioner and ultimately to independent practitioner.

INDICATIVE SKILLS FOR DEMONSTRATING COMPETENCY IN OMFS

Condition	Core operative skill(s)
Management of a patient with dentoalveolar pathology.	Surgical extraction of unerupted or impacted teeth and roots. Apical surgery or excision of jaw cyst.
Management of infections of the head and neck.	Drainage of tissue space infection.
Management of patient with a compromised airway.	Surgical access to airway (tracheostomy or cricothyroidotomy).
Management of maxillofacial trauma.	Repair of facial lacerations. Reduction and fixation of fracture of mandible. Fracture of mandibular condyle – open reduction and fixation. Elevation and fixation of fractured zygoma. Fracture of orbital floor – repair and graft.
Management of salivary gland swellings.	Submandibular gland excision. Parotidectomy.
Management of orofacial pain and temporomandibular joint dysfunction.	Temporomandibular joint arthrocentesis.
Management of a patient with a benign jaw tumour.	Resection of odontogenic tumour or fibro-osseous lesion. Harvest of bone graft.
Management of potentially malignant and malignant epithelial tumours of the mucosa and skin.	Excision of malignant skin tumour. Local skin flaps.
Management of a patient with a neck lump or swelling.	Neck dissection(s).
Management of a patient with a developmental or acquired deformity of the facial skeleton.	Mandibular ramus osteotomy. Maxillary osteotomy. Rhinoplasty.

The training programme provides opportunities for exposure to a wide range of oral and maxillofacial surgical problems. The aim is to acquire competency in the generality of the specialty by the end of year 5. This includes the opportunity to pursue an area of subspecialization in the latter period of training that may be further developed after the award of a CCT.

The award of a CCT depends on a satisfactory annual ARCP and is given at the completion of training and success in the intercollegiate specialty Fellowship of the Royal College of Surgeons (FRCS) examination. Trainees are normally expected to acquire the Membership of the Faculty of Dental Surgery/ Diploma of membership of the Joint Dental Faculty of the Royal College of Surgeons of England (MFDS/MJDF) of one of the UK Dental Faculties of the Royal Colleges of Surgeons (part C) or equivalent at some stage during training.

Specialist training in Germany

Germany has the highest number of oral and maxillofacial Surgeons in Europe. Since 2009, the specialty has grown by 50 members on average per year. Currently there are more than 1700 members registered in the German Society of Oral- and Maxillofacial Surgery, 1400 of whom are working under the status of specialist.

The society was founded in 1950 and has representation at all 34 medical university faculties in the country. From its inception, dual qualification in medicine and dentistry has been mandatory for admission.

Currently entry to specialist training is achieved by personal job application for a training position after completion of medical and/or dental studies. In general, German trainees start their specialist training after completion of both studies, but there exists the possibility to start specialist training after completion of medicine or dentistry only (exception in Bavaria). If the candidate enters dentistry with a medical degree, this will allow transfer of 'credits' that can shorten the time to obtain the dental degree down from 5 to 4 years.

Studying dentistry in some parts of Germany can open up a career in oral surgery not dissimilar to the situation in the United Kingdom, although for the most part hospital (both university and nonuniversity) departments are double-degree oral and maxillofacial surgery led. In contrast to the United Kingdom, the entire training can be completed in only one unit. Rotations are not necessary; therefore, changes among different units are rather rare. Training occurs in the workplace by *oberarzt* – a group of specialists who range from a UK-type registrar to an old-style senior registrar to a consultant, depending on seniority working under a single 'Chief', the professor.

At the end of the 5 years of mandatory training, a Certificate of Completion of Training (CCT) in Oral and Maxillofacial Surgery is awarded. The administration of specialist training in Germany is different from that in the United Kingdom. Local governments (Medical Chambers) in the different regions of Germany are responsible for the trainee, as is the unit head of department. The scope and method of training depend on the head of the department and often that person's particular interest or expertise and concepts of training. These can differ widely from unit to unit.

In Bavaria, for example, specialization can be started only after completion of both degrees, whereas in all other 17 Medical Chambers of Germany, a double degree has to be proved at the latest at the time of examination.

The emphasis in the early years of specialist training is on dentoalveolar surgery and on basic trauma and emergency surgical skills such as performing a tracheostomy or acute abscess drainage via extraoral incisions. Tumour surgery, orthognathic surgery, cleft repair, reconstructive and microsurgery, craniofacial surgery, temporomandibular joint (TMJ) surgery and the entire spectrum comparable to training in the United Kingdom follow, but the content varies according to the chief's interests. Probably the greatest difference between the two countries is that competencies in other surgical specialties akin to UK basic surgical training are not required. The aim is to acquire competency in the generality of the specialty by the end of year 5. Operations are performed every day as day cases and as inpatients. The bed problem so familiar to the United Kingdom is much less of an issue in Germany. Evidence that a certain number of every operation in the specialty has been performed by the end of the training is required.

Summary

The specialist training programme in oral and maxillofacial surgery in Germany lasts for 5 years and is dependent on the selected unit, case mix and the department's profile in patients' treatment. The departments compete for the best trainees, and the trainees compete for the best departments. At each of the 34 university departments, a simultaneous academic career with achievement of a PhD is possible, and for becoming a chief it is mandatory. The programme in most of the 82 oral and maxillofacial surgery departments in Germany offers a broad and deep training with a considerable amount of operative surgical procedures. The training is planned to allow for early autonomy for those surgeons wishing to carry out independent practice after specialization (in which a combination office and hospital 'attending' practice is possible) and has a hierarchical structure within the hospital environment. Trainees and oral and maxillofacial surgeons who voluntarily stay at the hospital after specialization can benefit from this clear structure.

Specialist training in the United States and Canada

Oral and maxillofacial surgical training in the United States (and Canada) is based on a post–dental school model of residency training. An office with or without 'attending' status at a hospital model is the most usual endpoint, although academic careers in university hospitals are widely available.

There are currently two types of programme – certificate and degree. The degree programme includes the incorporation of the requirements to complete a medical degree (MD). Programmes in the United States are accredited by the Commission on Dental Accreditation (CODA) and require a minimum of 30 months of clinical oral and maxillofacial surgery training. There is extensive training in anesthesia (a minimum of 5 months) and rotations to surgical and medical services for a minimum of 13 total months off service.

Admission is by competitive interview, with applicants matched to residencies through a national matching programme. During the clinical training in oral and maxillofacial surgery, residents receive gradated experiences in dentoalveolar surgery, implantology, maxillofacial trauma, maxillofacial pathology, including TMJ surgery, reconstructive surgery and orthognathic surgery.

Much of the clinical training occurs in an ambulatory environment, with the residents performing both the procedural sedation and surgery. On completion of an accredited programme, residents are eligible to sit the examinations of the American Board of Oral and Maxillofacial Surgery to become board certified. This process currently involves successfully completing the written qualifying examination and the oral certifying examination. Recertification is required every 10 years and is by written examination.

In Canada, completion of an accredited programme provides eligibility to sit for the National Dental Specialty Examination (NDSE), successful completion of which is a prerequisite to becoming a Fellow in the Royal College of Dentists of Canada (FRCD(C)). Fellowship training in subspecialty areas, such as oncology and cosmetic surgery, is available.

Summary

The specialist training in the United States and Canada is post–dental school training that prepares residents for independent practice on completion of training in either an office-based or hospital environment. Further in-service training is available as fellowships for those wishing to subspecialize in an area compatible with a career that is hospital or university hospital based.

Research and oral and maxillofacial surgery training

In every specialty, including in oral and maxillofacial surgery, research can improve clinical outcomes. It is possible to master surgery at the highest level, but a career will be incomplete without exposure to and preferably experience of research.

Traditionally, trainees were in a position to publish short papers such as technical notes and short communications (case reports). More recently, the demands of the specialty have somewhat changed. There is a need for high-quality research. Journals have become more demanding.

The broad possibilities of the specialty allow young trainees to contribute to science and perform high-quality research, particularly if their training units have a research infrastructure. In the United Kingdom, this is the area most in need of development currently. Unfortunately, high-quality research requires appropriate funding, and this is subject to the vagaries of fashion – much though purist academics would deny they could be subject to such a petty concept. Currently, funding for anything that is not held to be 'translational' is very hard to come by.

All techniques are evolving and still need input from the clinical and laboratory areas of the specialty. The most productive opportunities lie with multidisciplinary activity, often allowing a less conventional approach to pertinent problems.

All trainees should develop the capacity for critical thinking to allow safe interpretation of the literature. A healthy scepticism based on understanding research methodology (rather than a simple reluctance to change one's established beliefs and bigotries) is an essential component of modern clinical practice. Methodology, particularly in study design, and basic statistics are the main fields worthy of study. A familiarity with the process of conducting a systematic review will almost certainly become mandatory.

It is important to differentiate a clinical from an academic career. The role of a surgeon, by definition, is to operate when indicated (that is, when you benefit the patient by causing no net harm). This role may be different from an academic with no access to clinical care. In contrast, a clinician with an academic interest can function independently at the highest clinical or academic level. There are clinicians internationally with unparalleled academic and research portfolios.

As a trainee, it can be difficult to produce research that can change clinical practice. This can be achieved only in teams and with supervisors with a proven track record of research. The advent of funded fellowships may produce a change. There is a shift in training worldwide from purely clinical to clinical with a significant research component. Some countries such as Germany mandate a PhD as a requirement for real progress in the hospital system. In other countries, a taught Master's degree or a track record of published work in peer-reviewed journals is the requirement. Although fellowships may be time consuming in some fields of research, these opportunities offer different ways of benefitting patients and progressing in your chosen field.

Comprehensive clinical and research training can be very demanding. This is because, apart from a degree in medicine and dentistry and the dental and surgical fellowships, a research degree such as an MD or a PhD is essential. Each of these formal qualifications stands separately from the skills training and hours of practice (which may need to be up to 10 000) to acquire the psychomotor abilities a comprehensively trained oral and maxillofacial surgeon should have.

Normally, this higher academic qualification can be completed at any stage of training. In our experience, a research degree will fit better once a trainee has acquired a range of surgical skills. This is normally after at least the early years in higher oral and maxillofacial surgical training.

This is a great vocation. Why would you want to do anything else?

Index

Imiquimod, 277
Immunosuppression, 11
Immunosuppressive drugs, 277
Impacted teeth, 108, 110*f*, 111*f*, 122–123
  canines, 125–129
  complications of, 123
  failure of incisor eruption, 123
  supernumerary, 124–125
Impetigo, 144
Implant-borne prostheses, 224*f*, 325, 397*f*
Implants, 218–219
  bony resculpting and, 409
  choice of, 218
  classification, 218
  complications for osseointegrated types, 224–225
  cover screws, 222*f*
  custom bar prostheses, 222–223
  exposed threads, 221*f*
  extraoral craniofacial, 223–224
  with genioplasty, 308–309, 406
  hearing aid anchoring and, 224
  individual placement, 221–222
  material for guided tissue regeneration, 222*f*
  principles for placement, 219–220
  Same Day Teeth, 222–223
  socket preparation, 221*f*
  submental approach for, 223*f*
  surgery for cancer patients, 224
  surgery for osseointegrated types, 220–222
  transmandibular implant, 223
  United States perspective, 225
Impregnated dressings, 14, 271
Impressions, 204, 252, 395
Inadine, 13, 14
Incised wounds, 260–261
Incisional biopsy, 156
Incision and drainage, 96
Incisors
  canine impaction and, 126
  class III relationships, 300*f*
  dilacerated, 123*f*
  failure of eruption, 123
  Hutchinson's, 149
  resorption, 126*f*
  transplantation, 130, 131*f*

Infected haematomas, 119
Infections, 11
  acute bacterial, 137–138, 139*f*, 140–143, 334–335
  anaerobic, 90, 137, 138
  chronic, 146–149
  common organisms, 12
  culturing, 57, 136, 263
  diagnosis of, 136
  fungal, 145–146
  host defence mechanisms, 136
  increased risk of, 188, 261, 262, 265, 271
  local anaesthetic injections and, 29
  microflora, 135, 136
  needle tract, 29
  postoperative, 271, 272
  from projectile injuries, 261–262
  prophylaxis, 60, 136–137
  salivary glands, 143–144, 334–335
  sinusitis, 180–181
  skin infections, 144–145
  transmission, 12, 63, 152
  viral, 144, 149–152
  wounds, 88, 265, 266, 272–273
Infectious mononucleosis, 150
Infective arthritis, 203
Infective endocarditis, 137
Inferior alveolar nerve
  block, 26–27
  branches, 161*f*
  lateralization, 225
  in third molar surgery, 115, 119
Inferior dental nerve
  block, 26–27
  injury to, 115, 118
Inferior rectus muscle release, 248
Inferior turbinectomy, 310
Infiltration analgesia, 28
Inflammation, 33, 96, 196, 203
Informed consent, 6–7, 8
Infraoccluded primary teeth, 129–130, 130*f*
Infraorbital nerve block, 28
Inhalation sedation, 30–31
Injectables, 201
Instruments, 5, 15–18
  exodontia, 80–82, 84*f*, 87*f*

surgical endodontics, 100*f*
  ultrasonic, 100
Insulin, 64
Intensity-modulated radiotherapy (IMRT), 357, 365
Intensive care, 67–68
Intermaxillary fixation (IMF), 237
Intermediate restorative material (IRM), 101
Internal oblique flap, 394*f*
International Association for the Study of Pain, 195
International Classification of Diseases (ICD), cleft deformity codes, 315–316
International normalized ratio (INR), 56, 78
Interpositional grafts, 215
Intra-arterial injections, 30
Intraligamentary analgesia, 28
Intraoral anaesthetics, 25
Intraradicular radiculectomy and crush, 210, 211*f*
Intravenous cannula insertion, 32*f*, 57–58
Intravenous fluids, 61, 228–229
Intravenous sedation, 31–32
Intubation, 230–231
Inverted-L osteotomy, 307–308
Investigations, 54
Iodine, 13, 14, 266
Iodoform, 5, 13
Iron deficiency, 196, 198
Irritation hyperplasia, 166, 211–213, 213*f*

J
Jannetta procedure, 197
Jaw exercises, 200
Jaw thrust manoeuvre, 230
Jelonet, 14, 271
Jigs, surgical positioning, 413*f*
Joint noises, TMJ, 193
Joint replacement, 203, 204, 206
Jugular venous pressure (JVP), 46

K
Keratoacanthoma (KA), 277
Keratoconjunctivitis sicca, 335